The Sports Medicine Patient Advisor

LOMBLUT

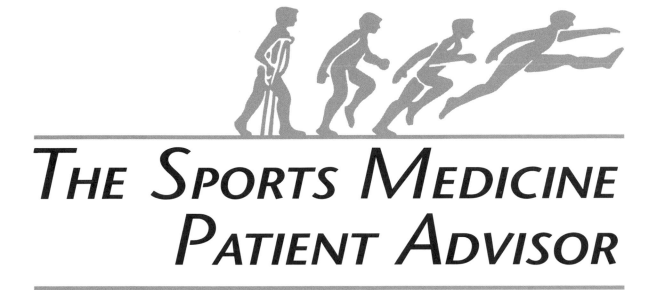

THE SPORTS MEDICINE
PATIENT ADVISOR

PIERRE ROUZIER, MD

Dedication

I am grateful to Lynette Edris for painstakingly helping me with this work at its earliest stages.

To the staff at Clinical Reference Systems, especially to Rick Thompson who listened to my first ideas, and to Susan Murphy who guided me along and made it the way it is.

To all my sports physicians and therapists who have helped with my own injuries - past, present and future.

And to my family—Arlene, Anthony and Nicholas, with whom I share a life of sports and sports medicine.

Acknowledgements

The author has developed the information contained in this book in conjunction with Clinical Reference Systems (CRS), which is now a part of McKesson HBOC Inc. CRS first published version 1.0 of the Sports Medicine Advisor as a software program in November, 1997. Version 2.0 was published in December, 1998. CRS has been developing and publishing patient education software products since 1982. The Sports Medicine Advisor, one of 8 programs in the Advisor series, is part of a comprehensive library of over 3,200 medical problems, surgical procedures, and parenting advice topics written and reviewed by healthcare professionals. Clinical Reference Systems can be reached by telephone at (800) 237-8401 or via the Internet at http://www.patienteducation.com.

Cover design: Joseph Savitch

Cover logo courtesy of Scott Coleman

Book design and layout: Jefferson Johnson

The Sports Medicine Patient Advisor

For information about this book, please contact:

SportsMed Press, 6 University Drive, Department 259, Amherst, Massachusetts 01004-6000 or via the Internet at www.sportsmedpress.com

ISBN 0-9671831-0-3

Manufactured in the United States of America

10 9 8 7 6 5 4 3 2 1

Contents

Introduction

The purpose of the Sports Medicine Patient Advisor is to give health care providers the resources with which to educate patients about sports injuries and to answer their sports medicine questions.

In an ideal setting, the patient would present to his or her provider after the initial injury or complaint and would receive the appropriate diagnosis. The patient would then be seen by a physical therapist or trainer and instructed in the proper rehabilitation exercises to aid in recovery and return to physical activity. Because of limitations in resources, it is often not feasible for our patients to see physical therapists or trainers.

The information contained in this book refers to the use of rehabilitation aids that can be found anywhere—weights in a high school gym or in a person's home, resistance bands that can be dispensed from a physician's office, or even soup cans that can be found in a patient's kitchen cabinet.

It is my hope that this book will be used frequently. No patient with a sports-related problem should leave your office without receiving one of these handouts.

Credits

Clinical Editor

Pierre Rouzier, MD

Dr. Pierre Rouzier is a family physician who practices sports medicine. He is a team physician at the University of Massachusetts at Amherst and assistant professor in the department of Family Medicine and Community Health , University of Massachusetts School of Medicine. Dr. Rouzier attended the University of Southern California School of Medicine and the University of Massachusetts Family Practice Residency. He has his certificate of added qualification in sports medicine. Dr. Rouzier has worked in the Indian Health Service with the White Mountain Apache tribe and has been been the assistant director of the St. Mary's Family Practice Residency in Grand Junction, Colorado.

Dr. Rouzier enjoys mountain biking, running, downhill and cross-country skiing, coaching children's sports, and traveling. He and his wife, Arlene, have two sons, Anthony and Nicholas.

Sports Medicine Advisor Contributors and Reviewers

Tammy White, MS, PT

Tammy White is the director of physical therapy at Heart of the Rockies Regional Medical Center in Salida, Colorado. She received her bachelor of science degree in sports science, with an emphasis in exercise physiology, in 1985 from the University of Denver, Denver, Colorado. She received her master of science degree in physical therapy from Duke University, Durham, North Carolina, in 1989. Ms. White's research includes long-distance running and its effects on the lumbar spine. Her athletic interests include backpacking, running, cross-country skiing, and swimming.

D. Jane Johnson

D. Jane Johnson is an artist living in Grand Junction, Colorado. She graduated from Mesa State College in 1993, with a BA in liberal arts and an emphasis on fine arts. She stays active primarily through her enjoyment of biking, volleyball, and the raising of her two sons, Conor and Julian.

Tom Gilfillan

Tom Gilfillan graduated from Adams State College in Alamosa, Colorado, with a BS in business administration. He is a professional research assistant doing cytogenetic laboratory work with the University of Colorado Health Sciences Center in Denver. Art is his hobby. He is married and has a daughter.

Michael E. Coblyn, EdD

Michael E. Coblyn, EdD, has been a professor of art at the University of Massachusetts at Amherst since 1982. He is director of the Department of Arts Foundations Program for incoming art students. He has a master's degree in painting from the University of Massachusetts (1981) and a doctorate in Museum Education from the University of Massachusetts (1997).

Scott Coleman, MA, PT

Scott Coleman is a 1977 graduate of the School of Physical Therapy at the University of Colorado Health Sciences Center. Mr. Coleman practiced for three years in a general physical therapy setting at Hilltop Rehabilitation Hospital in Grand Junction, Colorado. In 1980, he developed a sports medicine practice that served the athletic programs of local high schools, as well as those of Mesa State College in Grand Junction.

In 1990, Mr. Coleman started Foresight Physical Therapy. In 1998, he joined with St. Mary's Hospital in Grand Junction, where he is director of outpatient services. In 1995, he was named Colorado's Physical Therapist of the Year. He is married and has four children. He enjoys many sports, including skiing, tennis, baseball, and cycling, and has a home woodworking shop.

Jacqueline (Jackie) R. Berning, PhD, RD

Dr. Berning's education includes a bachelor of science degree in clinical dietetics from Northern Arizona University in Flagstaff, Arizona, and a master of science degree in exercise physiology from the University of Colorado in Boulder, Colorado. She received her PhD in nutrition from Colorado State University in Fort Collins, Colorado. Currently, she is assistant professor at the University of Colorado in Colorado Springs, where she teaches in the biology department.

Her expertise is in sport nutrition and teaching students and athletes how to make wise food choices for increased performance. She has worked with athletes at the University of Colorado, the Denver Broncos, the Denver Nuggets, the Cleveland Indians minor league teams, and the United States Swimming (USS) olympic and national teams.

Dr. Berning's research interests lie with nutritional requirements for sport and exercise and the bone mineral content of young female athletes.

She lives in Castle Rock, Colorado, with her husband and their two young sons.

Richard T. Caldwell, MD

Dr. Caldwell is a practicing U.S. Public Health Service physician. Dr. Caldwell attended Kansas State University in Manhattan, Kansas, and the University of Texas Medical Branch, in Galveston, Texas. He did his family practice residency at Brookhaven Memorial Hospital in East Patchogue, New York, and at the University of Texas Health Science Center in Houston. He is a diplomate of the American Board of Family Practice and a fellow of the American Academy of Family Physicians. Dr. Caldwell has his certificate of added qualification in sports medicine.

He has been a high school team physician in New Mexico, Colorado and Arizona and was the team physician at Haskell Indian Nations University in Lawrence, Kansas. He has been the U.S.A. 100 Kilometer Team physician since 1995. Among his personal athletic achievements are setting the U.S. 100-mile run road record in 1979 and winning the U.S. national championship for the 100-mile run in both 1984 and 1986. Dr. Caldwell estimates he has run more than 70,000 miles in the last 20 years.

Daniel G. McBride, MD

Dr. Daniel G. McBride is an orthopedic surgeon at Hampshire Orthopedics & Sports Medicine in Northampton, Massachusetts, and team orthopedic surgeon for the University of Massachusetts at Amherst, Amherst College, and Smith College. He completed sports medicine Fellowships at American Sports Medicine Institute in Birmingham, Alabama, and Sportsmed SA in Adelaide, South Australia.

Jeffrey M. Anderson, MD

Dr. Jeffrey Anderson is the director of Sports Medicine in the University of Connecticut Division of Athletics. He also has an appointment as clinical assistant professor of family medicine at the University of Connecticut Health Center. Dr. Anderson graduated from the University of Michigan Medical School and completed a residency in family medicine and a fellowship in primary care sports medicine at the University of Connecticut Health Center. He and his wife Christine have two sons, Erik and Luke.

Priscilla M. Clarkson, PhD, FACSM

Priscilla M. Clarkson is a professor of exercise science and associate dean for the School of Public Health and Health Sciences at the University of Massachusetts, Amherst. She is a fellow in the American College of Sports Medicine (ASCM) and has served as a member of the board of trustees. She has been president of the New England regional ACSM Chapter and is a former vice president of the national ACSM. She is the 1997 recipient of the ACSM Citation Award.

Professor Clarkson has published over 100 scientific research articles and has given numerous national and international presentations. The major focus of her research is on exercise-induced muscle damage and repair in humans. She has also published in the area of sport nutrition and has focused on micronutrient requirements and the problem of eating disorders in female athletes. Professor Clarkson is currently the editor for the International Journal of Sport Nutrition.

Professor Clarkson serves on the Research Review Board of the Gatorade Sports Science Institute and the Nutritional Advisory Council for Nabisco, and is a member of the Exercise Countermeasures Working Group for NASA (Johnson Space Center) to design and evaluate exercise programs during space flight. She is a member of the Science Working Group at NASA to develop laboratories for the space station. Professor Clarkson also serves as a member of the NCAA Competitive and Medical Safeguards Committee.

Robin E. Levine, MA, RD, CDE

Robin E. Levine is associate director of the Center for Nutrition in Sport and Human Performance, a member of the faculty of the Department of Nutrition, and sports nutritionist for the Department of Athletics at the University of Massachusetts in Amherst.

She received her bachelor's degree from George Washington University and her master's degree from Goddard College, during which time she was mentored by D. Mark Hegsted, PhD, of the Harvard School of Public Health. She is a registered dietician and is board-certified as a diabetes educator. She served as senior clinical nutritionist and coordinator of Nutrition, Eating Disorders, and Diabetes Care Services at the University Health Services of the University of Massachusetts for 15 years before joining the nutrition faculty and the Department of Athletics.

Ms. Levine has presented widely on the topics of eating disorders, sport nutrition, and medical nutrition therapy for diabetes. She co-chairs two regional conferences on eating disorders. She is a member of the American Diabetes Association (and a member of SCAN, the sport nutrition and cardiovascular health and wellness practice group of that organization) and a member of the American Association of Diabetes Educators.

Ron Laham

Ron Laham is the athletic trainer for the University of Massachusetts' basketball and baseball teams. Ron graduated from Northeastern University and received his Maser's degree in athletic training / sports medicine at the University of Virginia. He has been head athletic trainer at State University of New York at Plattsburgh and has served as athletic trainer for the U.S. Under-22 basketball team in international competitions. He is a certified athletic trainer and a member of the National Athletic Trainers Association.

Additional Contributors

Phyllis G. Cooper, RN, MN
Cooper Consulting, Woodland Hills, California.

Dee Ann DeRoin, MPH, MD
Indian Health Service, Haskell Indian Nations University, Lawrence, Kansas.

Judith M. Mathias, RN, MA
Aurora, Colorado.

Peter Scott
Informational Medical Systems, Minneapolis, Minnesota.

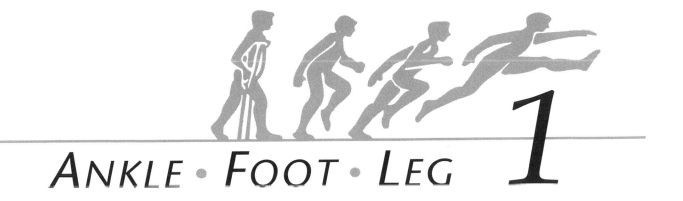

ANKLE · FOOT · LEG 1

Achilles Tendon injury

What is an Achilles tendon injury?

The Achilles tendon is a band of tissue that connects the heel bone to the calf muscle of the leg. Injury to the tendon may cause it to become inflamed or torn.

Achilles tendonitis is the term used when the tendon is inflamed. The inflammation causes pain at the back of your leg near the heel. A tear of the tendon is called a rupture. It also causes pain near your heel.

How does it occur?

Achilles tendonitis can be caused by:

- overuse of the Achilles tendon
- tight calf muscles
- tight Achilles tendons
- lots of uphill running
- increasing the amount or intensity of sports training, sometimes along with switching to racing flats, which are racing shoes with less heel lift
- over-pronation, a problem where your feet roll inward and flatten out more than normal when you walk or run
- wearing high heels at work and then switching to lower-heeled shoes for exercise.

An Achilles tendon may tear during sudden activity. For example the tendon might tear when you jump or start sprinting.

What are the symptoms?

Achilles tendonitis causes pain and may cause swelling over the Achilles tendon. The tendon is tender and may be swollen. You will have pain when you rise up on your toes and pain when you stretch the tendon. The range of motion of your ankle may be limited.

When the tendon tears or ruptures, you may feel a pop. If there is a complete tear, you will be unable to lift your heel off the ground or point your toes.

How is it diagnosed?

Your health care provider will examine your leg, looking for tenderness and swelling. Your provider will watch your feet when you walk or run to see if you over-pronate.

How is it treated?

- Put ice packs on the Achilles tendon for 20 to 30 minutes every 3 to 4 hours for the first 2 or 3 days or until the pain goes away.
- Raise your lower leg on a pillow when you are lying down.

- Take anti-inflammatory medication as prescribed by your health care provider.
- If your health care provider prescribes a heel lift insert for your shoe, wear it at least until your tendon heals and possibly longer. The lift prevents extra stretching of your Achilles tendon.
- While you are recovering from your injury, change your sport or activity to one that does not make your condition worse.

Achilles Tendonitis

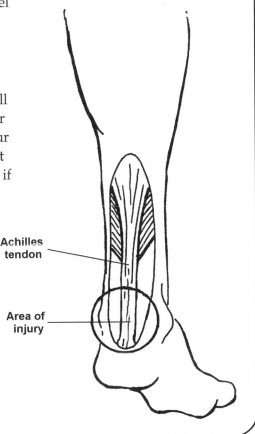

Achilles tendon

Area of injury

Achilles Tendon Injury

For example, you may need to swim instead of run.

- Do any exercises your health care provider gives you to stretch and strengthen your Achilles tendon.

- If you over-pronate, your health care provider may prescribe custom-made shoe inserts, called orthotics, which help keep your foot stable.

- In some severe cases of Achilles tendonitis, your foot may be put in a cast for several weeks.

- A tear of the tendon may require surgery. Or your foot may be put in a cast for 6 to 10 weeks.

When can I return to my sport or activity?

The goal of rehabilitation is to return you to your sport or activity as soon as is safely possible. If you return too soon you may worsen your injury, which could lead to permanent damage. Everyone recovers from injury at a different rate. Return to your activity is determined by how soon your Achilles tendon area recovers, not by how many days or weeks it has been since your injury occurred. In general, the longer you have symptoms before you start treatment, the longer it will take to get better.

You may safely return to your sport or activity when, starting from the top of the list and progressing to the end, each of the following is true:

- You have full range of motion in the injured leg compared to the uninjured leg.

- You have full strength of the injured leg compared to the uninjured leg.

- You can jog straight ahead without pain or limping.

- You can sprint straight ahead without pain or limping.

- You can do 45-degree cuts, first at half-speed, then at full-speed.

- You can do 20-yard figures-of-eight, first at half-speed, then at full-speed.

- You can do 90-degree cuts, first at half-speed, then at full-speed.

- You can do 10-yard figures-of-eight, first at half-speed, then at full-speed.

- You can jump on both legs without pain and you can jump on the injured leg without pain.

How can I prevent Achilles tendonitis?

The best way to prevent Achilles tendon injury is to stretch your calf muscles and Achilles tendons before exercise. If you have tight Achilles tendons or calf muscles, stretch them twice a day whether or not you are doing any sports activities that day.

If you have a tendency to get Achilles tendonitis, avoid running uphill a lot.

Achilles Tendonitis Rehabilitation Exercises

You can do the towel stretch right away. When the towel stretch is too easy, try the standing calf stretch, soleus stretch, and plantar fascia stretch. When you no longer have sharp pain in your calf or tendon, start exercises 5, 6, and 7.

1. Towel stretch: Sit on a hard surface with your injured leg stretched out in front of you. Loop a towel around the ball of your foot and pull the towel toward your body, keeping your knee straight. Hold this position for 30 seconds and repeat 3 times.

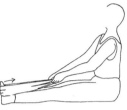

Towel stretch

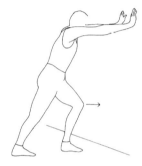

Standing calf stretch

2. Standing calf stretch: Facing a wall, put your hands against the wall at about eye level. Keep the injured leg back, the uninjured leg forward, and the heel of your injured leg on the floor. Turn your injured foot slightly inward (as if you were pigeon-toed) as you slowly lean into the wall until you feel a stretch in the back of your calf. Hold for 30 seconds. Do this several times a day.

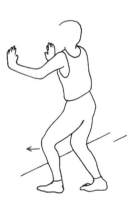

3. Standing soleus stretch: Stand facing a wall with your hands at about chest level. With both knees slightly bent and the injured foot back, gently lean into the wall until you feel a stretch in your lower calf. Once again, slightly toe in with the injured foot and keep your heel down on the floor. Hold this for 30 seconds. Return to the starting position. Repeat 3 times.

Standing soleus stretch

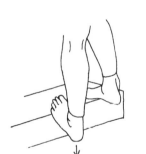

Plantar fascia stretch

4. Plantar fascia stretch: Standing with the ball of your injured foot on a stair and slightly toed out, reach for the bottom of the step with your heel until you feel a stretch in the arch of your foot. Hold this position for 30 seconds. Relax and then repeat 3 times.

5. Toe raises: Stand in a normal weight-bearing position. Rock back on your heels so that your toes come off the ground. Hold this position for 5 seconds. Repeat 10 times. Do 3 sets of 10.

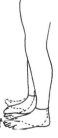

Toe raises

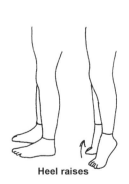

Heel raises

6. Heel raises: Standing, balance yourself on both feet behind a chair. Rise up on your toes, hold for 5 seconds and then lower yourself down. Repeat 10 times. Do 3 sets of 10.

Achilles Tendonitis Rehabilitation Exercises

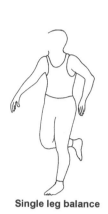

Single leg balance

7. Single leg balance: Stand without any support and attempt to balance on your injured leg. Begin with your eyes open and then try to perform the exercise with your eyes closed. Hold the single-leg position for 30 seconds. Repeat 3 times.

Ankle Sprain

What is an ankle sprain?

An ankle sprain is an injury that causes a stretch or tear of one or more ligaments in the ankle joint. Ligaments are strong bands of tissue that connect bones at the joint.

Sprains may be graded I, II, or III depending on their severity:

- grade I sprain: pain with minimal damage to the ligaments
- grade II sprain: more ligament damage and mild looseness of the joint
- grade III sprain: complete tearing of the ligament and the joint is very loose or unstable.

Sometimes sprains are just classified as mild or severe, depending on the amount of ligament damage.

Most sprains occur on the outside part of the ankle, but they can occur on the inside as well.

How does it occur?

A sprain is caused by twisting your ankle. Your foot usually turns in or under but may turn to the outside.

What are the symptoms?

Symptoms of a sprained ankle include:

- mild aching to sudden pain
- swelling

- discoloration
- inability to move the ankle properly
- pain in the ankle even when you are not putting any weight on it.

How is it diagnosed?

To diagnose a sprained ankle, the doctor will review how the injury occurred and consider your symptoms. He or she will examine your ankle carefully. X-rays may be taken of your ankle.

How it is treated?

Treatment may include:

- Applying ice packs to your ankle for 20 to 30 minutes every 3 to 4 hours for the first 2 to 3 days or until the pain goes away. Thereafter, ice your ankle at least once a day until the other symptoms are gone.
- Elevating your ankle by placing a pillow underneath your foot. Try to keep your ankle above the level of your heart.
- Wrapping an elastic bandage around your ankle to keep the swelling from getting worse.
- Wearing a lace-up brace or ankle stirrup (an Aircast or Gelcast).

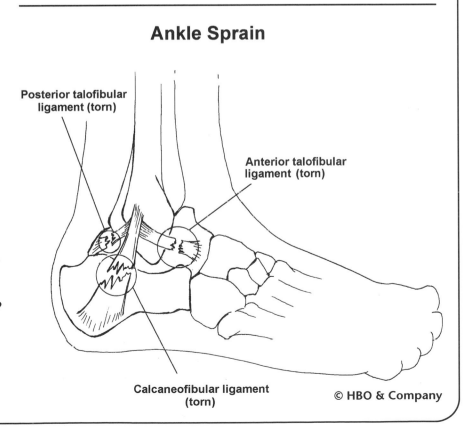

Ankle Sprain

Posterior talofibular ligament (torn)

Anterior talofibular ligament (torn)

Calcaneofibular ligament (torn)

© HBO & Company

— Ankle Sprain —

- Using crutches until you can walk without pain.
- Taking anti-inflammatory medication or other pain medication prescribed by your doctor.
- Doing ankle exercises to improve your ankle strength and range of motion. The exercises will help you return to your normal activity or sports.

Rarely, severe ankle sprains with complete tearing of the ligaments need surgery. After surgery your ankle will be in a cast for 4 to 8 weeks.

How long will the effects last?

The length of recovery depends on many factors:

- age
- health
- severity of injury and previous injuries to that joint.

When can I return to my sport or activity?

The goal of rehabilitation is to return you to your sport or activity as soon as is safely possible. If you return too soon you may worsen your injury, which could lead to permanent damage. Everyone recovers from injury at a different rate. Return to your sport or activity will be determined by how soon your ankle recovers, not by how many days or weeks it has been since your injury occurred. In general, the longer you have symptoms before you start treatment, the longer it will take to get better.

You may safely return to your sport or activity when, starting from the top of the list and progressing to the end, each of the following is true:

- You have full range of motion in the injured ankle compared to the uninjured ankle.
- You have full strength of the injured ankle compared to the uninjured ankle.
- You can jog straight ahead without pain or limping.
- You can sprint straight ahead without pain or limping.
- You can do 45-degree cuts, first at half-speed, then at full-speed.

- You can do 20-yard figures-of-eight, first at half-speed, then at full-speed.
- You can do 90-degree cuts, first at half-speed, then at full-speed.
- You can do 10-yard figures-of-eight, first at half-speed, then at full-speed.
- You can jump on both legs without pain and you can jump on the injured leg without pain.

How can I help prevent an ankle sprain?

To help prevent an ankle sprain, follow these guidelines:

- Wear proper, well-fitting shoes when you exercise.
- Stretch gently and adequately before and after athletic or recreational activities.
- Avoid sharp turns and quick changes in direction and movement.
- Consider taping the ankle or wearing a brace for strenuous sports, especially if you have a previous injury.

Ankle Sprain Rehabilitation Exercises

As soon as you can tolerate pressure on the ball of your foot, begin stretching your ankle using the towel stretch. When this stretch is too easy, try the standing calf stretch and soleus stretch. You can do exercises 4 and 5 when your ankle swelling has stopped increasing. You may do exercises 6 through 10 when you can stand on your injured ankle without pain.

1. Towel stretch: Sit on a hard surface with your injured leg stretched out in front of you. Loop a towel around the ball of your foot and pull the towel toward your body, keeping your knee straight. Hold this position for 30 seconds. Repeat 3 times.

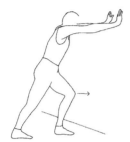

Standing calf stretch

2. Standing calf stretch: Facing a wall, put your hands against the wall at about eye level. Keep the injured leg back, the uninjured leg forward, and the heel of your injured leg on the floor. Turn your injured foot slightly inward (as if you were pigeontoed). Slowly lean into the wall until you feel a stretch in the back of your calf. Hold for 30 seconds. Do this several times a day.

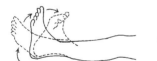

Towel stretch

3. Standing soleus stretch: Stand facing a wall with your hands at about chest level. With both knees slightly bent and the injured foot back, gently lean into the wall until you feel a stretch in your lower calf. Once again, angle the toes of your injured foot slightly inward and keep your heel down on the floor. Hold this for 30 seconds. Return to the starting position. Repeat 3 times.

Standing soleus stretch

Ankle range of motion

4. Ankle range of motion: You can do this exercise sitting or lying down. Pretend you are writing each of the letters of the alphabet with your foot. This will move your ankle in all directions. Do this twice.

5. Thera-Band exercises

   A. Resisted dorsiflexion: Sitting with your leg out straight and your foot near a door, wrap the tubing around the ball of your foot. Anchor the other end of the tubing to the door by tying a knot in the tubing, slipping it between the door and the frame, and closing the door. Pull your toes toward your face. Return slowly to the starting position. Repeat 10 times. Do 3 sets of 10.

   B. Resisted plantar flexion: Sitting with your leg outstretched, loop the middle section of the tubing around the ball of your foot. Hold the ends of the tubing in both hands. Gently press the ball of your foot down and point your toes, stretching the Thera-Band. Return to the starting position. Repeat 10 times. Do 3 sets of 10.

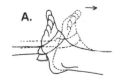

A.

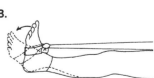

B.

Theraband exercises

Ankle Sprain Rehabilitation Exercises

C. Resisted inversion: Sit with your legs out straight and cross your un-injured leg over your injured ankle. Wrap the tubing around the ball of your injured foot and then loop it around your uninjured foot so that the Thera-Band is anchored at one end. Hold the other end of the Thera-Band in your hand. Turn your injured foot inward and upward. This will stretch the tubing. Return to the starting position. Repeat 10 times. Do 3 sets of 10.

C.

D.

Theraband exercises

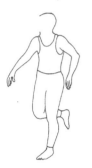

Heel raises

D. Resisted eversion: Sitting with both legs out stretched and the tubing looped around both feet, slowly turn your injured foot upward and outward. Hold this position for 5 seconds. Repeat 10 times. Do 3 sets of 10.

6. Heel raises: Standing, balance yourself on both feet behind a chair. Rise up on your toes, hold for 5 seconds and then lower yourself down. Repeat 10 times. Do 3 sets of 10.

7. Toe raises: Stand in a normal weight-bearing position. Rock back on your heels so that your toes come off the ground. Hold this position for 5 seconds. Repeat 10 times. Do 3 sets of 10.

Toe raises

Single leg balance

8. Single leg balance: Stand without any support and attempt to balance on your injured leg. Begin with your eyes open and then try to perform the exercise with your eyes closed. Hold the single-leg position for 30 seconds. Repeat 3 times.

9. Jump rope: Jump rope landing on both legs for 5 minutes, then on only the injured leg for 5 minutes.

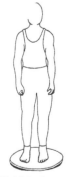

Wobble board

10. Wobble board: This exercise is important to restore balance and coordination to your ankle. Make a wobble board by cutting a circle of plywood two feet across. Place it on top of a 5 or 10 pound weight from a barbell set. Stand on the wobble board. Balance first on both legs, then on the injured leg. Do this for 2 to 5 minutes 3 times a day. You may need to hold onto a chair or table for balance.

Jump rope

© HBO & Company

Broken Ankle

What is a broken ankle?

A broken ankle is a break in one or both of the bones that make up the ankle joint. These bones are the tibia and the fibula.

How does it occur?

Ankle breaks, or fractures, can occur in many ways: for example, by falls, contact sports and exercise injuries, and force from a blow.

There are many types of fractures, which determine the severity of the injury and its treatment:

- nondisplaced fracture: the broken pieces of bone remain properly aligned

- displaced fracture: the broken pieces of bone are not properly aligned

- comminuted fracture: there are more than two pieces of bone at the fracture.

- compound (open) fracture: one end of the broken bone has broken through the skin.

- closed fracture: neither end of the broken bone has pierced the skin.

- impacted fracture: the ends of the broken bone are driven into each other.

- avulsion fracture: the muscle or ligament has pulled a portion of the bone away from where it was originally attached.

- pathological fracture: the bone has been weakened or destroyed by disease (such as osteoporosis) so that the bone breaks easily.

What are the symptoms?

Symptoms of an ankle fracture include:

- a snapping or popping sound at the time of the injury

- loss of function (hurts to move the ankle)

- pain

- tenderness

- swelling

- deformity (sometimes)

- discolored skin, or bruising, which appears hours to days after the injury.

Rarely, you may have an open wound with an ankle fracture.

How is it diagnosed?

To diagnose an ankle fracture, the doctor will review your symptoms, ask about how the injury occurred, and examine you. The doctor will also order x-rays. Several different views of the bone may be taken to pinpoint the fracture.

How is it treated?

The immediate emergency treatment for a fractured ankle is immobilization (keeping it from moving), elevation, compression (wrapping it with an elastic or Ace bandage), and the application of ice packs.

The doctor may need to set your ankle bone back into its proper place and put you in a cast for 6 to 8 weeks. If the fracture is not too severe, you may be able to walk in the cast after a short period.

If the ankle bone cannot be aligned perfectly before it is ready for a cast, surgery will be necessary.

In the first 2 to 3 weeks after the injury, be sure to keep your ankle elevated on pillows and place ice packs on top of the cast for 20 to 30 minutes every 3 to 4 hours to help reduce swelling.

You should also:

- Make sure the cast does not get wet. Cover the cast with plastic when you bathe.

- Use crutches or a cane, as directed by your doctor. Your doctor will tell you how much weight you can put on your leg, if any.

- Not scratch the skin around the cast or poke things down the cast.

How can I take care of myself?

To help take care of yourself, follow the full course of treatment your doctor prescribes. Also, follow these guidelines:

Broken Ankle

- Eat a variety of nutritious foods.
- Get plenty of rest.
- Elevate the leg when possible to reduce any swelling.

Call the doctor immediately if:

- You have swelling above or below the fracture.
- Your toenails or feet turn grey or blue and stay grey or blue even when your leg is elevated.
- You have numbness or complete loss of feeling in the skin below the fracture.
- You have lingering pain at the site of the fracture under the cast, or increasing pain not helped by elevation or pain medication.
- You have burning pain under the cast.

When can I return to my sport or activity?

The goal of rehabilitation is to return you to your sport or activity as soon as is safely possible. If you return too soon you may worsen your injury, which could lead to permanent damage. Everyone recovers from injury at a different rate. Return to your sport or activity will be determined by how soon your ankle recovers, not by how many days or weeks it has been since your injury occurred. Some people return within a few days after the cast is removed, some in several weeks. Your ankle will be healing while you are doing your rehabilitation exercises. These exercises will help improve your ankle strength and range of motion.

You may safely return to your sport or activity when, starting from the top of the list and progressing to the end, each of the following is true:

- You have full range of motion in the injured leg compared to the uninjured leg.
- You have full strength of the injured leg compared to the uninjured leg.
- You can jog straight ahead without pain or limping.
- You can sprint straight ahead without pain or limping.

- You can do 45-degree cuts, first at half-speed, then at full-speed.
- You can do 20-yard figures-of-eight, first at half-speed, then at full-speed.
- You can do 90-degree cuts, first at half-speed, then at full-speed.
- You can do 10-yard figures-of-eight, first at half-speed, then at full-speed.
- You can jump on both legs without pain and you can jump on the injured leg without pain.

How can I help prevent an ankle fracture?

To help prevent an ankle fracture, follow these guidelines:

- Wear proper shoes that fit correctly when you exercise.
- Gently stretch before and after physical activities such as aerobics, running, and sports.
- Avoid playing recreational sports when you are fatigued.
- Think about safety.

Broken Ankle Rehabilitation Exercises

As soon as you can tolerate pressure on the ball of your foot, begin stretching your ankle using the towel stretch. When this stretch is too easy, try the standing calf stretch and soleus stretch. You can do exercises 4 and 5 when your ankle swelling has stopped increasing. You may do exercises 6 through 9 when you can stand on your injured ankle without pain.

1. Towel stretch: Sit on a hard surface with your injured leg stretched out in front of you. Loop a towel around the ball of your foot and pull the towel toward your body, keeping your knee straight. Hold this position for 30 seconds. Repeat 3 times.

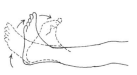

Towel stretch

2. Standing calf stretch: Facing a wall, put your hands against the wall at about eye level. Keep the injured leg back, the uninjured leg forward, and the heel of your injured leg on the floor. Turn your injured foot slightly inward (as if you were pigeon-toed). Slowly lean into the wall until you feel a stretch in the back of your calf. Hold for 30 seconds. Do this several times a day.

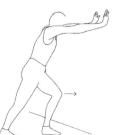

Standing calf stretch

3. Standing soleus stretch: Stand facing a wall with your hands at about chest level. With both knees slightly bent and the injured foot back, gently lean into the wall until you feel a stretch in your lower calf. Once again, angle the toes of your injured foot slightly inward and keep your heel down on the floor. Hold this for 30 seconds. Return to the starting position. Repeat 3 times.

Towel stretch

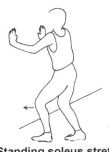

Standing soleus stretch

4. Ankle range of motion: You can do this exercise sitting or lying down. Pretend you are writing each of the letters of the alphabet with your foot. This will move your ankle in all directions. Do this twice.

Ankle range of motion

5. Thera-Band exercises

   A. Resisted dorsiflexion: Sitting with your leg out straight and your foot near a door, wrap the tubing around the ball of your foot. Anchor the other end of the tubing to the door by tying a knot in the tubing, slipping it between the door and the frame, and closing the door. Pull your toes toward your face. Return slowly to the starting position. Repeat 10 times. Do 3 sets of 10.

   B. Resisted plantar flexion: Sitting with your leg outstretched, loop the middle section of the tubing around the ball of your foot. Hold the ends of the tubing in both hands. Gently press the ball of your foot down and point your toes, stretching the Thera-Band. Return to the starting position. Repeat 10 times. Do 3 sets of 10.

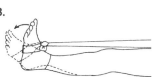

Theraband exercises

Broken Ankle Rehabilitation Exercises

C. Resisted inversion: Sit with your legs out straight and cross your uninjured leg over your injured ankle. Wrap the tubing around the ball of your injured foot and then loop it around your uninjured foot so that the Thera-Band is anchored at one end. Hold the other end of the Thera-Band in your hand. Turn your injured foot inward and upward. This will stretch the tubing. Return to the starting position. Repeat 10 times. Do 3 sets of 10.

D. Resisted eversion: Sitting with both legs outstretched and the tubing looped around both feet, slowly turn your injured foot upward and outward. Hold this position for 5 seconds. Repeat 10 times. Do 3 sets of 10.

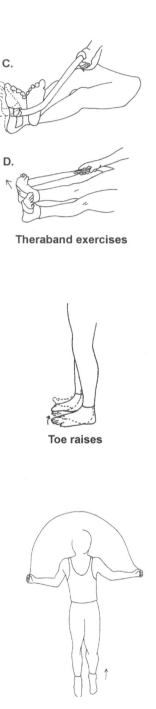

Theraband exercises

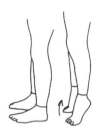

Heel raises

6. Heel raises: Standing, balance yourself on both feet behind a chair. Rise up on your toes, hold for 5 seconds and then lower yourself down. Repeat 10 times. Do 3 sets of 10.

7. Toe raises: Stand in a normal weight-bearing position. Rock back on your heels so that your toes come off the ground. Hold this position for 5 seconds. Repeat 10 times. Do 3 sets of 10.

Toe raises

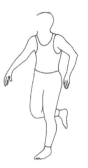

Single leg balance

8. Single leg balance: Stand without any support and attempt to balance on your injured leg. Begin with your eyes open and then try to perform the exercise with your eyes closed. Hold the single-leg position for 30 seconds. Repeat 3 times.

9. Jump rope: Jump rope landing on both legs for 5 minutes, then only on the injured leg for 5 minutes.

10. Wobble board: This exercise is important to restore balance and coordination to your ankle. Make a wobble board by cutting a circle of plywood two feet across. Place it on top of a 5 or 10 pound weight from a barbell set. Stand on the wobble board. Balance first on both legs, then on the injured leg. Do this for 2 to 5 minutes 3 times a day. You may need to hold onto a chair or table for balance.

Jump rope

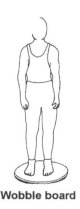

Wobble board

Arch Pain

What is arch pain?

There are two arches in your foot. The longitudinal arch runs the length of your foot, and the transverse arch runs across the width of your foot. The arches are made up of ligaments, which keep the bones of your feet in place. Arch pain can occur in one or both arches but occurs most commonly in the longitudinal arch.

How does it occur?

Arch pain most often occurs as a result of overuse in activities such as running, hiking, walking, and jumping. People who have flat feet, or people whose feet flatten and roll inward when walking (a problem called over-pronation) are more prone to arch pain. Arch pain usually comes on slowly. However, it can occur suddenly if the ligaments are stretched or torn during a forceful activity such as sprinting or jumping.

What are the symptoms?

The symptom is pain along the arch of the foot.

How is it diagnosed?

Your doctor will examine your foot for pain and tenderness along the arch.

How is it treated?

You should place ice packs on your arch for 20 to 30 minutes every 3 to 4 hours for 2 or 3 days or until the pain goes away. Your doctor may prescribe an anti-inflammatory medication.

Your arch needs extra support. Taping your arch or using an extra arch support in your shoe may give you the support you need. Your doctor may prescribe custom-made arch supports called orthotics.

When can I return to my sport or activity?

The goal of rehabilitation is to return you to your sport or activity as soon as is safely possible. If you return too soon you may worsen your injury, which could lead to permanent damage. Everyone recovers from injury at a different rate.

Return to your activity will be determined by how soon your foot recovers, not by how many days or weeks it has been since your injury occurred. In general, the longer you have symptoms before you start treatment, the longer it will take to get better.

You may safely return to your sport or activity when, starting from the top of the list and progressing to the end, each of the following is true:

- You have full range of motion in the injured foot compared to the uninjured foot.

- You have full strength of the injured foot compared to the uninjured foot.

- You can jog straight ahead without pain or limping.

- You can sprint straight ahead without pain or limping.

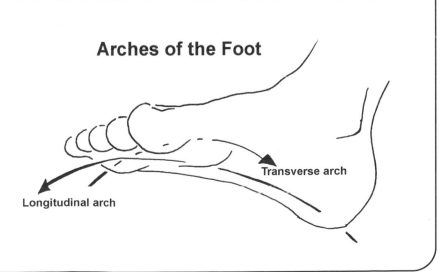

Arches of the Foot

Transverse arch

Longitudinal arch

Arch Pain

- You can do 45-degree cuts, first at half-speed, then at full-speed.
- You can do 20-yard figures-of-eight, first at half-speed, then at full-speed.
- You can do 90-degree cuts, first at half-speed, then at full-speed.
- You can do 10-yard figures-of-eight, first at half-speed, then at full-speed.

- You can jump on both feet without pain and you can jump on the injured foot without pain.

How can I prevent arch pain?

Arch pain can be prevented by wearing shoes that fit properly and have proper arch support. Stretching your feet and arches before your activity will also help prevent this injury. You may need orthotics. Some people will need to wear orthotics all the time and others only during sporting activities.

Arch Pain Rehabilitation Exercises

You may begin exercising the muscles of your foot right away by gently stretching them with the towel stretch. When the towel stretch becomes too easy, you may begin doing the standing calf stretch, plantar fascia stretch, and sitting toe raise. Next, you can begin strengthening the muscles of your foot and lower leg by doing exercises 5 and 6.

1. Towel stretch: Sit on a hard surface with leg on your injured side stretched out in front of you. Loop a towel around the ball of your foot and pull the towel toward your body, stretching the back of your calf muscle. Hold this position for 30 seconds. Repeat 3 times.

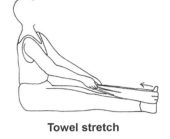

Towel stretch

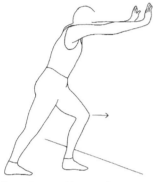

Standing calf stretch

2. Standing calf stretch: Stand facing a wall with your hands against the wall at about eye level. Place the leg on your injured side about 12 to 18 inches behind your other leg. Gently lean into the wall by bending your forward knee and keeping your back knee straight. Keep your rear heel on the floor. You will feel a stretch in the calf muscle. Hold this position for 30 to 60 seconds. Repeat 3 times. When you can stand comfortably on your injured foot, you can begin stretching the planter fascia (the bottom of your foot).

3. Plantar fascia stretch: Standing with the ball of your injured foot on a stair, reach for the bottom step with your heel until you feel a stretch in the arch of your foot. Hold this position for 30 to 60 seconds and then relax. Repeat 3 times. After you have stretched the bottom muscles of your foot, you can begin strengthening the top muscles of your foot.

Plantar fascia stretch

4. Frozen can roll: Roll your bare injured foot back and forth from your heel to your mid-arch over a frozen juice can. Repeat for 3 to 5 minutes. This exercise is particularly helpful if done first thing in the morning.

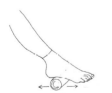

Frozen can roll

5. Sitting toe raise: Sit in a chair with your feet flat on the floor. Raise the toes and the ball of your injured foot off the floor while keeping your heel on the floor. Hold for 5 seconds. Repeat 10 times. Do 3 sets of 10.

Towel pickup

6. Towel pickup: With your heel on the ground, pick up a towel with your toes. Release. Repeat 10 to 20 times.

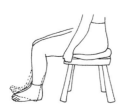

Sitting toe raise

Arch Pain Rehabilitation Exercises

6. Resisted Thera-Band exercises for the lower leg

A. Resisted dorsiflexion: Sit with the leg on your injured side out straight injured out straight and your foot facing a doorway. Tie a loop in one end of the Thera-Band. Put your foot through the loop so that the tubing goes around the arch of your foot. Tie a knot in the other end of the Thera-Band and shut the knot in the door. Move backward until there is tension in the tubing. Keeping your knee straight, pull your foot toward your face, stretching the tubing. Slowly return to the starting position. Repeat 10 times. Do 3 sets of 10.

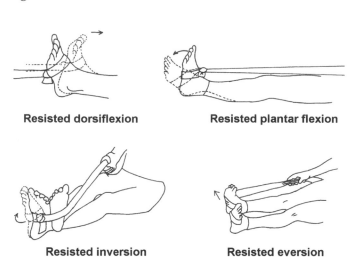

Resisted dorsiflexion   Resisted plantar flexion

Resisted inversion   Resisted eversion

B. Resisted plantar flexion. Sitting with your leg outstretched, loop the middle section of the tubing around the ball of your foot. Hold the ends of the tubing in both hands. Gently press the ball of your foot down and point your toes, stretching the Thera-Band. Return to the starting position. Repeat 10 times. Do 3 sets of 10.

C. Resisted inversion: Sit with your legs out straight and cross the leg on your uninjured side over the ankle of your injured foot. Wrap the tubing around the ball of your injured foot and then loop it around your uninjured foot so that the Thera-Band is anchored there at one end. Hold the other end of the Thera-Band in your hand. Turn your injured foot inward and upward. This will stretch the tubing. Return to the starting position. Repeat 10 times. Do 3 sets of 10.

D. Resisted eversion: Sit with both legs stretched out in front of you, with your feet about a shoulder's width apart. Tie a loop in one end of the Thera-Band. Put your injured foot through the loop so that the tubing goes around the arch of that foot. Then, wrap the Thera-Band around the outside of the uninjured foot. Hold onto the other end of the tubing with your hand to provide tension. Turn your injured foot up and out. Make sure you keep your uninjured foot still so that it will allow the tubing to stretch as you move your injured foot. Return to the starting position. Repeat 10 times. Do 3 sets of 10.

Athlete's Foot

What is athlete's foot?

Athlete's foot is a common skin problem caused by a fungus. Usually beginning on the skin between the toes, the fungus infection becomes scaly and itchy. Over time it may cause a break in the skin and become sore. Another term for athlete's foot is tinea pedis.

How does it occur?

The fungus that causes athlete's foot is everywhere in the environment. It is commonly picked up from the floors of showers, locker rooms, and exercise facilities. The fungus is more likely to grow on sweaty, constantly wet, or improperly dried feet (especially in shoes or socks with poor ventilation).

What are the symptoms?

Symptoms include:
- itching
- cracking and peeling skin, usually between the last two toes
- soreness
- blisters (occasionally).

How is it diagnosed?

Your health care provider can usually diagnose athlete's foot after examining your skin. Sometimes he or she may swab or scrape off a skin sample to test for fungus. If your provider suspects that you may also have a bacterial infection, the skin sample may be tested for bacteria.

How is it treated?

The infection may clear up without treatment, but most fungal infections are treated with medicine put on the skin. If the infection is severe or widespread, your provider may prescribe a medication to take by mouth.

How long will the effects last?

The acute stage of the infection usually lasts 1 to 10 days. Chronic infection may persist for months or years. If a severe case of athlete's foot is not treated, it may develop into a serious bacterial infection. The infection may eventually affect the toenails, which are harder to treat.

How can I help prevent athlete's foot?

Follow these guidelines:
- Wear cotton socks when you exercise.
- Change your socks every day.
- Wear sandals or shoes with ventilation holes or porous upper material (a natural material such as canvas or leather rather than man-made material).
- Air out your shoes when you aren't wearing them.
- Wear thongs or sandals when you take a shower in a locker room.
- Dry your feet very well, especially between the toes.
- Apply an antifungal powder on the affected area.
- Disinfect shower and locker room floors.

Athlete's Foot

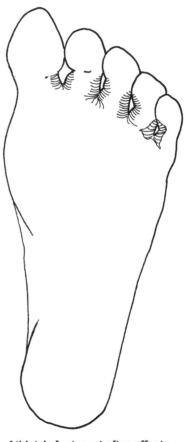

Athlete's foot most often affects the areas between the toes

© HBO & Company

Bunion (Hallux Valgus)

What is a bunion?

A bunion is an abnormal bony bump that forms on the joint at the base of the big toe. The big toe joint becomes enlarged to the inside, with the toe turned and pointing inward. The medical term for the deformity where the big toe angles toward the other toes is hallux valgus.

People with weak or flat feet and women who wear high heels a lot tend to develop bunions.

How does it occur?

Bunions most often result from wearing shoes that don't fit properly or from wearing high-heeled shoes with narrow, pointed toes. When a shoe rubs against the toe joint it irritates the area and makes it swollen, red, and painful. A tough, calloused covering grows over the site.

The tendency to have bunions may be inherited.

What are the symptoms?

Symptoms include:

- a bony bump at the base of the big toe
- swelling, redness, and soreness of the big toe joint
- thickening of the skin at the base of the big toe.

How is it diagnosed?

Your doctor will examine the affected foot. He or she may want to take x-rays of the joint.

How is it treated?

Often nonsurgical treatment is sufficient. You can usually relieve pressure on the big toe by:

- wearing roomy, comfortable shoes
- wearing a corrective device that pushes the big toe back into the right position and holds it in place
- placing a pad on the bunion.

In addition, take anti-inflammatory medication (such as aspirin or ibuprofen) for pain relief. Custom-made arch supports called orthotics may help reduce bunion pain. If the bunion gets worse and causes too much discomfort, your doctor may suggest surgery (called bunionectomy) to:

- take out the swollen tissue
- straighten the toe by taking out part of the bone
- permanently join the bones of the affected joint.

How long will the effects last?

A bunion is a permanent problem. You'll continue to have it unless you have surgery to remove it. Recovery from bunion surgery may take 2 months or more.

How can I take care of myself?

If you have swelling, redness, or pain in the big toe joint:

Bunion

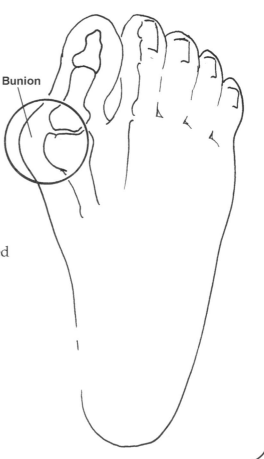

Bunion

Bunion (Hallux Valgus)

- Keep pressure off the affected toe.
- Wear comfortable shoes that fit well and allow enough room for your toes.

- See your doctor or a foot specialist if your condition doesn't improve or if new symptoms develop.
- Follow your doctor's instructions for taking prescribed medication.

What can be done to help prevent bunions?

You can help prevent bunions from developing by wearing comfortable shoes that fit well. Be sure your shoes don't cramp or irritate your toes. This is especially important if your family has a history of weak or flat feet, conditions that may be inherited.

Calcaneal Apophysitis
(Sever's Disease)

What is calcaneal apophysitis?

The heel bone is called the calcaneus. In children, there is an area on the heel bone where the bone grows that is called the growth plate, or apophysis. Calcaneal apophysitis, also called Sever's disease, is inflammation of the calcaneal growth plate that causes pain in the heel. It is the most common cause of heel pain in children, adolescents, and teenagers.

How does it occur?

This inflamed heel growth plate is caused by overusing the foot with repetitive heel strikes. It may also occur from wearing shoes with poor heel padding or poor arch supports.

What are the symptoms?

A child will complain of heel pain. Running and jumping usually increase the symptoms.

How is it diagnosed?

The doctor will find tenderness over the bottom part of your child's heel. In severe cases of calcaneal apophysitis, the doctor may order an x-ray to be sure there is no damage to the growth plate.

How is it treated?

Your child may need to rest or do activities that do not cause heel pain. It is very important that your child wear shoes with padded heel surfaces and good arch supports. Extra heel pads may be placed in your child's shoe. Orthotics (custom-made arch supports) may be helpful. Your doctor may also prescribe an anti-inflammatory medication for your child.

When can my child return to his or her sport or activity?

The goal of treatment is to return your child to his or her sport or activity as soon as is safely possible. If your child returns too soon the injury may be made worse, which could lead to permanent damage. Everyone recovers from injury at a different rate. Return to his or her activity will be determined by how soon your child's heel recovers, not by how many days or weeks it has been since the injury occurred. In general, the longer your child has symptoms before starting treatment, the longer it will take to get better.

If the heel hurts, your child needs to rest from his or her sport or activity. Your child should rest for several days at a time and then go back gradually. Before returning, he or she should be able to jog painlessly, then sprint painlessly, and be able to hop on the injured foot painlessly. If at any time during this process your child develops further heel pain, he or she should rest for 3 to 4 more days until the pain is gone before trying to return again.

How calcaneal apophysitis be prevented?

Calcaneal apophysitis is best prevented by having your child wear shoes that fit properly. The heel portion of the shoe should not be too tight, and there should be good padding in the heel. You may want to put extra heel pads in your child's shoes.

© HBO & Company

Calcaneal Apophysitis (Sever's Disease)

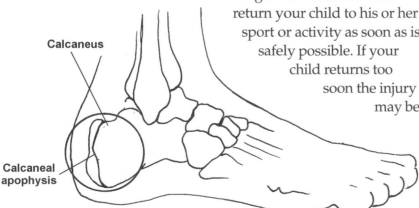

Calcaneus

Calcaneal apophysis

Calf Strain

What is a calf strain?

A strain is an injury in which muscle fibers or tendons are stretched or torn. People commonly call such an injury a "pulled" muscle. A calf strain is an injury to the muscles and tendons in the back of your leg below your knee.

How does it occur?

A strain of your calf muscles can occur during a physical activity where you push off forcefully from your toes. It may occur in running, jumping, or lunging.

What are the symptoms?

A calf muscle strain may cause immediate pain in the back of your lower leg. You may hear or feel a pop or a snap.

You may get the feeling that someone has hit you in the back of the leg. It will be hard to rise up on your toes. Your calf may be swollen and bruised.

How is it diagnosed?

Your doctor will examine your lower leg. Your calf muscles will be tender.

How is it treated?

Treatment may include:

- applying ice packs to your calf for 20 to 30 minutes every 3 to 4 hours for 2 or 3 days or until the pain goes away

- elevating your leg on a pillow while you are lying down
- wrapping an elastic bandage around your calf to keep the swelling from getting worse
- using crutches, if it is too painful to walk.
- taking anti-inflammatory medications
- getting physical therapy, which may include treatment of the muscle tissue by a therapist using ultrasound or muscle stimulation.
- having your doctor or therapist tape the injured muscles while they are healing to help you to return to athletic activities
- doing rehabilitation exercises.

While you are recovering from your injury, you will need to change your sport or activity to one that does not make your condition worse. For example, you may need to swim instead of run.

When can I return to my sport or activity?

The goal of rehabilitation is to return you to your sport or activity as soon as is safely possible. If you return too soon you may worsen your injury, which could lead to permanent damage. Everyone recovers

from injury at a different rate. Return to your activity will be determined by how soon your calf recovers, not by how many days or weeks it has been since your injury occurred. In general, the longer you have symptoms before you start treatment, the longer it will take to get better.

Calf Strain/Tear

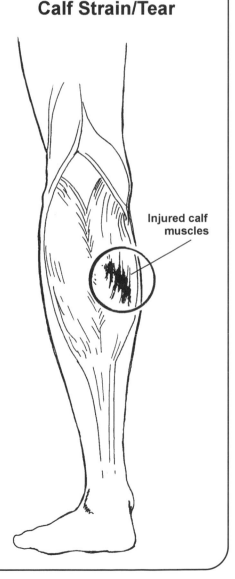

Injured calf muscles

Calf Strain

You may safely return to your sport or activity when, starting from the top of the list and progressing to the end, each of the following is true:

- You have full range of motion in the injured leg compared to the uninjured leg.
- You have full strength of the injured leg compared to the uninjured leg.
- You can jog straight ahead without pain or limping.
- You can sprint straight ahead without pain or limping.

- You can do 45-degree cuts, first at half-speed, then at full-speed.
- You can do 20-yard figures-of-eight, first at half-speed, then at full-speed.
- You can do 90-degree cuts, first at half-speed, then at full-speed.
- You can do 10-yard figures-of-eight, first at half-speed, then at full-speed.
- You can jump on both legs without pain and you can jump on the injured leg without pain.

How can calf strains be prevented?

Calf strains are best prevented by warming up properly and doing calf-stretching exercises before your activity. This is especially important if you are doing jumping or sprinting sports.

Calf Strain Rehabilitation Exercises

You can begin gently stretching your calf muscle using the towel stretch right away. Make sure you only get a gentle pull and not a sharp pain while you are doing this stretch. After you can do the towel stretch easily, you can start the standing calf stretch. After a couple days of stretching, you can begin strengthening your calf and lower leg muscles by using a Thera-Band as in exercises 3 and 4. You may do exercises 5, 6, and 7 when you can stand on your toes without pain.

1. Towel stretch: Sit on a hard surface with your injured leg stretched out in front of you. Loop a towel around the ball of your foot and pull the towel toward your body, keeping the knee straight and stretching the calf muscle. Hold this position for 30 seconds and then relax. Repeat 3 times. You should get an uncomfortable feeling but it should not be a sharp pain.

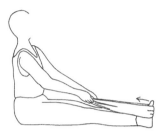

Towel stretch

2. Standing calf stretch: Stand facing a wall with your hands on the wall at about chest level. Your injured leg should be about 12 to 18 inches behind your uninjured leg. Keep your injured leg straight with your heel on the floor and lean into the wall. Bend your front knee until you feel a stretch in the back of the calf muscle of your injured leg. Hold this position for 30 to 60 seconds. Repeat 3 times.

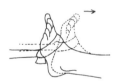

Resisted dorsiflexion

3. Resisted dorsiflexion: Sit with your injured leg out straight and your foot facing a doorway. Tie a loop in one end of the Thera-Band. Put your foot through the loop so that the tubing goes around the arch of your foot. Tie a knot in the other end of the Thera-Band and shut the knot in the door near the bottom. Move backward until there is tension in the tubing. Keeping your knee straight, pull your foot toward your face, stretching the tubing. Slowly return to the starting position. Repeat this 10 times. Do 3 sets of 10.

Standing calf stretch

4. Resisted plantar flexion. Sitting with your leg outstretched, loop the middle section of the tubing around the ball of your foot. Hold the ends of the tubing in both hands. Gently press the ball of your foot down and point your toes, stretching the Thera-Band. Return to the starting position. Repeat this 10 times. Do 3 sets of 10.

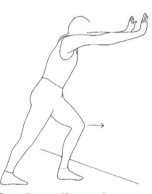

Resisted plantar flexion

5. Standing heel raise: Balance yourself while standing behind a chair or other stable object. Raise your body up onto your toes, lifting your heels off the floor. Hold this for about 2 seconds and then slowly lower your heels back down to the floor. Repeat 10 times. Do 3 sets of 10.

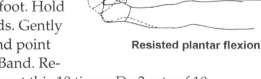

Heel raises

Calf Strain Rehabilitation Exercises

You can challenge yourself by standing only on your injured leg and lifting your heel off the ground.

6. Single leg balance: Attempt to balance on your injured leg while not letting the arch of that foot flatten. Don't curl your toes. Try to hold this position for 30 seconds. After this becomes easy, do it with your eyes closed.

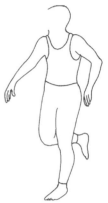

Single leg balance

As your balance becomes better and you are able to balance for 30 seconds on your injured leg you can challenge yourself.

7. Wall jump: Face a wall and place a piece of masking tape about 2 feet above your head. Jump up with your arms above your head and try to touch the piece of tape. Make sure you do a "spring" type of motion and do not land hard onto your feet. Progress to taking off and landing on one foot.

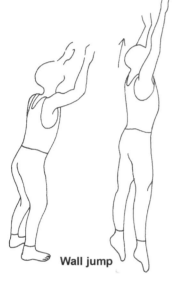

Wall jump

Another good exercise is hopping. You can start at one end of the room and try to hop as high as you can across the room on one foot. Jumping rope is also a good exercise.

Ingrown Toenail

What is an ingrown toenail?

An ingrown toenail is a toenail that grows into the surrounding skin or tissue of the toe. The toenail on the big toe is the one that is most commonly ingrown.

How does it occur?

An ingrown toenail usually occurs as a result of improper nail trimming. If a nail is cut curved instead of straight across, it may grow into the flesh at the edge of the nail and become ingrown.

Nails may also become ingrown as a result of direct blows or from wearing shoes or boots that are too tight.

What are the symptoms?

An area around the corners and edges of the toenail is painful. The toe may be swollen and red. There may be drainage. A toe with an ingrown toenail that becomes infected will be red and swollen and will have pus.

How is it diagnosed?

Your health care provider will examine your toe.

How is it treated?

Discomfort may be relieved by soaking your foot in a basin of warm water two or three times a day. If only a small part of your toenail is ingrown, the corner of the nail can be lifted up with a pair of tweezers and a small piece of cotton placed underneath this part of the nail.

Your health care provider may remove all or part of the ingrown nail. He or she will use numbing medicine before doing this. To prevent the nail from becoming ingrown again your provider may put a chemical on the nail growth area or may surgically remove the growth area.

Your health care provider may prescribe antibiotics if your toe is infected.

When can I return to my sport or activity after an ingrown toenail?

You may return to your sport or activity when you no longer have pain in your toe. It is important that your shoes fit well.

How can I prevent an ingrown toenail?

- Trim your toenails straight across without curving the edges.
- Wear shoes that do not cramp your toes.
- Cushion a nail that presses into the skin by putting cotton under the corners and edges that tend to become ingrown.

Ingrown Toenail

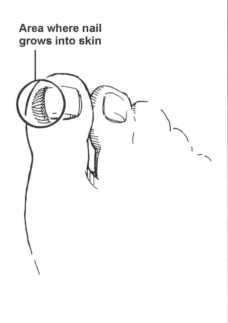

Area where nail grows into skin

Metatarsalgia

What is metatarsalgia?

The metatarsal bones are the long bones of the feet. They are located between the bones that form the ankle (tarsal bones) and the bones of the toes (phalanges). Metatarsalgia is pain in the long bones of the feet, especially located at the heads, or tips, of these bones.

How does it occur?

Metatarsalgia typically occurs from doing too much of a weight-bearing activity such as running, jumping, or walking. It may occur if you start wearing a new type of shoes, especially high-heeled shoes. In some people, the tips of some metatarsals point further down than in others, making these bones more likely to hurt.

What are the symptoms?

You will have pain in the middle of the foot, especially over the bones. You will have pain when the bones move and tenderness over the bony surfaces.

How is it diagnosed?

Your doctor will examine your foot and may order an x-ray to see if a foot bone is fractured. If you have metatarsalgia, the x-ray will show no break.

How is it treated?

You may be treated with an anti-inflammatory medication. Your doctor may prescribe a pad to put underneath the tender metatarsal. Custom-made arch supports (orthotics) are often prescribed for metatarsalgia.

While you are recovering from your injury, you will need to change your sport or activity to one that does not make your condition worse. For example, you may need to swim or bicycle instead of run or walk.

When can I return to my sport or activity?

The goal of rehabilitation is to return you to your sport or activity as soon as is safely possible. If you return too soon you may worsen your injury, which could lead to permanent damage. Everyone recovers from injury at a different rate. Return to your sport or activity will be determined by how soon your foot recovers, not by how many days or weeks it has been since your injury occurred. In general, the longer you have symptoms before you start treatment, the longer it will take to get better.

You may safely return to your sport or activity when, starting from the top of the list and progressing to the end, each of the following is true:

- You have full range of motion in the injured foot compared to the uninjured foot.

Metatarsalgia

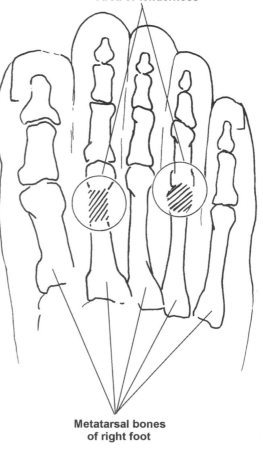

Area of tenderness

Metatarsal bones of right foot

Metatarsalgia

- You have full strength of the injured foot compared to the uninjured foot.
- You can jog straight ahead without pain or limping.
- You can sprint straight ahead without pain or limping.
- You can do 45-degree cuts, first at half-speed, then at full-speed.

- You can do 20-yard figures-of-eight, first at half-speed, then at full-speed.
- You can do 90-degree cuts, first at half-speed, then at full-speed.
- You can do 10-yard figures-of-eight, first at half-speed, then at full-speed.
- You can jump on both feet without pain and you can

jump on the injured foot without pain.

How can I prevent metatarsalgia?

Metatarsalgia is best prevented by wearing good shoes that fit well.

Morton's Neuroma

What is a Morton's neuroma?

Nerves run between the bones in the foot and along the toes. A neuroma is a benign (not cancerous) tumor of nerve tissue. A Morton's neuroma most commonly occurs between the bones of the third and fourth toes or those of the second and third toes.

How does it occur?

A neuroma may be caused by running or walking too much, but often it just occurs on its own. The pain is made worse by running on hard surfaces and by wearing shoes that are too tight.

What are the symptoms?

Your foot will be painful. The pain is usually worse when your toes are pointed up. You may get numbness or tingling in the affected area. You will have tenderness between the bones of the third and fourth toes or between the bones of the second and third toes.

How is it diagnosed?

Your doctor will examine your foot and review your symptoms.

How is it treated?

Treatment may include:

- wearing properly fitting shoes
- taking anti-inflammatory drugs
- wearing a pad below one of the bones in your foot or custom-made arch supports (orthotics)
- getting an injection of a cortisonelike medication if the above treatments fail.

Surgery may be required to remove the neuroma.

How can I prevent a Morton's neuroma?

It is not known how to prevent a Morton's neuroma. However, wearing properly fitting shoes with good padding will help decrease the pain of a Morton's neuroma.

Morton's Neuroma

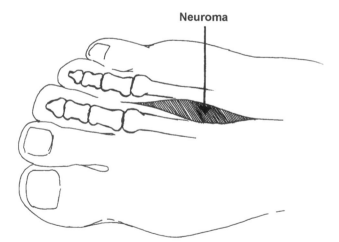

Neuroma

© HBO & Company

Peroneal Tendon Strain

What is a peroneal tendon strain?

A strain is an injury in which muscle fibers or tendons are stretched or torn. The peroneal muscles are on the outer side of the lower leg and their tendons attach to the foot. These muscles and tendons help move your foot to the outside.

How does it occur?

During an injury when the foot and ankle are rolled inward, a movement called inversion, the peroneal tendons may be stretched or torn. They also may be injured when your foot is forced upward toward your shin. Peroneal tendon strain can result from running on sloped surfaces or running in shoes with excessive wear on the outside of the heel.

What are the symptoms?

You will have pain on the outer side of your lower leg and ankle. You may hear a pop or a snap when the injury occurs. You may have swelling around your ankle.

How is it diagnosed?

Your doctor will examine your ankle and lower leg. He or she will move your ankle and leg to test these tendons. X-rays may be taken to see if there is a break in your ankle or in one of the bones in your feet.

How is it treated?

Treatment may include:

- applying ice packs to your ankle for 20 to 30 minutes every 3 to 4 hours for 2 or 3 days or until the pain goes away

- elevating your ankle to help the swelling go away by lying down and placing your foot and ankle on a pillow

- wrapping an elastic bandage around your ankle to help keep the swelling down

- wearing a stirrup splint (called an Aircast or Gelcast) or a lace-up ankle brace as prescribed by your doctor

- doing exercises to strengthen your peroneal muscles and tendons and to strengthen your ankle joint.

While you are recovering from your injury, you will need to change your sport or activity to one that will not make your condition worse. For example, you may need to bicycle or swim instead of run.

When can I return to my sport or activity?

The goal of rehabilitation is to return you to your sport or activity as soon as is safely possible. If you return too soon you may worsen your injury, which could lead to permanent damage. Everyone recovers from injury at a different rate. Return to your sport or activity will be determined by how soon your ankle recovers, not

Peroneal Tendon Strain

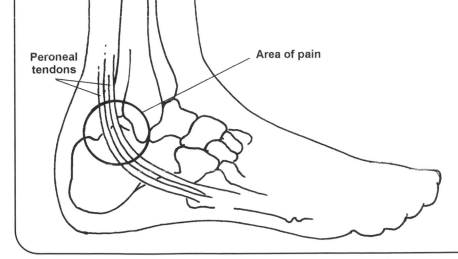

Peroneal tendons

Area of pain

Peroneal Tendon Strain

by how many days or weeks it has been since your injury occurred. In general, the longer you have symptoms before you start treatment, the longer it will take to get better.

You may safely return to your sport or activity when, starting from the top of the list and progressing to the end, each of the following is true:

- You have full range of motion in the injured leg compared to the uninjured leg.
- You have full strength of the injured leg compared to the uninjured leg.
- You can jog straight ahead without pain or limping.
- You can sprint straight ahead without pain or limping.
- You can do 45-degree cuts, first at half-speed, then at full-speed.
- You can do 20-yard figures-of-eight, first at half-speed, then at full-speed.
- You can do 90-degree cuts, first at half-speed, then at full-speed.
- You can do 10-yard figures-of-eight, first at half-speed, then at full-speed.
- You can jump on both legs without pain and you can jump on the injured leg without pain.

For rehabilitation exercises for peroneal tendon strain, press

How can I prevent a peroneal tendon strain?

- Keep your ankles and peroneal muscles strong.
- Wear high-top athletic shoes or a supportive ankle brace.
- Warm up properly before starting your sport or activity.
- When running, choose level surfaces and avoid rocks or holes.

Peroneal Tendon Strain Rehabilitation Exercises

You may start these exercises when you can stand comfortably on your injured leg with your heel resting on the floor and your full weight evenly distributed on both legs.

1. Towel stretch: Sit on a hard surface with your injured leg stretched out in front of you. Loop a towel around the ball of your foot and pull the towel toward your body, stretching the back of your calf muscle. Hold this position for 30 seconds. Repeat 3 times.

   When you don't feel much of a stretch using the towel, you can start the standing calf stretch.

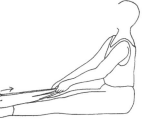

Towel stretch

2. Standing calf stretch: Facing a wall, place your hands against the wall at about eye level. Keep the injured leg back and the uninjured leg forward and the heel of your injured leg on the floor. Turn your injured foot slightly inward (as if you were pigeon-toed). Slowly lean into the wall until you feel a stretch in the back of your calf. Hold for 30 to 60 seconds. Do this 3 times.

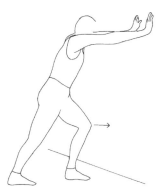

Standing calf stretch

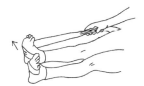

Resisted dorsiflexion

3. Thera-Band exercises

   A. Resisted dorsiflexion: Sitting with your leg out straight and your foot near a door, wrap the tubing around the ball of your foot. Anchor the other end of the tubing to the door by tying a knot in the tubing, slipping it between the door and the frame, and closing the door. Pull your toes toward your face. Return slowly to the starting position. Repeat 10 times. Do 3 sets of 10.

   B. Resisted eversion: Sitting with both legs outstretched and the tubing looped around both feet, slowly turn both feet upward and outward. Hold this position for 5 seconds. Repeat 10 times. Do 3 sets of 10.

Resisted eversion

4. Toe raises: Stand in a normal weight-bearing position. Rock back on your heels so that your toes come off the ground. Hold this position for 5 seconds. Repeat 10 times. Do 3 sets of 10.

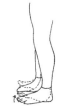

Standing toe raise

5. Single leg balance: Standing without support, attempt to balance on your injured leg while maintaining a good arch in your foot and not curling your toes. Begin doing this exercise with your eyes open and then attempt to do it with your eyes closed. Repeat 3 times.

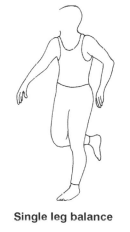

Single leg balance

Peroneal Tendon Strain Rehabilitation Exercises

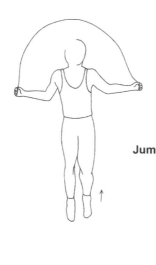

Jump rope

6. Jump rope: Jump rope landing on both legs for 5 minutes, then only on the injured leg for 5 minutes.

Plantar Fasciitis

What is plantar fasciitis?

Plantar fasciitis is a painful inflammation of the bottom of the foot between the ball of the foot and the heel.

How does it occur?

There are several possible causes of plantar fasciitis, including:

- wearing high heels
- gaining weight
- increased walking, standing, or stair-climbing.

If you wear high-heeled shoes, including western-style boots, for long periods of time, the tough, tendonlike tissue of the bottom of your foot can become shorter. This layer of tissue is called fascia. Pain occurs when you stretch fascia that has shortened. This painful stretching might happen, for example, when you walk barefoot after getting out of bed in the morning.

If you gain weight, you might be more likely to have plantar fasciitis, especially if you walk a lot or stand in shoes with poor heel cushioning. Normally there is a pad of fatty tissue under your heel bone. Weight gain might break down this fat pad and cause heel pain.

Runners may get plantar fasciitis when they change their workout and increase their mileage or frequency of

workouts. It can also occur with a change in exercise surface or terrain, or if your shoes are worn out and don't provide enough cushion for your heels.

If the arches of your foot are abnormally high or low, you are more likely to develop plantar fasciitis than if your arches are normal.

What are the symptoms?

The main symptom of plantar fasciitis is heel pain when you walk. You may also feel pain when you stand and possibly even when you are resting. This pain typically occurs first thing in the morning after you get out of bed, when your foot is placed flat on the floor. The pain occurs because you are stretching the plantar fascia. The pain usually lessens with more walking, but you may have it again after periods of rest.

You may feel no pain when you are sleeping because the position of your feet during rest allows the fascia to shorten and relax.

How is it diagnosed?

Your health care provider will ask about your symptoms. He or she will ask if the bottom of your heel is tender and if you have pain when you stretch the bottom of your foot. An x-ray of your heel may be done.

How is it treated?

Give your painful heel lots of rest. You may need to stay completely off your foot for several days when the pain is severe.

Your health care provider may recommend or prescribe anti-inflammatory medications, such as aspirin or ibuprofen. These drugs decrease

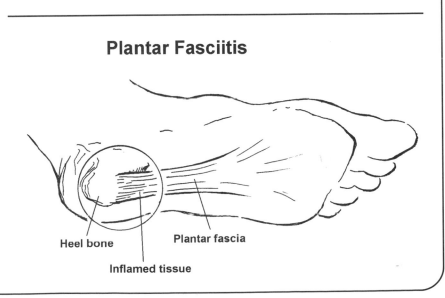

Plantar Fasciitis

Heel bone

Plantar fascia

Inflamed tissue

Plantar Fasciitis

pain and inflammation. Resting your heel on an ice pack for a few minutes several times a day can also help. Try to cushion your foot. You can do this by wearing athletic shoes, even at work, for awhile. Heel cushions can also be used. The cushions should be worn in both shoes. They are most helpful if you are overweight or elderly.

An orthotics sole support, specially molded to fit your foot, may be part of your treatment. These supports can be particularly helpful if you have flat feet or high arches.

If your heel pain is not relieved by the treatments described above, your health care provider may recommend physical therapy. The goals of physical therapy are to stretch the plantar fascia and to strengthen the lower leg muscles, which stabilize the ankle and heel. Sometimes physical therapists recommend athletic taping to support the bottom of the foot. A splint may be fitted to the calf of your leg and foot, to be worn at night to keep your foot stretched during sleep. Another possible treatment is injection of cortisone in the heel. Surgery is rarely necessary.

How long will the effects last?

You may find that the pain is sometimes worse and sometimes better over time. If you get treatment soon after you notice the pain, the symptoms should stop after several weeks. If, however, you have had plantar fasciitis for a long time, it may take many weeks to months for the pain to go away.

When can I return to my sport or activity?

The goal of rehabilitation is to return you to your sport or activity as soon as is safely possible. If you return too soon you may worsen your injury, which could lead to permanent damage. Everyone recovers from injury at a different rate. Return to your sport will be determined by how soon your foot recovers, not by how many days or weeks it has been since your injury occurred. In general, the longer you have symptoms before you start treatment, the longer it takes to get better.

You may safely return to your sport or activity when, starting from the top of the list and progressing to the end, each of the following is true:

- You have full range of motion in the injured foot compared to the uninjured foot.
- You have full strength of the injured foot compared to the uninjured foot.

- You can jog straight ahead without pain or limping.
- You can sprint straight ahead without pain or limping.
- You can do 45-degree cuts, first at half-speed, then at full-speed.
- You can do 20-yard figures-of-eight, first at half-speed, then at full-speed.
- You can do 90-degree cuts, first at half-speed, then at full-speed.
- You can do 10-yard figures-of-eight, first at half-speed, then at full-speed.
- You can jump on both feet without pain and you can jump on the injured foot without pain.

For rehabilitation exercises for plantar fasciitis, press

How do I prevent plantar fasciitis?

The best way to prevent plantar fasciitis is to wear shoes that are well made and fit your feet. This is especially important when you exercise or walk a lot or stand for a long time on hard surfaces. Get new athletic shoes before your old shoes stop supporting and cushioning your feet. You should also:

- Avoid repeated jarring to the heel.
- Maintain a healthy weight.

© HBO & Company

Plantar Fasciitis Rehabilitation Exercises

You may begin exercising the muscles of your foot right away by gently stretching them as follows:

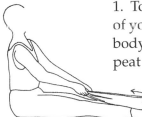

Towel stretch

1. Towel stretch: Sit on a hard surface with your injured leg stretched out in front of you. Loop a towel around the ball of your foot and pull the towel toward your body, stretching the back of your calf muscle. Hold this position for 30 seconds. Repeat 3 times. When the towel stretch becomes too easy, you may begin doing the standing calf stretch.

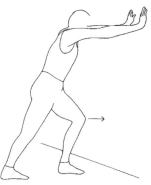

Standing calf stretch

2. Standing calf stretch: Facing a wall, put your hands against the wall at about eye level. Keep the injured leg back, the uninjured leg forward, and the heel of your injured leg on the floor. Turn your injured foot slightly inward (as if you were pigeon-toed) as you slowly lean into the wall until you feel a stretch in the back of your calf. Hold for 30 to 60 seconds. Repeat 3 times. When you can stand comfortably on your injured foot, you can begin stretching the planter fascia at the bottom of your foot.

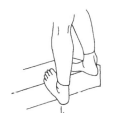

Plantar fascia stretch

3. Plantar fascia stretch: Stand with the ball of your injured foot on a stair. Reach for the bottom step with your heel until you feel a stretch in the arch of your foot. Hold this position for 30 to 60 seconds and then relax. Repeat 3 times.

After you have stretched the bottom muscles of your foot, you can begin strengthening the top muscles of your foot.

Frozen can roll

4. Frozen can roll: Roll your bare injured foot back and forth from your heel to your mid-arch over a frozen juice can. Repeat for 3 to 5 minutes. This exercise is particularly helpful if done first thing in the morning.

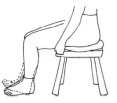

Sitting toe raise

5. Sitting toe raise: Sit in a chair with your feet flat on the floor. Raise the toes and the ball of your injured foot off the floor while keeping your heel on the floor. Hold for 5 seconds. Repeat 10 times. Do three sets of 10.

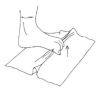

Towel pickup

6. Towel pickup: With your heel on the ground, pick up a towel with your toes. Release. Repeat 10 to 20 times.

Plantar Fasciitis Rehabilitation Exercises

Next, you can begin strengthening the muscles of your foot and lower leg by using a Thera-Band.

7. Resisted Thera-Band exercises for the lower leg

A. Resisted dorsiflexion: Sit with your injured leg out straight and your foot facing a doorway. Tie a loop in one end of the Thera-Band. Put your foot through the loop so that the tubing goes around the arch of your foot. Tie a knot in the other end of the Thera-Band and shut the knot in the door. Move backward until there is tension in the tubing. Keeping your knee straight, pull your foot toward your face, stretching the tubing. Slowly return to the starting position. Repeat 10 times. Do 3 sets of 10.

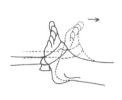

Resisted dorsiflexion

B. Resisted plantar flexion. Sit with your leg outstretched and loop the middle section of the tubing around the ball of your foot. Hold the ends of the tubing in both hands. Gently press the ball of your foot down and point your toes, stretching the Thera-Band. Return to the starting position. Repeat 10 times. Do 3 sets of 10.

Resisted plantar flexion

C. Resisted inversion: Sit with your legs out straight and cross your un-injured leg over your injured ankle. Wrap the tubing around the ball of your injured foot and then loop it around your uninjured foot so that the Thera-Band is anchored there at one end. Hold the other end of the Thera-Band in your hand. Turn your injured foot inward and upward. This will stretch the tubing. Return to the starting position. Repeat 10 times. Do 3 sets of 10.

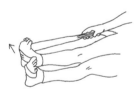

Resisted inversion

D. Resisted eversion: Sit with both legs stretched out in front of you, with your feet about a shoulder's width apart. Tie a loop in one end of the Thera-Band. Put your injured foot through the loop so that the tubing goes around the arch of that foot and wraps around the outside of the uninjured foot. Hold onto the other end of the tubing with your hand to provide tension. Turn your injured foot up and out. Make sure you keep your uninjured foot still so that it will allow the tubing to stretch as you move your injured foot. Return to the starting position. Repeat 10 times. Do 3 sets of 10.

Resisted eversion

Over-Pronation

What is over-pronation?

In normal walking or running, the first part of the foot to strike the ground is usually the heel. As a person's body weight is transferred to the middle of the foot, the arch of the foot will naturally flatten out a small amount. This flattening is called pronation. If your foot flattens more than is normal, it is called over-pronation. Over-pronation can cause many problems, such as Achilles tendonitis and heel pain, and can contribute to knee problems.

How does it occur?

Over-pronation occurs when you are walking or running and your foot hits the ground and the arch and the bones in your feet flatten out and roll inward. This can occur because of looseness in the ligaments or tendons that attach to your foot bones. You can be born with this type of problem or it can result from injuries or overuse.

What are the symptoms?

Over-pronation can cause pain in your arch, heel, shin, ankle, knee, hip, or back.

How is it diagnosed?

Your doctor will examine your feet and watch you walk or run. He or she will notice that the motion of your feet when they strike the ground is not normal. Your running shoes may show an abnormal pattern of wear.

How is it treated?

Over-pronation and the problems that go with it are best treated with custom-made arch supports called orthotics. Orthotics are usually made by making a mold of your feet so your specific foot problem can be taken care of. Orthotics are made from several types of material, ranging from spongy rubber to hard plastic.

How can I prevent over-pronation?

Over-pronation is usually caused by a problem with your feet that you were born with. However, the problems associated with over-pronation can be prevented by wearing orthotics in your shoes.

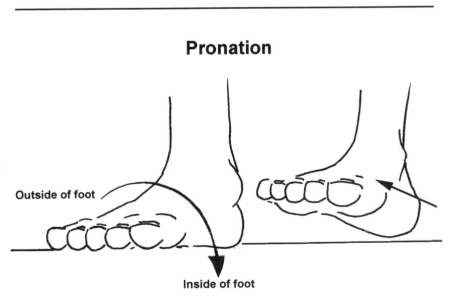

Pronation

Outside of foot

Inside of foot

The arch flattens out as the foot strikes the ground.

© HBO & Company

Shin Pain (Shin Splints)

What is shin pain?

Shin pain is pain on the front of the lower leg below the knee and above the ankle. It can hurt over the shin bone (tibia) or over the muscles on either side of the shin bone. Shin pain is also called shin splints.

How does it occur?

Shin pain generally occurs from overuse. This problem can come from stress fractures of the tibia or fibula or from irritation of the muscles or other tissues in the lower leg. It can occur in runners who increase their mileage or the intensity of their running, or who change the surface on which they are running. When you walk or run, your foot normally flattens out a small amount when it strikes the ground. If your foot flattens out more than normal, it is called over-pronation. Over-pronation can contribute to shin pain.

What are the symptoms?

You have pain over the front part of your lower leg. You may have pain at rest, during exercise, or both.

How is it diagnosed?

Your doctor examine your lower leg. He or she will look for tenderness over the front of your shin. Your doctor may watch you walk or run to see if you have problems with over-pronation. Your doctor may order x-rays or a bone scan to check for stress fractures.

How is it treated?

Treatment may include:

- applying ice packs to your shin for 20 to 30 minutes every 3 to 4 hours for 2 or 3 days or until the pain goes away

- doing ice massage (Freeze water in a Styrofoam cup. Peel the top of the cup away to expose the ice and hold onto the bottom of the cup while you rub ice into your leg for 5 to 10 minutes.)

- taking anti-inflammatory medication prescribed by your doctor

- wearing prescribed, custom-made arch supports

Shin Pain

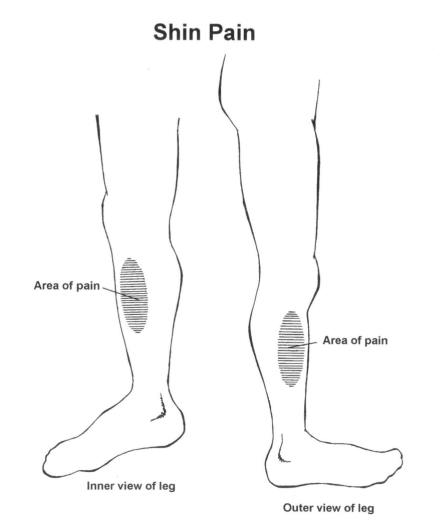

Area of pain

Area of pain

Inner view of leg

Outer view of leg

Shin Pain (Shin Splints)

(orthotics) to correct over-pronation

- doing rehabilitation exercises.

While you are recovering from your injury, you will need to change your sport or activity to one that does not make your condition worse. For example, you may need to bicycle or swim instead of run. When you begin to run again, you should wear good shoes and run on soft surfaces.

When can I return to my sport or activity?

The goal of rehabilitation is to return you to your sport or activity as soon as is safely possible. If you return too soon you may worsen your injury, which could lead to permanent damage. Everyone recovers from injury at a different rate. Return to your sport or activity will be determined by how soon your leg recovers, not by how many days or weeks it has been since your injury occurred. In general, the longer you have symptoms before you start treatment, the longer it will take to get better.

You may safely return to your sport or activity when, starting from the top of the list and progressing to the end, each of the following is true:

- You have full range of motion in the injured leg compared to the uninjured leg.
- You have full strength of the injured leg compared to the uninjured leg.
- You can jog straight ahead without pain or limping.
- You can sprint straight ahead without pain or limping.
- You can do 45-degree cuts, first at half-speed, then at full-speed.
- You can do 20-yard figures-of-eight, first at half-speed, then at full-speed.
- You can do 90-degree cuts, first at half-speed, then at full-speed.
- You can do 10-yard figures-of-eight, first at half-speed, then at full-speed.
- You can jump on both legs without pain and you can jump on the injured leg without pain.

How can I prevent shin pain?

- Since shin pain usually occurs from overuse, be sure to begin your activities gradually.
- Wear shoes with proper padding.
- Run on softer surfaces.
- Warm up properly and stretch the muscles in the front of your leg and in your calf.

Shin Pain (Shin Splints) Rehabilitation Exercises

Start these exercises when your pain has decreased by about 25% from the time when your injury was most painful.

1. Calf stretch

A. Calf stretch with towel: Sitting on a firm surface with your injured leg straight in front of you, take a towel and loop it around the ball of your foot. Pull the towel toward you. Hold this position for 30 seconds. Relax. Repeat 3 times. When you don't feel much of a stretch anymore using the towel, start stretching the calf in the standing position described below.

B. Standing calf stretch: Facing a wall, place both hands at about eye level on the wall. Keep your uninjured leg forward and your injured leg back about 12 to 18 inches behind your uninjured leg. Keep your injured leg straight and your heel on the floor. Next, do a slight lunge by bending the knee of the forward leg. Lean into the wall until you feel a stretch in your calf muscle. Hold this for 30 to 60 seconds. Repeat 3 times.

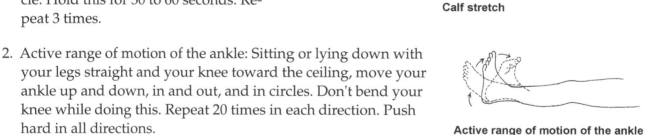

A.   **B.**

Calf stretch

2. Active range of motion of the ankle: Sitting or lying down with your legs straight and your knee toward the ceiling, move your ankle up and down, in and out, and in circles. Don't bend your knee while doing this. Repeat 20 times in each direction. Push hard in all directions.

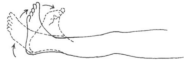

Active range of motion of the ankle

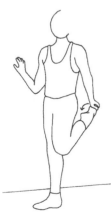

Anterior compartment stretch

3. Anterior compartment stretch: Stand with one hand against a wall or chair for balance. Bend your knee and grasp the front of the foot of your injured leg. Bend the front of the foot toward the heel. You should feel a stretch in the front of your shin. Hold for 10 seconds. Repeat 10 times.

4. Thera-Band strengthening exercises for the lower leg

A. Resisted dorsiflexion flexion: Sit in front of a doorway with your legs outstretched. Anchor the Thera-Band in a door by tying knots in the ends and closing the knots in the door. Next, loop the Thera-Band around the forefoot of your injured leg. Pull your foot toward your face with the Thera-Band supplying resistance. Return slowly to the starting position. Repeat 10 times. Do 3 sets of 10.

Shin Pain (Shin Splints) Rehabilitation Exercises

B. Resisted plantar flexion: Sitting with your legs outstretched, put the tubing around the foot of your injured leg and hold the ends of the tubing in your hands. Gently press your foot down stretching the Thera-Band. Return to the starting position. Repeat 10 times. Do 3 sets of 10.

C. Resisted inversion: Sit on the floor with your uninjured leg crossed over your injured ankle. Hold one end of the Thera-Band in your hand and tie the other end in a loop. Place the loop around the forefoot of the injured leg and have the band wrapped around the uninjured foot to provide an anchor. Move your injured foot inward with the Thera-Band providing resistance. Return your foot to the starting position. Repeat 10 times. Do 3 sets of 10.

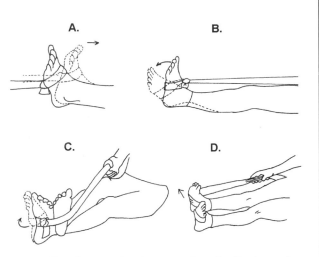

Thera-Band strengthening exercises for the lower leg

D. Resisted eversion: Sitting on the floor with both legs straight out, have the Thera-Band looped around both feet. Slowly turn the injured foot outward, keeping the uninjured foot still. Return to the starting position. Repeat 10 times. Do 3 sets of 10.

5. Heel raises: Balance yourself while standing behind a chair or counter. Raise your body up onto your toes, then slowly lower it. Repeat 10 times. Do 2 sets of 10.

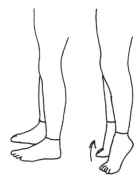

Heel raises

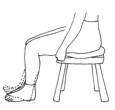

Sitting toe raise

6. Toe raises

A. Sitting: Sit on a firm surface with your feet flat on the floor. Keep your heel on the floor and raise your toes off the floor. Repeat 10 times. Do 3 sets of 10. When the sitting exercise becomes easy, progress to standing, as described below.

B. Standing: Standing with your feet flat on the floor, rock back onto your heels and lift your toes off the floor. Hold this for 5 seconds. Repeat 10 times. Do 3 sets of 10.

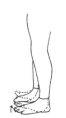

Standing toe raise

Stress Fractures

What is a stress fracture?

A stress fracture is a hairline crack that can occur in bones from repeated or prolonged use. The most common sites for stress fracture are the foot bones (metatarsals), shin bone (tibia), outer lower leg bone (fibula), thigh bone (femur), and back bones (vertebrae).

How does it occur?

Stress fractures are overuse injuries. The majority of leg injuries occur during activities such as running, jumping, or dancing. Stress fractures of the feet were originally called march fractures because they were commonly seen in military personnel.

What are the symptoms?

You have pain with activity. You may have swelling and bruising.

How is it diagnosed?

Your doctor will examine you and may order an x-ray. However, x-rays do not always show a stress fracture. Your doctor may order a more specialized test called a bone scan.

How is it treated?

The most important treatment for a stress fracture is rest. Other treatment may include:

- applying ice packs over your injury for 20 to 30 minutes every 3 to 4 hours for 2 to 3 days or until the pain goes away
- if you are a runner, running only if there is no pain
- changing your activity, such as from running to swimming
- taking anti-inflammatory medication prescribed by your doctor
- wearing a cast for 3 to 6 weeks while your bone heals.

Stress Fractures in Leg and Foot

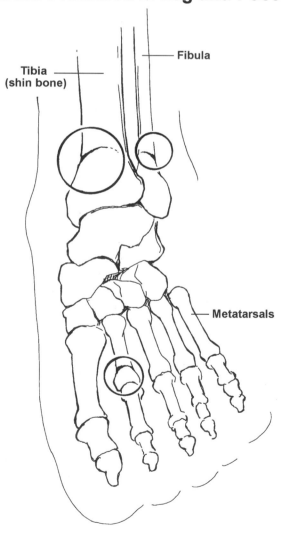

Tibia (shin bone)

Fibula

Metatarsals

Stress Fractures

When can I return to my sport or activity?

The goal of rehabilitation is to return you to your sport or activity as soon as is safely possible. If you return too soon you may worsen your injury, which could lead to permanent damage. Everyone recovers from injury at a different rate. Return to your sport or activity will be determined by how soon the fracture heals, not by how many days or weeks it has been since your injury occurred. In general, the longer you have symptoms before you start treatment, the longer it will take to get better.

After a stress fracture you may do sports or activities that do not cause pain. It is very important not to "run through the pain" because this may cause further injury. You should vary your activity for one week at a time. For instance, if you have a stress fracture from running, you should either rest or swim for a week, then attempt to run short distances. If there is no pain, you can gradually increase your distance.

How can I prevent a stress fracture?

Stress fractures are caused by overuse. The best way to avoid getting a stress fracture is to listen to your body and not force yourself to do activities while you are in pain.

© HBO & Company

Turf Toe

What is turf toe?

Turf toe is pain at the joint where the big toe attaches to the rest of the foot.

How does it occur?

Turf toe can result from excessive pushing off of the big toe when you run or jump. Jamming the toe into a hard surface can also cause turf toe.

What are the symptoms?

You have pain where your big toe attaches to your foot. You may have difficulty bending and straightening your toe. Your toe joint may be swollen.

How is it diagnosed?

Your doctor will ask about your symptoms and examine your toe. He or she may order an x-ray to be sure you did not break your toe.

Turf toe can sometimes look like gout, a type of arthritis of the big toe. Your doctor may order tests to be sure you do not have gout.

How is it treated?

Treatment may include the following:

- putting ice packs on your toe for 20 to 30 minutes every 3 to 4 hours for the first 2 to 3 days or until the pain goes away

- elevating your foot on a pillow
- taking anti-inflammatory medications prescribed by your doctor.

One of the keys to treating turf toe is keeping the toe from moving too much. Your toe can be taped to restrict how much it moves. You may have a special insole placed in your shoe that will reduce the movement of your big toe.

When can I return to my sport or activity?

The goal of rehabilitation is to return you to your sport or activity as soon as is safely possible. If you return too soon you may worsen your injury, which could lead to permanent damage. Everyone recovers from injury at a different rate. Return to your sport or activity will be determined by how soon your toe recovers, not by how many days or weeks it has been since your injury occurred. In general, the longer you have symptoms before you start treatment, the longer it will take to get better.

You may safely return to your sport or activity when, starting from the top of the list and progressing to the end, each of the following is true:

- You have full range of motion in the injured toe

compared to the uninjured toes.
- You have full strength of the injured toe compared to the uninjured toes.
- You can jog straight ahead without pain or limping.
- You can sprint straight ahead without pain or limping.
- You can do 45-degree cuts, first at half-speed, then at full-speed.

Turf Toe

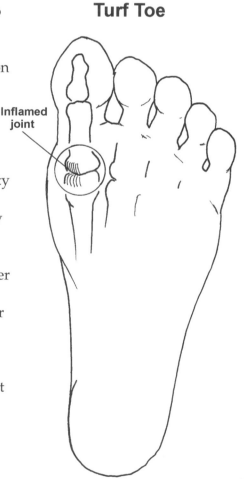

Inflamed joint

Turf Toe

- You can do 20-yard figures-of-eight, first at half-speed, then at full-speed.
- You can do 90-degree cuts, first at half-speed, then at full-speed.
- You can do 10-yard figures-of-eight, first at half-speed, then at full-speed.
- You can jump on both feet without pain and you can jump on the foot with the injured toe without pain.

How can I prevent turf toe?

Turf toe is best prevented by wearing good shoes that fit properly and by avoiding jamming your big toe into a hard surface.

© HBO & Company

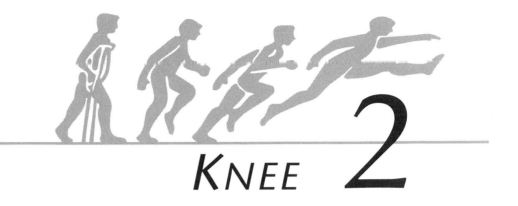

KNEE 2

Anterior Cruciate Ligament (ACL) Sprain

What is an anterior cruciate ligament (ACL) sprain?

A sprain is a joint injury that causes a stretch or a tear in a ligament. Ligaments are strong bands of tissue that connect one bone to another. The anterior cruciate ligament (ACL) is one of the major ligaments in the middle of the knee. It connects the thigh bone (femur) to the shin bone (tibia). This ligament, along with the posterior cruciate ligament, helps keep the knee stable and protects the femur from sliding or turning on the tibia.

Sprains are graded I, II, or III depending on their severity:

- grade I sprain: pain with minimal damage to the ligaments
- grade II sprain: more ligament damage and mild looseness of the joint
- grade III sprain: the ligament is completely torn and the joint is very loose or unstable.

How does it occur?

The anterior cruciate ligament is frequently injured in forced twisting motions of the knee. It may also become injured when the knee is straightened further than it normally can straighten (hyperextended). It sometimes occurs when the thigh bone is forcefully pushed across the shin bone, such as with a sudden stop while you are running or a sudden transfer of weight while you are skiing.

What are the symptoms?

There is usually a loud, painful pop when the joint is first injured. This is often followed by a lot of swelling of the knee within the first several hours after the injury. This swelling is called an effusion and is made up of blood in the knee joint.

If you have torn your anterior cruciate ligament in an injury that occurred months or years ago and you haven't had reconstructive surgery, you may have the feeling that the knee is giving way during twisting or pivoting movements.

How is it diagnosed?

Your doctor will examine your knee and may find that your knee has become loose. If you have swelling in the joint, your doctor may decide to remove the blood in your knee with a needle and syringe. You may need x-rays to see if there is an injury to the bones in your knee. An MRI (magnetic resonance imaging) scan may

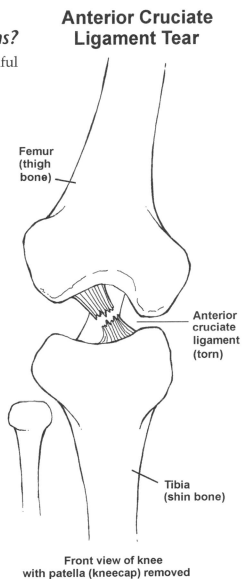

Anterior Cruciate Ligament Tear

Femur (thigh bone)

Anterior cruciate ligament (torn)

Tibia (shin bone)

Front view of knee with patella (kneecap) removed

Anterior Cruciate Ligament (ACL) Sprain

also be done and should clearly show the condition of your ACL (as well as that of other ligaments and cartilage).

How is it treated?

Treatment includes the following:

- Put an ice pack on your knee for 20 to 30 minutes every 3 to 4 hours for 2 or 3 days or until the pain goes away.
- Keep your knee elevated whenever possible by placing a pillow underneath it until the swelling goes away.
- Do the exercises recommended by your doctor or physical therapist.

Your doctor may recommend that you:

- Wrap an elastic bandage around your knee to keep the swelling from getting worse.
- Use a knee immobilizer initially to protect the knee.
- Use crutches.

For complete tears, you and your doctor will decide if you should have intense rehabilitation or if you should have surgery followed by rehabilitation. The torn anterior cruciate ligament cannot be sewn back together. The ligament must be reconstructed by taking ligaments or tendons from another part of your leg and connecting them to the tibia and femur.

You may consider having reconstructive ACL surgery if:

- Your knee is unstable and gives out during routine or athletic activity.
- You are a high-level athlete and your knee could be unstable and give out during your sport (for example, basketball, football, or soccer).
- You are a younger person who is not willing to give up an athletic lifestyle.
- You want to prevent further injury to your knee. An unstable knee may lead to injuries of the meniscus and arthritis.

You may consider not having the surgery if:

- Your knee is not unstable and is not painful and you are able to do your chosen activities without symptoms.
- You are willing to give up sports that put extra stress on your knee.
- You are not involved in sports.

If a growing child tears an ACL, the doctor may recommend that surgery be postponed until the child has stopped growing.

When can I return to my sport or activity?

The goal of rehabilitation is to return you to your sport or activity as soon as is safely possible. If you return too soon you may worsen your injury, which could lead to permanent damage. Everyone recovers from injury at a different rate. Return to your activity will be determined by how soon your knee recovers, not by how many days or weeks it has been since your injury occurred. In general, the longer you have symptoms before you start treatment, the longer it will take to get better.

You may safely return to your sport or activity when, starting from the top of the list and progressing to the end, each of the following is true:

- Your injured knee can be fully straightened and bent without pain.
- Your knee and leg have regained normal strength compared to the uninjured knee and leg.
- The effusion is gone.
- You are able to jog straight ahead without limping.
- You are able to sprint straight ahead without limping.
- You are able to do 45-degree cuts.
- You are able to do 90-degree cuts.
- You are able to do 20-yard figure-of-eight runs.
- You are able to do 10-yard figure-of-eight runs.

Anterior Cruciate Ligament (ACL) Sprain

- You are able to jump on both legs without pain and jump on the injured leg without pain.

If you feel that your knee is giving way or if you develop pain or have swelling in your knee, you should see your doctor. If you've had surgery, be sure that your doctor has told you that you can return to your sport.

How can I prevent an anterior cruciate ligament sprain?

Unfortunately, most injuries to the anterior cruciate ligament occur during accidents that are not preventable. However, you may be able to avoid these injuries by having strong thigh and hamstring muscles and maintaining a good leg stretching routine. In activities such as skiing, make sure your ski bindings are set correctly by a trained professional so that your skis will release when you fall.

Anterior Cruciate Ligament Sprain (ACL) Rehabilitation Exercises

You may begin exercising your knee when the swelling has gone down and you are able to stand with equal weight on both legs.

1. Heel slide: Sit on a firm surface with your legs straight in front of you. Slowly slide the heel of your injured leg toward your buttock by pulling your knee to your chest as you slide. Return to the starting position. Repeat this 20 times.

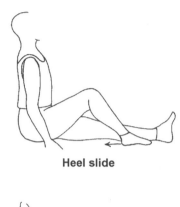

Heel slide

2. Prone knee flexion: Lying on your stomach, bend your injured knee and try to touch your buttock with your heel. Slowly return to the starting position. As this gets easier, you can add an ankle weight of 3 to 5 pounds. Repeat 10 times. Do 3 sets of 10.

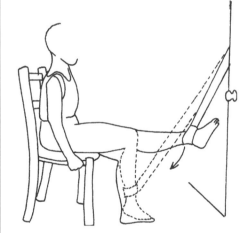

Theraband hamstring curls

3. Thera-Band hamstring curls: Sit in a chair facing a door and about 3 feet from the door. Loop and tie one end of the tubing around the ankle of your injured leg. Tie a knot in the other end of the Thera-Band and shut the knot in the door. Bend your knee so that your foot slides along the floor and moves back underneath the chair, stretching the tubing. Slowly let your foot slide forward again. Repeat this 10 times. Do 3 sets of 10.

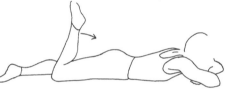

Prone knee flexion

You can challenge yourself by moving the chair farther away from the door and increasing the resistance of the Thera-Band.

4. Heel raises: Stand on both feet, raise your heels off the floor and come up onto your toes. Hold this position for 2 seconds and slowly lower yourself back down. Do 3 sets of 10 repetitions.

To challenge yourself, stand only on your injured leg and raise up on your toes, lifting your heel off the floor. Do 3 sets of 10.

After your hamstrings have become stronger and you feel your leg is stable, you can begin strengthening the quadriceps (a large muscle in the front of the thigh). A good way to do this is to do a wall squat with a ball.

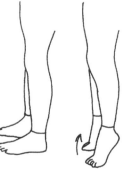

Heel raises

Anterior Cruciate Ligament Sprain (ACL) Rehabilitation Exercises

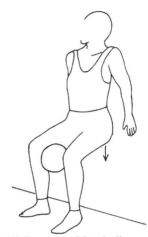

Wall squat with a ball

5. Wall squat with a ball: Stand with your back, shoulders, and head against a wall and look straight ahead. Keep your shoulders relaxed and your feet 1 foot away from the wall and a shoulder-width apart. Place a rolled up pillow or a Nerf ball between your thighs. Keeping your head against the wall, slowly squat while squeezing the pillow or ball at the same time. Squat down until your thighs are parallel to the floor. Hold this position for 10 seconds. Slowly stand back up. Make sure you keep squeezing the pillow or ball throughout this exercise. Repeat 20 times.

Anterior Cruciate Ligament (ACL) Reconstruction

What is the anterior cruciate ligament (ACL)?

Ligaments are strong bands of tissue that connect one bone to another. The anterior cruciate ligament (ACL) is one of four major ligaments in the knee. It is in the center of the knee joint, connecting the thigh bone (femur) to the shin bone (tibia). The ACL helps keep the knee stable by limiting twisting and forward sliding motions of the knee.

The ACL is commonly injured in sports when there is a forced twisting motion of the knee or when the knee is hit while the foot is planted. It may also be injured during a sudden stop when the femur moves forcefully over the tibia.

What is an ACL reconstruction?

A torn ACL will not heal by itself. In the past, doctors tried to repair the ACL by sewing the torn ends of the ligament together, but this did not work. The ACL must be reconstructed by using ligaments or tendons from another part of the body to replace the torn ACL. Tendons are connective tissue bands that attach muscles to bones. The replacement tissue is called a graft.

The grafts can come from several places. Most often the graft is taken from the patellar tendon, which attaches your kneecap (patella) to your shin bone (tibia). The graft is made up of the middle third of the patellar tendon and small pieces of bone from the kneecap and the shin bone. A graft may also come from your hamstring tendon. The hamstring muscles are in the back of your thigh.

If the graft comes from your own body, it is called an autograft. If the graft comes from someone who has died, it is called an allograft. Doctors have tried using some types of

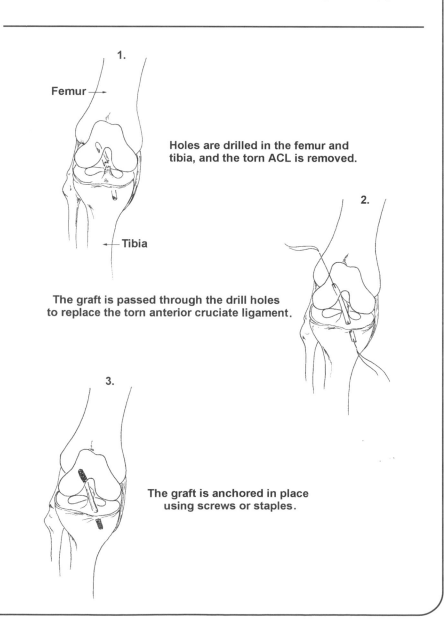

1.

Femur

Tibia

Holes are drilled in the femur and tibia, and the torn ACL is removed.

2.

The graft is passed through the drill holes to replace the torn anterior cruciate ligament.

3.

The graft is anchored in place using screws or staples.

— Anterior Cruciate Ligament (ACL) Reconstruction —

synthetic grafts but so far these have not worked well. Research is being done to see if there are better types of grafts that can be used.

Your doctor will discuss the options with you and will help you decide which procedure is best for you.

You may consider having reconstructive ACL surgery if:

- Your knee is unstable and gives out during routine or athletic activity.

- You are a high-level athlete and your knee could be unstable and give out during your sport (for example, basketball, football, or soccer).

- You are a younger person who is not willing to give up an athletic lifestyle.

- You want to prevent further injury to your knee. An unstable knee may lead to injuries of the meniscus and arthritis.

You may consider not having the surgery if:

- Your knee is not unstable and is not painful and you are able to do your chosen activities without symptoms.

- You are willing to give up sports that put extra stress on your knee.

- You are not involved in sports.

If a growing child tears an ACL, the doctor may recom-mend that surgery be post-poned until the child has stopped growing.

How do I prepare for an ACL reconstruction?

Plan for your care and recov-ery after surgery. Allow time to rest, and try to find people to help you for a few days.

Follow your doctor's instructions. You may be asked not to take aspirin for a week or so before your surgery. Do not eat or drink anything after midnight or the morning before surgery. You may have physical therapy before surgery to begin your rehabili-tation.

What happens during surgery?

You will have either general or spinal anesthesia. A general anesthetic will relax your mus-cles and make you feel as if you are in a deep sleep. A spinal anesthetic leaves you awake but unable to feel any-thing from the waist down.

Your doctor will prepare the graft. If your patellar tendon is to be used, the doctor will make an incision 1 to 3 inches below your kneecap. Then he or she will remove your torn ACL using an arthroscope. An arthroscope is a thin tube through which your doctor can view the inside of your knee joint. Various thin, small instruments are used to per-form surgery in the knee. Your doctor will drill holes in your femur and tibia where the graft will be attached. The graft will be passed through the holes and anchored in place by screws or staples. The incisions from the graft site and the arthroscopy will be closed with stitches, tape, or staples.

During your surgery, your doctor may also treat any other knee injuries such as torn cartilage.

What happens after the surgery?

You may be allowed to go home a few hours after surgery or you may have to spend the night in the hospi-tal. Treatment after surgery may include:

- elevating your knee on a pillow several times a day as long as it is swollen and painful

- putting ice packs on your knee for 20 to 30 minutes 3 to 4 times a day for a few weeks

- taking medication prescribed by your doctor for pain and swelling

- having physical therapy to rehabilitate your knee.

You may be on crutches for a week or two after surgery. You may not be able to drive for at least a few weeks.

© HBO & Company

Anterior Cruciate Ligament (ACL) Reconstruction

What are the complications?

Complications may include:

- loss of range of motion in your knee, joint stiffness
- persistent pain
- a blood clot in the leg
- bleeding
- infection.

When should I call the doctor?

Call the doctor immediately if:

- You have a lot of bleeding or a discolored drainage from the puncture sites.
- You have a lot of pain in your knee.

- You get a fever.
- You have swelling in your calf or thigh that does not improve when you elevate your leg.

Call your doctor during office hours if:

- You have questions about the surgery or its result.

When can I return to my sport or activity?

The goal of rehabilitation is to return you to full participation in your sport or activity as soon as is safely possible. If you return too soon you may worsen your injury, which could lead to permanent damage. Everyone recovers from injury at a different rate. Return to your activity will be determined by how soon your knee recovers, not how many days or weeks it has been since your surgery.

Rehabilitation from ACL surgery is very complex. Your doctor and therapist will watch your progress very carefully and gradually allow you to be more active. It may take 4 to 9 months of rehabilitation to get back to some activities. It may take 12 months or more for your knee to feel the way it did before your injury.

Arthroscopic Meniscectomy

What is an arthroscopic meniscectomy?

An arthroscopic meniscectomy is a procedure in which the doctor uses an arthroscope and other tools to remove all or part of a damaged meniscus in the knee or, if possible, to repair a meniscus. A meniscus is a piece of rubbery tissue (fibrocartilage) between the bones of the knee joint. An arthroscope is a tube with a light at the end that projects an image of the inside of your knee onto a TV monitor. The arthroscope is about the diameter of a pencil.

When is it used?

The procedure is used when you have damaged cartilage in your knee.

Examples of alternatives are:

- limiting your activity
- taking drugs to reduce the swelling
- having physical therapy
- having open knee surgery
- choosing not to have treatment, while recognizing the risks of your condition.

You should ask your doctor about these choices.

How do I prepare for an arthroscopic meniscectomy?

Plan for your care and recovery after the operation, especially if you are to have general anesthesia. Allow for time to rest and try to find other people to help you with your day-to-day duties.

Follow instructions provided by your doctor. Do not eat or drink anything after midnight or the morning before the procedure. Do not even drink coffee, tea, or water.

What happens during the procedure?

You will be given a general, regional, or local anesthetic. Which type depends on you, your anesthesiologist, and your surgeon. A general anesthetic will relax your muscles and make you feel as if you are in a deep sleep. Both local and regional anesthetics numb part of the body while you remain awake. All three types of anesthesia should keep you from feeling pain during the operation.

The doctor will put an arthroscope and one or two tools into the knee joint through small incisions (cuts). Fluid is injected into the knee to expand the joint so that the structures and cartilage can be seen. The doctor will examine the knee to find any damage. She or he may repair any torn cartilage or shave down the cartilage in the knee and remove the pieces of cartilage. The doctor will then remove the arthroscope and the tools and close the small openings with stitches.

What happens after the procedure?

You will go home the same day. You should keep your leg elevated. Take it easy for at least the next 2 to 3 days. Do not take part in strenuous activities until the doctor feels you are ready.

After arthroscopy:

- Use crutches for 1 to 2 days or until you can walk nearly normally.
- Elevate your leg so that your ankle is higher than your knee and your knee is higher than your hip.
- Put ice on your knee for 20 to 30 minutes 3 or 4 times a day until symptoms are gone.
- Bend your knee when symptoms have decreased.
- Change your bandage after 4 days and cover the cuts with band-aids or gauze.
- If you have a brace or splint, consult your doctor.
- If the cartilage is repaired and not trimmed, your doctor may want you to use crutches longer and to not put weight on your leg.

Ask your doctor what other

Arthroscopic Meniscectomy

steps you should take and when you should come back for a checkup.

What are the benefits of this procedure?

The arthroscopy may treat the knee without the need for open knee surgery with bigger incisions. There is more rapid recovery than with open knee surgery.

What are the risks associated with this procedure?

- There are some risks when you have general anesthesia. Discuss these risks with your doctor.
- Local anesthesia may not numb the area quite enough

and you may feel some minor discomfort. Also, in rare cases, you may have an allergic reaction to the drug used in this type of anesthesia. Local anesthesia is considered safer than general anesthesia in older people and in people with certain medical conditions.

- The blood vessels and nerves around the knee may be injured causing numbness or weakness in the leg below the knee.
- There is a risk of deep vein thrombosis, a condition in which a blood clot forms within a deep-lying vein.
- There is a risk of infection and bleeding.

You should ask your doctor how these risks apply to you.

When should I call the doctor?

Call your doctor immediately if:

- There is excessive drainage from the puncture sites.
- There is unusual pain.
- Your knee locks.
- You develop a fever.
- You develop signs of deep vein thrombosis.
- You develop signs of infection.

Call your doctor during office hours if:

- You have questions about the procedure or its result.
- You want to make an appointment for a follow-up examination.

Baker's Cyst

What is a Baker's cyst?

A bursa is a fluid-filled sac that acts as a cushion between tendons, bones, and skin. A Baker's cyst is an abnormal swelling of a bursa located in the space behind the knee (the popliteal space). The cyst connects to the membrane covering the knee joint.

How does it occur?

No one really knows what causes Baker's cysts. However, the cysts can occur when the lining of the knee joint produces too much fluid, as in rheumatoid arthritis, or after an injury.

What are the symptoms?

You may have pain, swelling, or a feeling of fullness in the area behind the knee.

How is it diagnosed?

Your doctor will examine your knee and find a bulge in the back of your knee. You may need to have a magnetic resonance image (MRI) or an arthrogram to help the doctor determine if you have a Baker's cyst. For an arthrogram, dye is injected into your knee and then an x-ray is taken to look at the joint capsule, the membrane surrounding the joint.

How is it treated?

The initial discomfort of a Baker's cyst may be treated by wearing an elastic bandage. Your doctor may prescribe anti-inflammatory medications, the cyst may be drained, or an operation may be performed to remove the cyst. Sometimes the cyst goes away on its own. If the cyst does not cause bothersome symptoms, it may not be treated.

How can a Baker's cyst be prevented?

There is really no way to prevent a Baker's cyst from forming.

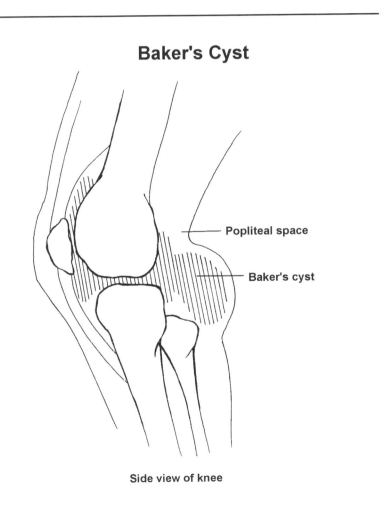

Baker's Cyst

Popliteal space

Baker's cyst

Side view of knee

Iliotibial Band Syndrome

What is iliotibial band syndrome?

Iliotibial band syndrome is inflammation and pain on the outer side of the knee. The iliotibial band is a layer of connective tissue. It begins at a muscle near the outer side of your hip, travels down the outer side of your thigh, crosses the outer side of the knee, and attaches to the outer side of your upper shin bone (tibia).

How does it occur?

Iliotibial band syndrome occurs when this band repeatedly rubs over the bump of the thigh bone (femur) near the knee, causing the band to be irritated. This most often occurs in running.

This condition can result from:

- having a tight iliotibial band
- having tight muscles in your hip, pelvis, or leg
- your legs not being the same length
- running on sloped surfaces
- running in shoes with a lot of wear on the outside of the heel.

What are the symptoms?

The symptom is pain on the outer side of the knee.

How is it diagnosed?

Your doctor will examine your knee and find tenderness where the band passes over the bump on the outer side of your knee. Your iliotibial band may be tight.

How is it treated?

Treatment includes the following:

- Place an ice pack over your iliotibial band for 20 to 30 minutes every 3 or 4 hours for 2 to 3 days or until the pain goes away.
- You can also do ice massage. Massage your knee with ice by freezing water in a Styrofoam cup. Peel the top of the cup away to expose the ice and hold onto the bottom of the cup while you rub ice over your knee for 5 to 10 minutes.

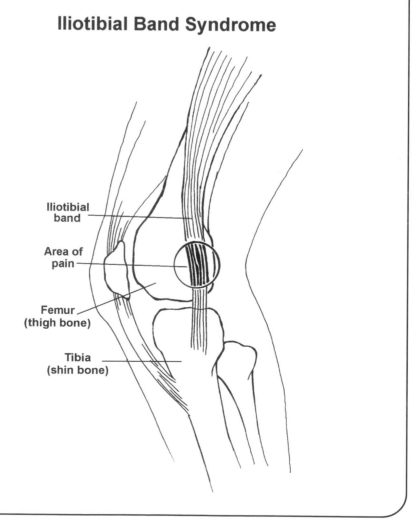

Iliotibial Band Syndrome

Iliotibial band

Area of pain

Femur (thigh bone)

Tibia (shin bone)

Iliotibial Band Syndrome

- Take an anti-inflammatory medication, according to your doctor's prescription.
- Do the stretching exercises recommended by your doctor or physical therapist.

Your doctor may give you an injection of a corticosteroid medication to reduce the inflammation and pain.

While your knee is healing, you will need to change your sport or activity to one that does not make your condition worse. For example, you may need to bicycle instead of run.

When can I return to my sport or activity?

The goal of rehabilitation is to return you to your sport or activity as soon as is safely possible. If you return too soon you may worsen your injury, which could lead to

permanent damage. Everyone recovers from injury at a different rate. Return to your sport or activity will be determined by how soon your knee recovers, not by how many days or weeks it has been since your injury occurred. In general, the longer you have symptoms before you start treatment, the longer it will take to get better.

You may safely return to your sport or activity when, starting from the top of the list and progressing to the end, each of the following is true:

- Your injured knee can be fully straightened and bent without pain.
- Your knee and leg have regained normal strength compared to the uninjured knee and leg.
- You are able to jog straight ahead without limping.

- You are able to sprint straight ahead without limping.
- You are able to do 45-degree cuts.
- You are able to do 90-degree cuts.
- You are able to do 20-yard figure-of-eight runs.
- You are able to do 10-yard figure-of-eight runs.
- You are able to jump on both legs without pain and jump on the injured leg without pain.

How can I prevent iliotibial band syndrome?

Iliotibial band syndrome is best prevented by warming up properly and doing stretching exercises before sports or other physical activity.

Iliotibial Band Syndrome Rehabilitation Exercises

You may do stretching exercises 1 through 5 and strengthening exercises 6 through 10 right away.

1. Iliotibial band stretch (standing): Cross your uninjured leg over your injured leg and bend down to touch your toes. Hold this position for 30 seconds. Come up to the starting position. Repeat 3 times.

2. Iliotibial band stretch (side-leaning): Stand sideways to a wall, your injured leg toward the inside. Place the hand nearest the wall on the wall for support. Cross your uninjured leg over the injured leg, keeping the foot the injured leg stable. Lean into the wall. Hold the stretch for 10 seconds and repeat. Do 2 sets of 10.

Iliotibial band stretches

3. Standing calf stretch: Face a wall and put your hands against the wall at about eye level. Keep your injured leg back, your uninjured leg forward, and the heel of your injured leg on the floor. Turn the foot on your injured leg slightly inward (as if you were pigeon-toed) as you slowly lean into the wall until you feel a stretch in the back of your calf. Hold for 30 seconds. Do this several times a day.

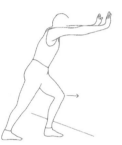

Standing calf stretch

4. Hamstring stretch: Lie on your back with your buttocks close to a doorway and extend your legs straight out in front of you. Raise your injured leg and rest it against the wall next to the door frame. Hold this position for 30 to 60 seconds, feeling a stretch in the back of your thigh. Repeat 3 times.

Hamstring stretch

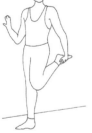

5. Quadriceps stretch: Stand sideways to a wall, about an arm's length away from the wall, your injured leg toward the outside. Facing straight ahead, keep the hand nearest the wall against the wall for support. With your other hand, grasp the ankle of your injured leg and pull your heel up toward your buttocks. Don't arch or twist your back. Hold this position for 30 seconds. Repeat 3 times.

Quadriceps stretch

6. Vastus medialis oblique quadricep sets: Sit on the floor with your injured leg straight in front of you. Press the back of your knee down while tightening the muscles on the top of your thigh. Concentrate on tightening the muscles on the inner side of your kneecap. Hold this position for 5 seconds. Repeat 20 times.

Oblique quadricep sets

Iliotibial Band Syndrome Rehabilitation Exercises

7. Straight leg raise: Sit on the floor with the injured leg straight and the other leg bent, foot flat on the floor. Pull the toes of your injured leg toward you as far as you can, while pressing the back of your knee down and tightening the muscles on the top of your thigh. Raise your leg 6 to 8 inches off the floor and hold for 5 seconds. Slowly lower it back to the floor. Repeat this 20 times.

8. Hip adduction, sidelying: Lie on your injured side with your top leg bent and that foot placed in front of the injured leg, which should be kept straight. Raise your injured leg as far as you can comfortably and hold it for 5 seconds. Keep your hips still while you are lifting your leg. Hold this position for 5 seconds and then slowly lower your leg. Repeat 20 times.

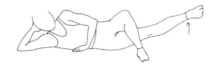

Hip adduction, sidelying

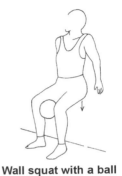

Wall squat with a ball

9. Wall squat with a ball: Stand with your back, shoulders, and head against a wall and look straight ahead. Keep your shoulders relaxed and your feet 1 foot away from the wall and a shoulder's width apart. Place a rolled up pillow or a Nerf ball between your thighs. Keeping your head against the wall, slowly squat while squeezing the pillow or ball at the same time. Squat down until you are almost in a sitting position. Your thighs will not yet be parallel to the floor. Hold this position for 10 seconds. Slowly stand back up. Make sure you keep squeezing the pillow or ball throughout this exercise. Repeat 20 times.

10. Hip adduction with Thera-Band: Stand sideways with your injured leg toward a door. Loop the tubing around the ankle of your injured leg. Anchor the other end of the tubing by tying a knot in the tubing, slipping it between the door and the frame about 8 to 10 inches above the floor, and closing the door. Keeping your injured knee straight, bring your injured leg across your body. Return to the starting position. Repeat 20 times.

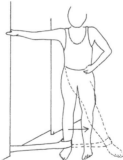

Hip adduction with Theraband

Knee Arthroscopy

What is knee arthroscopy?

Knee arthroscopy is a procedure in which the doctor examines your knee with an instrument called an arthroscope. An arthroscope is a tube with a light on the end that is inserted in your knee and projects an image of the inside of your knee onto a TV monitor. The arthroscope is about the diameter of a pencil.

When is it used?

This procedure is used to diagnose the cause of pain, swelling, tenderness, or weakness in your knee.

Examples of alternatives are:

- Limit your activity.
- Take anti-inflammatory drugs to reduce swelling.
- Wear a brace.
- Have physical therapy.
- Have open knee surgery.
- Have MRI (magnetic resonance imaging).
- Choose not to have treatment, recognizing the risks of your condition.

You should ask your doctor about these choices.

How do I prepare for knee arthroscopy?

Plan for your care and recovery after the operation, especially if you are to have general anesthesia. Allow for time to rest and try to find other people to help you with your day-to-day duties.

Follow any instructions your doctor may give you. Do not eat or drink anything after midnight or the morning before the procedure. Do not even drink coffee, tea, or water after midnight.

What happens during the procedure?

The doctor will give you a general, regional, or local anesthetic. A general anesthetic will relax your muscles and make you feel as if you are in a deep sleep. Both local and regional anesthetics numb part of the body while you remain awake. All three types of anesthesia should keep you from feeling pain during the operation.

The doctor will then insert the arthroscope, a tube containing a saltwater solution, and a probe instrument into the lower part of your knee. He or she will inject fluid into the knee.

Your doctor may find loose material in the knee or a tear in the cartilage or ligaments. Sometimes the doctor can repair the tears and remove loose pieces of cartilage using small instruments and the arthroscope. If the problem cannot be fixed by this procedure, the doctor may recommend open knee surgery.

After the procedure the doctor will close the small openings with one or two stitches or sticky tape.

What happens after the procedure?

- You can go home the day of the procedure.
- You should take it easy for at least the next 2 or 3 days.
- Keep your leg elevated, with your foot higher than your knee and your knee higher than your hip.
- Start bending the knee as soon as possible.
- Use your crutches until you can walk nearly normally.
- Do light strengthening exercises if instructed to do so by your doctor.
- Ask your doctor when you can resume full activity. Your recovery time will depend on what was done and how much arthritis you have in your knee.

Ask your doctor what other steps you should take and when you should come back for a checkup.

Knee Arthroscopy

What are the benefits of knee arthroscopy?

Your knee problem may be corrected without a large incision, which requires a longer stay in the hospital, more discomfort, and greater expense.

What are the risks associated with this procedure?

- There are some risks when you have general anesthesia. Discuss these risks with your doctor.

- A local or regional anesthetic may not numb the area quite enough and you may feel some minor discomfort. Also, in rare cases, you may have an allergic reaction to the drug used in this type of anesthesia. Local or regional anesthesia is considered safer than general anesthesia in people who are older or have certain medical conditions.

- Nerve injury can occur, causing numbness around the small incisions.

- During repair of the cartilage, nerve or artery damage can occur, which can cause numbness, weakness, or pain in your leg and foot. This rarely happens.

- Infection and bleeding may occur.

You should ask your doctor how these risks apply to you.

When should I call the doctor?

Call the doctor immediately if:

- There is excessive drainage from the puncture sites.

- There is unusual pain in your knee.

- You develop swelling in your calf or thigh that is not relieved by elevating your leg.

- You develop a fever.

Call the doctor during office hours if:

- You have questions about the procedure or its result.

- You want to make another appointment.

Lateral Collateral Ligament Sprain

What is lateral collateral ligament sprain?

A sprain is a joint injury that causes a stretch or tear in a ligament, a strong band of tissue connecting one bone to another. The lateral collateral ligament is located on the outer side of the knee. It attaches the bottom portion of the thigh bone (femur) to the outside bone in the lower leg (fibula).

Sprains are graded I, II, or III depending upon the severity of the sprain:

- grade I sprain: pain with minimal damage to the ligaments
- grade II sprain: more ligament damage and mild looseness of the joint
- grade III sprain: complete tearing of the ligament and the joint is very loose or unstable.

How does it occur?

The lateral collateral ligament can be injured by a twisting motion or from a blow to the inner side of the knee.

What are the symptoms?

There will often be pain on the outer side of your knee. Your knee may be swollen and tender. You may have the feeling of your knee giving way. You might hear or feel a pop or snap at the time of injury.

How is it diagnosed?

Your doctor will examine your knee for tenderness over the outer side of your knee. Your doctor will gently move your knee around to see if the knee joint is stable and if the ligament is stretched or torn. Your doctor may order an x-ray or magnetic resonance image (MRI) of your knee.

How is it treated?

Treatment may include:

- applying ice packs to your knee for 20 to 30 minutes every 3 to 4 hours for 2 to 3

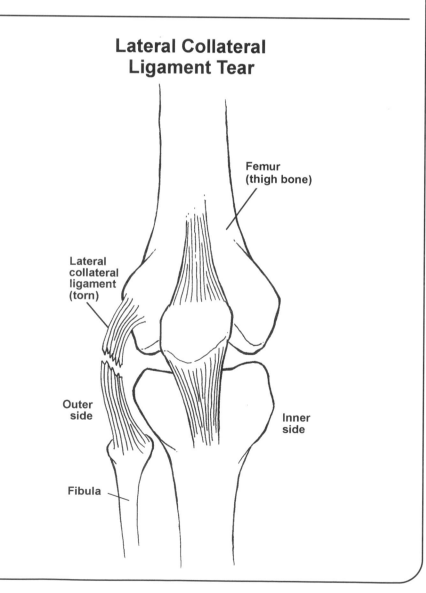

Lateral Collateral Ligament Tear

Femur (thigh bone)

Lateral collateral ligament (torn)

Outer side

Inner side

Fibula

Lateral Collateral Ligament Sprain

days or until the pain and swelling go away

- elevating your knee by placing a pillow underneath it
- wrapping an elastic bandage around your knee to keep the swelling from getting worse
- using crutches until you can walk without pain
- taking anti-inflammatory medication or a pain medication prescribed by your doctor
- doing rehabilitation exercises.

While you are recovering from your injury, you will need to change your sport or activity to one that does not make your condition worse. For example, you may need to swim instead of run.

When can I return to my sport or activity?

The goal of rehabilitation is to return you to your sport or activity as soon as is safely possible. If you return too soon you may worsen your injury, which could lead to

permanent damage. Everyone recovers from injury at a different rate. Return to your sport or activity will be determined by how soon your knee recovers, not by how many days or weeks it has been since your injury occurred. In general, the longer you have symptoms before you start treatment, the longer it will take to get better.

You may safely return to your sport or activity when, starting from the top of the list and progressing to the end, each of the following is true:

- Your injured knee can be fully straightened and bent without pain.
- Your knee and leg have regained normal strength compared to the uninjured knee and leg.
- Your knee is not swollen.
- You are able to jog straight ahead without limping.
- You are able to sprint straight ahead without limping.
- You are able to do 45-degree cuts.
- You are able to do 90-degree cuts.

- You are able to do 20-yard figure-of-eight runs.
- You are able to do 10-yard figure-of-eight runs.
- You are able to jump on both legs times without pain and jump on the injured leg without pain.

If you feel that your knee is giving way or if you develop pain or have swelling in your knee, you should see your doctor.

How can I prevent a lateral collateral ligament sprain?

Unfortunately, most injuries to the lateral collateral ligament occur during accidents that are not preventable. However, you may be able to avoid these injuries by having strong thigh and hamstring muscles, as well as by maintaining a good leg stretching routine. In activities such as skiing, be sure that your ski bindings are set correctly by a trained professional so that your skis will release when you fall.

Lateral Collateral Ligament Sprain ——— *Rehabilitation Exercises*

You may do exercises 1 through 4 right away. You may do exercise 5 when your knee pain has decreased.

1. Heel slide: Sit on a firm surface with your legs straight in front of you. Slowly slide the heel of your injured leg toward your buttocks by pulling your knee to your chest as you slide. Return to the starting position. Repeat 20 times.

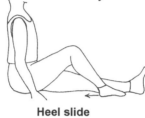

Heel slide

2. Hip abduction and adduction: Lie on your back with your legs straight out in front of you and your toes pointed toward the ceiling. Slide your injured leg out to the side as far as possible. Slide it back to the starting position. Repeat 10 times.

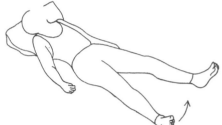

Hip abduction and adduction

3. Straight leg raise: Sit on the floor with your injured leg straight and your other leg bent, with your foot flat on the floor. Move the toes of your injured leg toward you as far as you can, while pressing the back of your knee down and tightening the muscles on the top of your thigh. Raise your leg 6 to 8 inches off the floor and hold for 5 seconds. Slowly lower it back to the floor. Repeat 20 times.

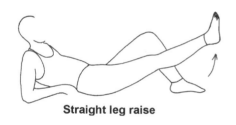

Straight leg raise

4. Prone knee flexion: Lie on your stomach with a towel rolled up underneath your injured thigh, just above your knee. Slowly bend your knee and try to touch your buttock with your heel. Return to the starting position. You can challenge yourself by wearing ankle weights. Repeat 20 times.

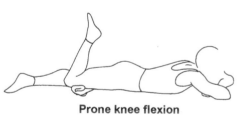

Prone knee flexion

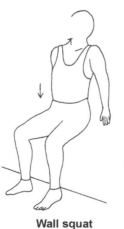

Wall squat

5. Wall squat: Stand with your back, shoulders, and head against a wall and look straight ahead. Keep your shoulders relaxed and your feet 1 foot away from the wall and a shoulder's width apart. Keeping your head against the wall, slowly squat until you are almost in a sitting position. Your thighs will not yet be parallel to the floor. Hold this position for 10 seconds. Slowly slide back up. Repeat 20 times.

Medial Collateral Ligament Sprain

What is a medial collateral ligament sprain?

A sprain is a joint injury that causes a stretch or a tear in a ligament, a strong band of tissue connecting one bone to the other. The medial collateral ligament is located on the inner side of the knee. It attaches the thigh bone (femur) to the shin bone (tibia).

Sprains are graded I, II, or III, depending upon the severity of the sprain:

- grade I sprain: pain with minimal damage to the ligaments

- grade II sprain: more ligament damage and mild looseness of the joint

- grade III sprain: complete tearing of the ligament and the joint is very loose or unstable.

How does it occur?

This injury usually occurs when a blow to the outer side of the knee causes stretching or tearing of the medial collateral ligament. It can also be caused by a twisting injury to the knee.

What are the symptoms?

Your will have pain on the innermost side of your knee. Your knee may be swollen and tender. You may have the feeling of the knee giving way. You might hear or feel a pop or snap at the time of injury.

How is it diagnosed?

Your doctor will examine your knee. Your doctor will gently move your knee around to see if the joint is stable and if the ligament is stretched or torn. He or she may order x-rays or a magnetic resonance image (MRI) of your knee.

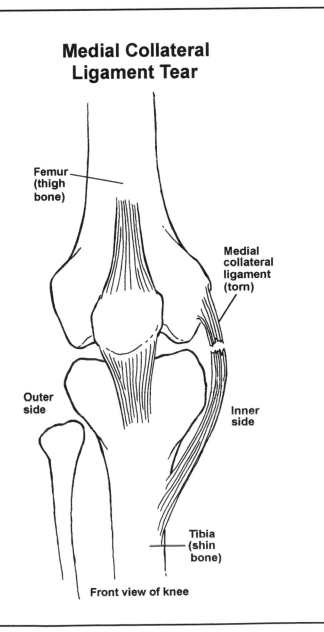

Medial Collateral Ligament Tear

Femur (thigh bone)

Medial collateral ligament (torn)

Outer side

Inner side

Tibia (shin bone)

Front view of knee

Medial Collateral Ligament Sprain

How is it treated?

Treatment may include:

- applying ice to your knee for 20 to 30 minutes every 3 to 4 hours for 2 to 3 days or until the pain and swelling go away
- elevating your knee by placing a pillow underneath it
- taking an anti-inflammatory medication or other drugs prescribed by your doctor
- wearing a knee immobilizer or knee brace to keep you from moving and further injuring your knee and to minimize the pain of moving your knee
- using crutches
- doing rehabilitation exercises.

While you are recovering from your injury, you will need to change your sport or activity to one that does not make your condition worse. For example, you may need to swim instead of run.

When can I return to my sport or activity?

The goal of rehabilitation is to return you to your sport or activity as soon as is safely possible. If you return too soon you may worsen your injury, which could lead to permanent damage. Everyone recovers from injury at a different rate. Return to your sport or activity will be determined by how soon your knee recovers, not by how many days or weeks it has been since your injury occurred. In general, the longer you have symptoms before you start treatment, the longer it will take to get better.

You may safely return to your sport or activity when, starting from the top of the list and progressing to the end, each of the following is true:

- Your injured knee can be fully straightened and bent without pain.
- Your knee and leg have regained normal strength compared to the uninjured knee and leg.
- Your knee is not swollen.
- You are able to jog straight ahead without limping.

- You are able to sprint straight ahead without limping.
- You are able to do 45-degree cuts.
- You are able to do 90-degree cuts.
- You are able to do 20-yard figure-of-eight runs.
- You are able to do 10-yard figure-of-eight runs.
- You are able to jump on both legs without pain and jump on the injured leg without pain.

If you feel that your knee is giving way or if you develop pain or have swelling in your knee, you should see your doctor.

How can I prevent a medial collateral ligament sprain?

Unfortunately, most injuries to the medial collateral ligament occur during accidents that are not preventable. However, you may be able to avoid these injuries by having strong thigh and hamstring muscles, as well as by maintaining a good leg stretching routine. In activities such as skiing, be sure your ski bindings are set correctly by a trained professional so that your skis will release when you fall.

Medial Collateral Ligament Sprain Rehabilitation Exercises

You may do exercises 1 through 5 right away. You may do exercises 6 and 7 when the pain in your knee has decreased.

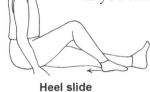

1. Heel slide: Sit on a firm surface with your legs straight in front of you, slowly slide the heel of your injured leg toward your buttocks by pulling your knee to your chest as you slide. Return to the starting position. Repeat 20 times.

Heel slide

2. Sitting hip adduction isometrics: Sit with your knees bent 90 degrees, a pillow placed between your knees, and your feet flat on the floor. Squeeze the pillow for 5 seconds and then relax. Repeat 20 times.

Sitting hip adduction isometrics

3. Straight leg raise: Sit on the floor with the injured leg straight and your other leg bent with your foot flat on the floor. Move the toes of your injured leg toward you as far as you can, while pressing the back of your knee down and tightening the muscles on the top of your thigh. Raise your leg 6 to 8 inches off the floor and hold for 5 seconds. Slowly lower it back to the floor. Repeat 20 times.

Straight leg raise

4. Hip adduction, sidelying: Lie on your injured side. Keep your injured leg straight. Bend your uninjured leg and place your foot in front of your injured leg. Raise your injured leg as far as you can comfortably and hold it for 5 seconds. Keep your hips still while you are lifting your leg. Hold this position for 5 seconds and then slowly lower your leg. Repeat 20 times.

Hip adduction, sidelying

5. Prone knee flexion: Lie on your stomach. Bend your injured knee and try to touch your buttock with your heel. Return to the starting position. Repeat 20 times.

Prone knee flexion

6. Wall slide: Stand with your back, shoulders, and head against a wall and look straight ahead. Keep your shoulders relaxed and your feet 1 foot away from the wall and a shoulder's width apart. Keeping your head against the wall, slowly squat. Hold this position for 10 seconds. Slowly slide back up. Repeat 20 times.

Wall slide

Medial Collateral Ligament Sprain Rehabilitation Exercises

7. Resisted Thera-Band exercises for the lower leg:

A. Resisted dorsiflexion: Sit with your injured leg out straight and your foot facing a doorway. Tie a loop in one end of the Thera-Band. Put your foot through the loop so that the tubing goes around the arch of your foot. Tie a knot in the other end of the Thera-Band and shut the knot in the door. Move backward until there is tension in the tubing. Keeping your knee straight, pull your foot toward your face, stretching the tubing. Slowly return to the starting position. Repeat 10 times. Do 3 sets of 10.

B. Resisted plantar flexion. Sit with your injured leg outstretched and loop the middle section of the tubing around the ball of your foot. Hold the ends of the tubing in both hands. Gently press the ball of your foot down and point your toes, stretching the Thera-Band. Return to the starting position. Repeat 10 times. Do 3 sets of 10.

C. Resisted inversion: Sit with your legs out straight and cross your uninjured leg over your injured leg. Wrap the tubing around the ball of the foot on your injured leg and then loop it around your other foot so that the Thera-Band is anchored there at one end. Hold the other end of the Thera-Band in your hand. Turn your foot on your injured leg inward and upward. This will stretch the tubing. Return to the starting position. Repeat 10 times. Do 3 sets of 10.

D. Resisted eversion: Sit with both legs stretched out in front of you, with your feet about a shoulder's width apart. Tie a loop in one end of the Thera-Band. Put the foot of your injured leg through the loop so that the tubing goes around the arch of that foot and the Thera-Band wraps around the outside of the foot on your uninjured leg. Hold onto the other end of the tubing with your hand to provide tension. Turn your injured foot up and out. Make sure you keep your other foot still so that it will allow the tubing to stretch as you move your injured foot. Return to the starting position. Repeat 10 times. Do 3 sets of 10.

Resisted Theraband exercises for the lower leg

Meniscal (Cartilage) Tear

What is a meniscal (cartilage) tear?

The meniscus is a piece of cartilage in the middle of your knee. Cartilage is tough, smooth, rubbery tissue that lines and cushions the surface of the joints. There is a meniscus on the inner side of your knee (the medial meniscus) and a meniscus on the outer side (the lateral meniscus). They attach to the top of the shin bone (tibia), make contact with the thigh bone (femur), and act as shock absorbers during weight-bearing activities.

How does it occur?

A meniscal tear can occur when the knee is forcefully twisted or occasionally with minimal or no trauma, such as when you are squatting.

What are the symptoms?

You may have pain in your knee joint. You may have immediate swelling with fluid in the joint, called an effusion. You may be unable to fully bend or straighten your leg. Your knee may lock or get stuck in one place. You may hear a snap or pop at the time of the injury.

A chronic (old) meniscal tear may give you pain on and off during activities, with or without swelling. Your knee may occasionally lock and you may have stiffness in the knee.

How is it diagnosed?

Your doctor will examine your knee and find that you have tenderness along the joint line. Your doctor will move your knee in several ways that may cause pain along the injured meniscal surface. Your doctor may order x-rays to see if there are injuries to the bones in your knee, but a meniscal tear will not show up on a x-ray. An MRI (magnetic resonance imaging) is sometimes useful in diagnosing a meniscal tear.

How is it treated?

Treatment may include:

- applying ice to your knee for 20 to 30 minutes every 3 to 4 hours for 2 or 3 days or until the pain and swelling are gone

Meniscal (Cartilage) Tear

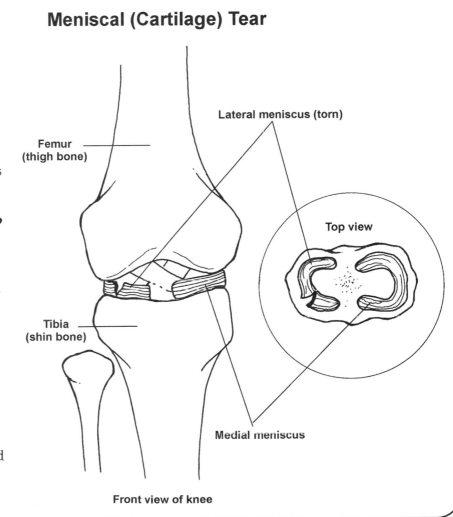

Femur (thigh bone)

Lateral meniscus (torn)

Top view

Tibia (shin bone)

Medial meniscus

Front view of knee

Meniscal (Cartilage) Tear

- elevating your knee by placing a pillow underneath your leg
- wrapping an elastic bandage around your knee to keep the swelling from getting worse
- wearing a knee immobilizer or other brace to prevent further injury
- using crutches
- taking anti-inflammatory or pain medication prescribed by your doctor.

Surgery is needed to repair or remove large torn pieces of cartilage.

While you are recovering from your injury, you will need to change your sport or activity to one that does not make your condition worse. For example, you may need to swim instead of run.

When can I return to my sport or activity?

The goal of rehabilitation is to return you to your sport or activity as soon as is safely possible. If you return too soon you may worsen your injury, which could lead to permanent damage. Everyone recovers from injury at a different rate. Return to your sport or activity will be determined by how soon your knee recovers, not by how many days or weeks it has been since your injury occurred. In general, the longer you have symptoms before you start treatment, the longer it will take to get better.

You may safely return to your sport or activity when, starting from the top of the list and progressing to the end, each of the following is true:

- Your injured knee can be fully straightened and bent without pain.
- Your knee and leg have regained normal strength compared to the uninjured knee and leg.
- Your knee is not swollen.
- You are able to jog straight ahead without limping.
- You are able to sprint straight ahead without limping.
- You are able to do 45-degree cuts.

- You are able to do 90-degree cuts.
- You are able to do 20-yard figure-of-eight runs.
- You are able to do 10-yard figure-of-eight runs.
- You are able to jump on both legs without pain and jump on the injured leg without pain.

If you feel that your knee is giving way or if you develop pain or have swelling in your knee, you should see your doctor.

How can a meniscal tear be prevented?

Unfortunately, most injuries to knee cartilage occur during accidents that are not preventable. However, you may be able to avoid these injuries by having strong thigh and hamstring muscles, as well as by maintaining a good leg-stretching routine. When skiing, be sure that your ski bindings are set correctly by a trained professional so that your skis will release when you fall.

Meniscal (Cartilage) Tear Rehabilitation Exercises

You may do exercises 1 through 3 right away. You may do exercises 4 through 6 when the pain in your knee has decreased.

1. Standing calf stretch: Facing a wall, put your hands against the wall at about eye level. Keep your injured leg back, your uninjured leg forward, and the heel of your injured leg on the floor. Turn your the foot of your injured leg slightly inward (as if you were pigeon-toed) as you slowly lean into the wall until you feel a stretch in the back of your calf. Hold for 30 seconds. Repeat 3 times.

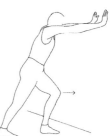

Standing calf stretch

2. Hamstring stretch: Lie on your back with your buttocks close to a doorway and extend your legs straight out in front of you along the floor. Raise your injured leg and rest it against the wall next to the door frame. Hold this position for 30 to 60 seconds. You will feel a stretch in the back of your thigh. Repeat 3 times.

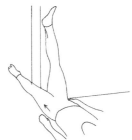

Hamstring stretch

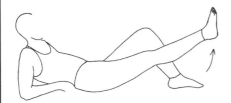

Straight leg raise

3. Straight leg raise: Sit on the floor with your injured leg straight, your other leg bent, and your foot flat on the floor. Move the toes of your injured leg toward you as far as you can, while pressing the back of your knee down and tightening the muscles on the top of your thigh. Raise your leg 6 to 8 inches off the floor and hold for 5 seconds. Slowly lower it back to the floor. Repeat 20 times.

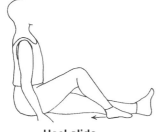

Heel slide

4. Heel slide: Sit on a firm surface with your legs straight in front of you. Slowly slide the heel of your injured leg toward your buttock by pulling your knee to your chest as you slide. Return to the starting position. Repeat 20 times.

5. Wall squat with a ball: Stand with your back, shoulders, and head against a wall and look straight ahead. Keep your shoulders relaxed and your feet 1 foot away from the wall and a shoulder's width apart. Place a rolled up pillow or a nerf ball between your thighs. Keeping your head against the wall, slowly squat while squeezing the pillow or ball at the same time. Squat down until your thighs are parallel to the floor. Hold this position for 10 seconds. Slowly stand back up. Make sure you keep squeezing the pillow or ball throughout this exercise. Repeat 20 times.

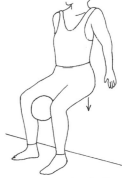
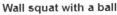

Wall squat with a ball

Meniscal (Cartilage) Tear Rehabilitation Exercises

6. Step-up: Stand with the foot of your injured leg on a support (like a block of wood) 3 to 5 inches high. Keep your other foot flat on the floor. Shift your weight onto the injured leg and straighten the knee as the uninjured leg comes off the floor. Lower your uninjured leg to the floor slowly. Repeat 10 times.

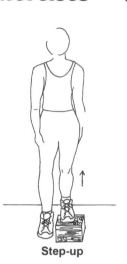

Step-up

Osgood-Schlatter Disease

What is Osgood-Schlatter disease?

Osgood-Schlatter disease is a painful enlargement of the bump of the shin bone (tibia) just below the knee. This bump is called the tibial tuberosity. The tendon from the kneecap (patella) inserts here. Osgood-Schlatter disease is most often seen in children between the ages of 10 and 15 and usually appears during a period of rapid growth.

How does it occur?

Osgood-Schlatter disease is caused by overuse of the knee in normal childhood and sporting activities. It is possible that muscles are too tight in the front of the thigh, the back of the thigh, or in the calf.

What are the symptoms?

Your child will complain of a painful bump below the kneecap. The parents or child may notice a bony enlargement at the top of the shin bone.

How is it diagnosed?

Your child's doctor will do a physical examination of the knee and review your child's symptoms. X-rays show an enlarged tibial tuberosity. An x-ray may also show irregular or loose bony fragments from the tibial tuberosity.

How is it treated?

Your child may need to rest or do activities that do not cause knee pain. Ice packs should be applied to the knee for 20 to 30 minutes every 3 to 4 hours for 2 to 3 days or until the pain goes away. If the knee is swollen, it should be elevated by placing a pillow under it. Your child's doctor may prescribe a special padded brace. The doctor may prescribe an anti-inflammatory medication and may recommend exercises.

When can my child return to his or her sport or activity?

The goal of rehabilitation is to return your child to his or her sport or activity as soon as is safely possible. If your child returns too soon the injury may worsen, which could lead to permanent damage. Everyone recovers from injury at a different rate. Return to his or her sport or activity will be determined by how soon your child's knee recovers, not

Osgood-Schlatter Disease

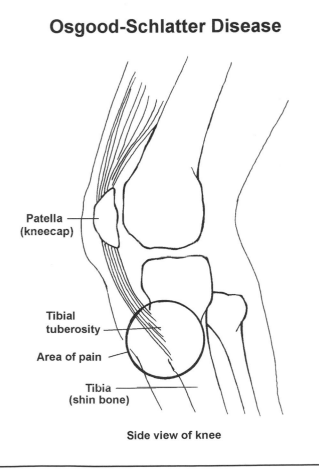

Patella (kneecap)

Tibial tuberosity

Area of pain

Tibia (shin bone)

Side view of knee

Osgood-Schlatter Disease

by how many days or weeks it has been since the injury occurred. In general, the longer your child has symptoms before starting treatment, the longer it will take to get better.

Your child may safely return to his or her sport or activity when, starting from the top of the list and progressing to the end, each of the following is true:

- Your child's tibial tuberosity is no longer tender.
- The injured knee can be fully straightened and bent without pain.

- The knee and leg have regained normal strength compared to the uninjured knee and leg.
- Your child is able to jog straight ahead without limping.
- Your child is able to sprint straight ahead without limping.
- Your child is able to do 45-degree cuts.
- Your child is able to do 90-degree cuts.
- Your child is able to do 20-yard figure-of-eight runs.
- Your child is able to do 10-yard figure-of-eight runs.

- Your child is able to jump on both legs without pain and jump on the injured leg without pain.

How can Osgood-Schlatter disease be prevented?

Osgood-Schlatter disease may be difficult to prevent. The most important thing to do is to have your child limit activity as soon as he or she notices the painful bump on the top of the shin bone. Proper warm-up and stretching exercises of the thigh, hamstring, and calf muscles may help prevent Osgood-Schlatter disease.

Osgood-Schlatter Disease Rehabilitation Exercises

You can start stretching the muscles in the back of your leg using exercises 1 and 2 right away. When you have only a little discomfort in the upper part of you lower leg bone (tibia), you can do exercises 3, 4, and 5.

1. Hamstring stretch: Lie on your back with your buttocks close to a doorway and extend your legs straight out in front of you along the floor. Raise your injured leg and rest it against the wall next to the door frame. Hold this position for 30 to 60 seconds. You will feel a stretch in the back of your thigh. Repeat 3 times.

Hamstring stretch

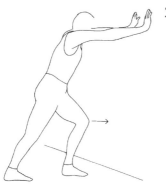

2. Calf stretch: Face a wall and put your hands against the wall at about eye level. Keep the injured leg back, the uninjured leg forward, and the heel of your injured leg on the floor. Turn your foot on your injured leg slightly inward (as if you were pigeon-toed) as you slowly lean into the wall until you feel a stretch in the back of your calf. Hold for 30 seconds. Repeat 3 times.

Calf stretch

3. Quadriceps stretch: Stand an arm's length away from a wall, facing straight ahead. Brace yourself by keeping the hand on the uninjured side against the wall. With your other hand, grasp the ankle of the injured leg and pull your heel up toward your buttocks. Don't arch or twist your back. Hold this position for 30 seconds. Repeat 3 times.

Quadriceps stretch

4. Straight leg raise: Sit on the floor with the injured leg straight and the other leg bent with your foot flat on the floor. Move the toes of your injured leg toward you as far as you can, while pressing the back of your knee down and tightening the muscles on the top of your thigh. Raise your leg 6 to 8 inches off the floor and hold for 5 seconds. Slowly lower it back to the floor. Repeat 10 times. Do 3 sets of 10.

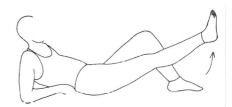

Straight leg raise

5. Prone hip extension: Lie on your stomach. Squeeze your buttocks together and raise your injured leg 5 to 8 inches off the floor. Keep your back straight. Hold your leg up for 5 seconds and then lower it. Repeat 10 times. Do 3 sets of 10.

Prone hip extension

Osteochondritis Dissecans (Bone Chips) of the Knee

What is osteochondritis dissecans of the knee?

Osteochondritis dissecans of the knee is a disorder in which fragments of bone or cartilage come loose and float around in the knee joint. Other terms for this condition are chondral fracture and osteochondral fracture. The fragments may also be referred to as a joint mouse or loose bodies.

How does it occur?

There has usually been a previous injury to the knee that caused a fragment of bone or cartilage to be chipped off the back of the kneecap or the top part of the knee joint.

What are the symptoms?

Your knee may lock up from time to time. You may see bulges along the joint surface. You may be able to feel these chips or loose bodies along the surface of your knee joint at various times.

How is it diagnosed?

Your doctor will examine your knee and may find that it clicks or locks. Fragments may be felt along the joint line. An x-ray or a magnetic resonance imaging (MRI) may show bony fragments.

How is it treated?

Loose bodies causing symptoms may need to be surgically removed. Large defects along the joint surface may need to be surgically corrected.

When can I return to my sport or activity?

The goal of rehabilitation is to return you to your sport or activity as soon as is safely possible. If you return too soon you may worsen your injury, which could lead to permanent damage. Everyone recovers from injury at a different rate. Return to your sport or activity will be determined by how soon your knee recovers, not by how many days or weeks it has been since your injury occurred. In general, the longer you have symptoms before you start treatment, the longer it will take to get better.

You may safely return to your sport or activity when, starting from the top of the list and progressing to the end, each of the following is true:

- Your injured knee can be fully straightened and bent without pain.

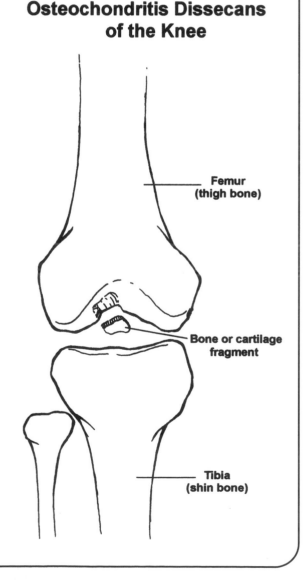

Osteochondritis Dissecans of the Knee

Femur (thigh bone)

Bone or cartilage fragment

Tibia (shin bone)

Osteochondritis Dissecans (Bone Chips) of the Knee

- Your knee and leg have regained normal strength compared to the uninjured knee and leg.

- Your knee is not swollen.

- You are able to jog straight ahead without limping.

- You are able to sprint straight ahead without limping.

- You are able to do 45-degree cuts.

- You are able to do 90-degree cuts.

- You are able to do 20-yard figure-of-eight runs.

- You are able to do 10-yard figure-of-eight runs.

- You are able to jump on both legs without pain and jump on the injured leg without pain.

If you feel that your knee is giving way or if you develop pain or have swelling in your knee, you should see your doctor. If your condition required surgery, ask your doctor when you can return to your sport or activity.

How can I prevent osteochondritis dissecans of the knee?

Osteochondritis dissecans is usually caused by trauma to the knee and is not preventable.

© HBO & Company

Patellar (Kneecap) Subluxation

What is a subluxing patella?

A subluxing patella (kneecap) is a temporary, partial dislocation of the kneecap from its normal position in the groove in the end of the thigh bone (femur). This groove is located between two bumps at the end of the thigh bone called the femoral condyles.

How does it occur?

This temporary dislocation of the kneecap usually happens during forced leg straightening, with the kneecap moving out of the groove to the outer side of the knee.

The cause is usually an abnormality in the way your legs are built. You may have an underdevelopment of the inner thigh muscle or an overdevelopment of the outer thigh muscle. Your kneecap may be higher in the leg than usual. You may be knock-kneed or have underdevelopment of the outer (lateral) femoral condyle.

What are the symptoms?

You may feel the kneecap moving out of position. You may have swelling and pain behind the kneecap. You may have pain when you bend or straighten your leg.

How is it diagnosed?

Your doctor will ask about your symptoms and examine your knee. He or she may be able to feel the kneecap slipping to the outside as you bend and straighten your leg. An x-ray may show underdevelopment of the lateral femoral condyle.

How is it treated?

Treatment may include:

- putting ice packs on your knee for 20 to 30 minutes every 3 to 4 hours for the first 2 or 3 days or until the pain goes away
- elevating your knee to help any swelling go away
- taking an anti-inflammatory medication
- wearing a brace prescribed by your doctor to keep your kneecap in place
- doing exercises to strengthen the inner side of the thigh muscle (quadriceps).

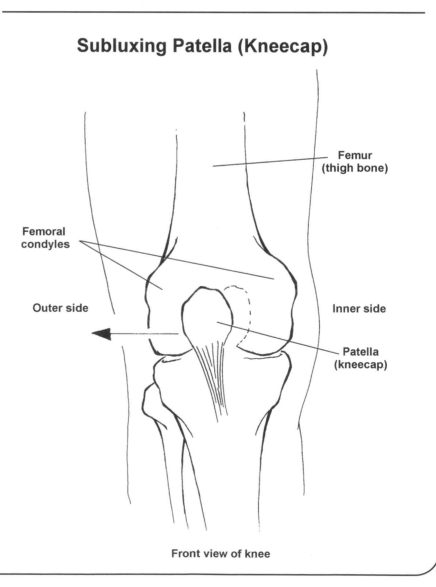

Subluxing Patella (Kneecap)

Femur (thigh bone)

Femoral condyles

Outer side

Inner side

Patella (kneecap)

Front view of knee

Patellar (Kneecap) Subluxation

Some people need surgery to keep the kneecap from subluxing.

While you are recovering from your injury you will need to change your sport or activity to one that will not make your condition worse. For example, you may need to bicycle instead of run.

When can I return to my sport or activity?

The goal of rehabilitation is to return you to your sport or activity as soon as is safely possible. If you return too soon you may worsen your injury, which could lead to permanent damage. Everyone recovers from injury at a different rate. Return to your sport or activity will be determined by how soon your knee recovers, not by how many days or weeks it has been since your injury occurred. In general, the longer you have symptoms before you start treatment, the longer it will take to get better.

You may safely return to your sport or activity when, starting from the top of the list and progressing to the end, each of the following is true:

- Your injured knee can be fully straightened and bent without pain.
- Your knee and leg have regained normal strength compared to the uninjured knee and leg.
- Your knee is not swollen.
- You are able to jog straight ahead without limping.
- You are able to sprint straight ahead without limping.
- You are able to do 45-degree cuts.
- You are able to do 90-degree cuts.
- You are able to do 20-yard figure-of-eight runs.
- You are able to do 10-yard figure-of-eight runs.
- You are able to jump on both legs without pain and jump on the injured leg without pain.

If you develop pain, swelling, or the feeling that your kneecap is moving out of place again, you need to contact your doctor.

How can I prevent a subluxing kneecap?

A subluxing kneecap is best prevented by keeping your thigh muscles strong, especially the group of muscles on the inner side of the thigh.

© HBO & Company

Patellar (Kneecap) Subluxation Rehabilitation Exercises

You may do all of these exercises right away. It is important to stretch the muscles in the back of your leg. It is also important to strengthen the muscles on the top of your thigh so your kneecap won't sublux again.

1. Hamstring stretch: Lie on your back with your buttocks close to a doorway and extend your legs straight out in front of you along the floor. Raise the injured leg and rest it against the wall next to the door frame. Hold this position for 30 to 60 seconds, feeling a stretch in the back of your thigh. Repeat 3 times.

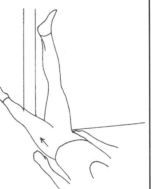

Hamstring stretch

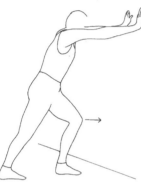

Calf stretch

2. Standing calf stretch: Facing a wall, put your hands against the wall at about eye level. Keep the injured leg back, the uninjured leg forward, and the heel of your injured leg on the floor. Turn the foot on your injured leg slightly inward (as if you were pigeon-toed) as you slowly lean into the wall until you feel a stretch in the back of your calf. Hold for 30 seconds. Do this several times a day.

3. Quadriceps set: Sit on the floor with the injured leg straight. Press the back of your knee down toward the floor while tightening the muscles on the top of your thigh. Concentrate on tightening the muscles on the inner side of your kneecap. Hold this position for 5 seconds. Repeat 20 times.

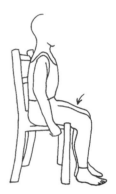

Quadriceps set

4. Straight leg raise: Sit on the floor with the injured leg straight and the other leg bent, foot flat on the floor. Pull the toes of your injured leg toward you as far as you can, while pressing the back of your knee down and tightening the muscles on the top of your thigh. Raise your leg 6 to 8 inches off the floor and hold for 5 seconds. Slowly lower it back to the floor. Repeat this 10 times. Do 3 sets of 10.

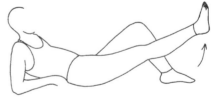

Straight leg raise

5. Prone hip extension: Lie on your stomach. Squeeze your buttocks together and raise the injured leg as far as you can comfortably, while keeping your back straight. Hold this leg in the air for 5 seconds and then lower it. Repeat 20 times.

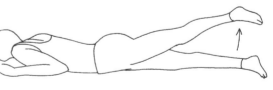

Prone hip extension

6. Weight lifting - leg extension: Do these if you have access to a weight lifting bench with a leg extension attachment. Sit on the bench with the weight attachment in front of your lower legs. Extend your knees by straightening your legs. Be sure your legs straighten completely. The last 15 degrees of extension are the most important. Use enough weight to cause fatigue but not pain. Do three sets of 10.

Patellar Tendonitis
(Jumper's Knee)

What is patellar tendonitis?

Patellar tendonitis, also call jumper's knee, is pain in the band of tissue (the patellar tendon) that connects the kneecap (patella) to the shin bone (tibia).

How does it occur?

The most common activity causing patellar tendonitis is too much jumping. Other repeated activities such as running, walking, or bicycling may lead to patellar tendonitis. All of these activities put repeated stress on the patellar tendon, causing it to be inflamed.

Patellar tendonitis can also happen to people who have problems with the way their hips, legs, knees, or feet are aligned. This alignment problem can result from having wide hips, being knock-kneed, or having feet with arches that collapse when you walk or run, a condition called over-pronation.

What are the symptoms?

Symptoms may include:

- pain and tenderness around the patellar tendon
- swelling in your knee joint or swelling where the patellar tendon attaches to the shin bone

- pain with jumping, running, or walking, especially downhill or downstairs
- pain with bending or straightening the leg
- tenderness behind the kneecap.

How is it diagnosed?

Your doctor will examine your knee to see if you have tenderness at the patellar tendon. He or she will also have you run, jump, or squat to see if this causes pain. Your feet will be examined to see if you have a problem with over-pronation. Your doctor may take x-rays of your knee.

How is it treated?

In the early stages you should apply ice packs for 20 to 30 minutes every 3 to 4 hours for 2 to 3 days or until the pain goes away. Your doctor may prescribe an anti-inflammatory medication. He or she

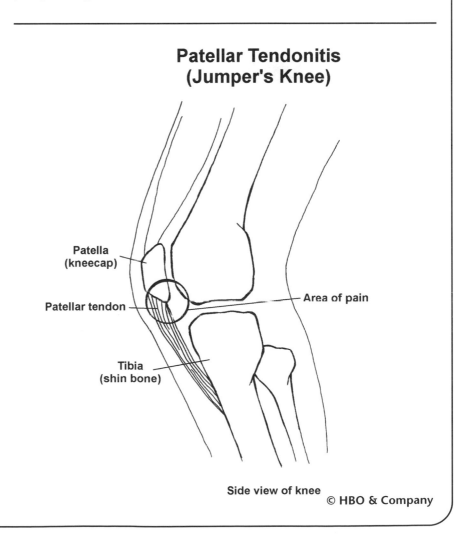

Patellar Tendonitis (Jumper's Knee)

Patella (kneecap)

Patellar tendon

Tibia (shin bone)

Area of pain

Side view of knee

© HBO & Company

Patellar Tendonitis (Jumper's Knee)

may also prescribe a band to wear across the patellar tendon, called an infra-patellar strap, or prescribe a special knee brace. The strap or brace will support your patellar tendon, preventing it from becoming overused or painful. If you have a problem with over-pronation, your doctor may prescribe custom-made arch supports called orthotics. You will be given rehabilitation exercises to help you return to your sport or activity.

While you are recovering from your injury you will need to change your sport or activity to one that does not make your condition worse. For example, you may need to swim instead of play basketball.

When can I return to my sport or activity?

The goal of rehabilitation is to return you to your sport or activity as soon as is safely possible. If you return too soon you may worsen your injury, which could lead to permanent damage. Everyone recovers from injury at a different rate. Return to your sport or activity will be determined by how soon your knee recovers, not by how many days or weeks it has been since your injury occurred. In general, the longer you have symptoms before you start treatment, the longer it will take to get better.

You may safely return to your sport or activity when, starting from the top of the list and progressing to the end, each of the following is true:

- Your injured knee can be fully straightened and bent without pain.
- Your knee and leg have regained normal strength compared to the uninjured knee and leg.
- Your knee is not swollen.

- You are able to jog straight ahead without limping.
- You are able to sprint straight ahead without limping.
- You are able to do 45-degree cuts.
- You are able to do 90-degree cuts.
- You are able to do 20-yard figure-of-eight runs.
- You are able to do 10-yard figure-of-eight runs.
- You are able to jump on both legs without pain and jump on the injured leg without pain.

How can I prevent patellar tendonitis?

Patellar tendonitis is usually caused by overuse during activities such as jumping or running. It can best be prevented by having strong thigh muscles.

© HBO & Company

Patellar Tendonitis (Jumper's Knee) Rehabilitation Exercises

You can start doing exercise 1 as soon as it is not too painful to move your kneecap. You can do the hamstring stretch (exercise 2) right away. When the pain in your knee has decreased, you can do the quadriceps stretch and start strengthening the thigh muscles using exercises 4 through 6.

1. Patellar mobility: Sit with your injured leg outstretched in front of you and the muscles on the top of your thigh relaxed. Take your index finger and thumb and gently press your kneecap down toward your foot. Hold this position for 10 seconds.

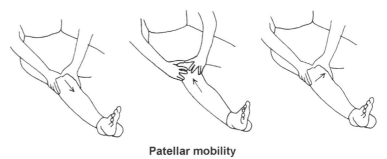

Patellar mobility

Return to the starting position. Next, pull your kneecap up toward your waist and hold it for 10 seconds. Return to the starting position. Then, try to gently push your kneecap inward toward your other leg and hold for 10 seconds. Repeat these for approximately 5 minutes.

2. Hamstring stretch: Stand with the heel of your injured leg resting on a stool that is about 15 inches high. Keep your knee straight. Gently lean forward from your hips, keeping your shoulders in line with your trunk, until you feel a stretch in the back of your thigh. Hold this position for 30 to 60 seconds. Return to the starting position. Do not round your shoulders and bring your head toward your toe. This will only stretch your low back and not your hamstrings. Repeat 3 times.

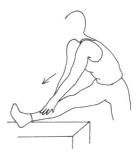

Hamstring stretch

3. Quadriceps stretch: Stand an arm's length away from a wall, facing straight ahead. Brace yourself by keeping the hand on the uninjured side against the wall. With your other hand, grasp the ankle of the injured leg and pull your heel up toward your buttocks. Don't arch or twist your back. Hold this position for 30 seconds. Repeat 3 times.

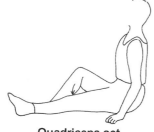

Quadriceps set

4. Quadriceps set: Sit on the floor with your injured leg straight out in front of you. Try to tighten the muscles at the top of your thigh by pushing the back of your knee down into the floor. Concentrate your contraction on the inside part of your thigh. Hold this position for 5 seconds. Repeat 10 times. Do 3 sets of 10.

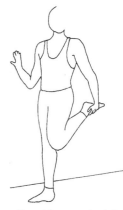

Quadriceps stretch

© HBO & Company

Patellar Tendonitis (Jumper's Knee) — *Rehabilitation Exercises*

5. Straight leg raise: Sit on the floor with your injured leg straight and the other leg bent so the foot is flat on the floor. Move the toes of your injured leg toward you as far as you can comfortably while tightening the muscles on the top of your thigh. Raise your leg 6 to 8 inches off the floor. Hold this position for 3 to 5 seconds and then slowly lower your leg. Repeat 10 times. Do 3 sets of 10.

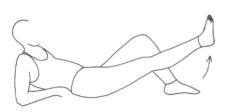

Straight leg raise

6. Weight lifting - leg extension: Do these if you have access to a weight lifting bench with a leg extension attachment. Sit on the bench with the weight attachment in front of your lower legs. Extend your knees by straightening your legs. Be sure your legs straighten completely. The last 15 degrees of extension are the most important. Use enough weight to cause fatigue but not pain. Do three sets of 10.

Patellofemoral Pain Syndrome
(Runner's Knee)

What is patellofemoral pain syndrome?

Patellofemoral pain syndrome is pain behind the kneecap. It has been given many names, including patellofemoral disorder, patellar malalignment, runner's knee, and chondromalacia.

How does it occur?

Patellofemoral pain syndrome can occur from overuse of the knee in sports and activities such as running, walking, jumping, or bicycling.

The kneecap (patella) is attached to the large group of muscles in the thigh called the quadriceps. It is also attached to the shin bone by the patellar tendon. The kneecap fits into grooves in the end of the thigh bone (femur) called the femoral condyle. With repeated bending and straightening of the knee, you can irritate the inside surface of the kneecap and cause pain.

Patellofemoral pain syndrome also may result from the way your hips, legs, knees, or feet are aligned. This alignment problem can be caused by your having wide hips or underdeveloped thigh muscles, being knock-kneed, or having feet with arches that collapse when walking or running (a condition called overpronation).

What are the symptoms?

The main symptom is pain behind the kneecap. You may have pain when you walk, run, or sit for a long time. The pain is generally worse when walking downhill or down stairs. Your knee may swell at times. You may feel or hear snapping, popping, or grinding in the knee.

How is it diagnosed?

Your doctor will review your symptoms, examine your knee, and may order knee x-rays.

How is it treated?

Treatment includes the following:

- Place an ice pack on your knee for 20 to 30 minutes every 3 to 4 hours for the first 2 to 3 days or until the pain goes away
- Elevate your knee by placing a pillow underneath your leg when your knee hurts.
- Take anti-inflammatory medication, such as ibuprofen, as prescribed by your doctor.

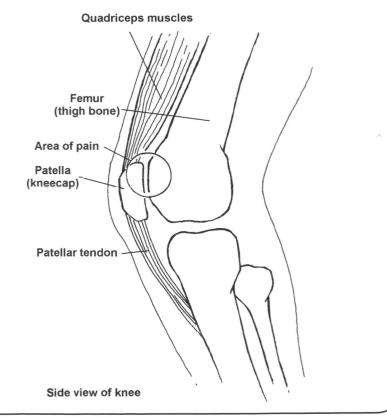

Patellofemoral Pain Syndrome (Runner's Knee)

Quadriceps muscles

Femur (thigh bone)

Area of pain

Patella (kneecap)

Patellar tendon

Side view of knee

Patellofemoral Pain Syndrome (Runner's Knee)

- Do the exercises recommended by your doctor or physical therapist.

Your doctor may recommend that you:

- Wear custom-made arch supports (orthotics) for over-pronation.

- Use an infrapatellar strap, a strap placed beneath the kneecap over the patellar tendon.

- Wear a neoprene knee sleeve, which will give support to your knee and patella.

While you are recovering from your injury, you will need to change your sport or activity to one that does not make your condition worse. For example, you may need to bicycle or swim instead of run. In cases of severe patellofemoral pain syndrome, surgery may be recommended. Your doctor will show you exercises to help decrease the pain behind your kneecap.

When can I return to my sport or activity?

The goal of rehabilitation is to return you to your sport or activity as soon as is safely possible. If you return too soon you may worsen your injury, which could lead to permanent damage. Everyone recovers from injury at a different rate. Return to your sport or activity will be determined by how soon your knee recovers, not by how many days or weeks it has been since you were injured. In general, the longer you have symptoms before you start treatment, the longer it will take to get better.

You may safely return to your sport or activity when, starting from the top of the list and progressing to the end, each of the following is true:

- Your injured knee can be fully straightened and bent without pain.

- Your knee and leg have regained normal strength compared to the uninjured knee and leg.

- You are able to jog straight ahead without limping.

- You are able to sprint straight ahead without limping.

- You are able to do 45-degree cuts.

- You are able to do 90-degree cuts.

- You are able to do 20-yard figure-of-eight runs.

- You are able to do 10-yard figure-of-eight runs.

- You are able to jump on both legs without pain and jump on the injured leg without pain.

How can I prevent patellofemoral pain syndrome?

Patellofemoral pain syndrome can best be prevented by strengthening your thigh muscles, particularly the inside part of this muscle group. It is also important to wear shoes that fit well and that have good arch supports.

© HBO & Company

Patellofemoral Pain Syndrome (Runner's Knee) Rehabilitation Exercises

You can do the hamstring stretch (exercise 1) right away. You can start doing exercise 2 as soon as it is not too painful to move your kneecap. When the pain in your knee has decreased, you can do the quadriceps stretch and start strengthening the thigh muscles using exercises 4 through 6.

1. Hamstring stretch: Stand with the heel of your injured leg resting on a stool that is about 15 inches high. Keep your knee straight. Gently lean forward from your hips, keeping your shoulders in line with your trunk, until you feel a stretch in the back of your thigh. Hold this position for 30 to 60 seconds. Return to the starting position. Do not round your shoulders and bring your head toward your toe. This will stretch your low back instead of your hamstrings. Repeat this exercise 3 times.

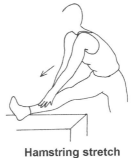

Hamstring stretch

2. Patellar mobility: Sit with your injured leg outstretched in front of you and the muscles on the top of your thigh relaxed. Take your index finger and thumb and gently press your kneecap down toward your foot. Hold this position for 10 seconds. Return to the starting position. Next, pull your kneecap up toward your waist and hold it for 10 seconds. Return to the starting position. Then, try to gently push your kneecap inward toward your other leg and hold for 10 seconds. Repeat these for approximately 5 minutes.

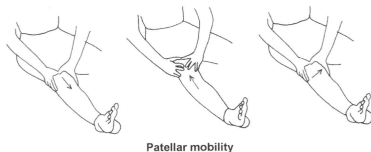

Patellar mobility

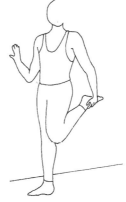

Quadriceps stretch

3. Quadriceps stretch: Stand an arm's length away from a wall, facing straight ahead. Brace yourself by keeping the hand on your uninjured side against the wall. With your other hand, grasp the ankle of the injured leg and pull your heel up toward your buttocks. Don't arch or twist your back. Hold this position for 30 seconds. Repeat 3 times.

4. Quadriceps set: Sit on the floor with your injured leg straight out in front of you. Try to tighten up the muscles at the top of your thigh by pushing the back of your knee down into the floor. Concentrate your contraction on the inside part of your thigh. It is very important to strengthen this part of your quadriceps muscle, called the vastus medialis, for your rehab to be successful. Hold this position for 5 seconds. Repeat 10 times. Do 3 sets of 10.

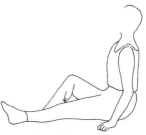

Quadriceps set

Patellofemoral Pain Syndrome (Runner's Knee) — *Rehabilitation Exercises*

5. Straight leg raise: Sit on the floor with your injured leg straight and the other leg bent so the foot is flat on the floor. Pull the toes of your injured leg toward you as far as you can comfortably while tightening the muscles on the top of your thigh. Raise your leg 6 to 8 inches off the floor. Hold this position for 3 to 5 seconds and then slowly lower your leg. Repeat 10 times. Do 3 sets of 10.

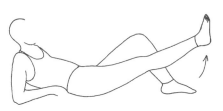

Straight leg raise

6. Weight lifting - leg extension: Do these if you have access to a weight lifting bench with a leg extension attachment. Sit on the bench with the weight attachment in front of your lower legs. Extend your knees by straightening your legs. Be sure your legs straighten completely. The last 15 degrees of extension are the most important. Use enough weight to cause fatigue but not pain. Do 3 sets of 10.

Pes Anserine Bursitis

What is pes anserine bursitis?

Pes anserine bursitis is an irritation or inflammation of a bursa in your knee. A bursa is a fluid-filled sac that acts as a cushion between tendons, bones, and skin.

The pes anserine bursa is located on the inner side of the knee just below the knee joint. Tendons of three muscles attach to the shin bone (tibia) over this bursa. These muscles act to bend the knee, bring the knees together, and cross the legs.

Pes anserine bursitis is common in swimmers who do the breaststroke and is sometimes called breaststroker's knee.

How does it occur?

Pes anserine bursitis can result from:

- overuse, as in breaststroke kicking or kicking a ball repeatedly
- repeated pivoting from a deep knee bend
- a direct blow to the area.

What are the symptoms?

Pes anserine bursitis causes pain on the inner side of the knee, just below the joint. You may have pain when you bend or straighten your leg.

How is it diagnosed?

Your doctor examines your knee for tenderness over the pes anserine bursa.

How is it treated?

Treatment may include:

- using ice packs on your knee for 20 to 30 minutes every 3 to 4 hours for 2 or 3 days or until the pain goes away
- wrapping an elastic bandage around your knee to reduce any swelling or to prevent swelling from occurring
- taking anti-inflammatory medication
- removal by your doctor of some of the fluid within the bursa if it is very swollen
- injection of a medication like cortisone into the swollen bursa
- leg stretching exercises.

When can I return to my sport or activity?

The goal of rehabilitation is to return you to your sport or

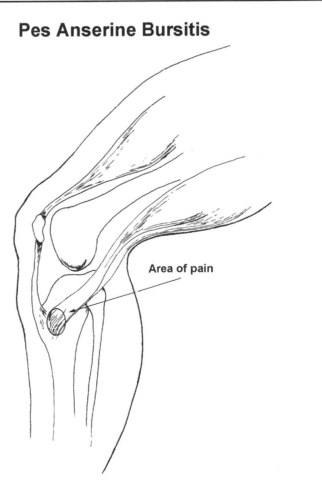

Pes Anserine Bursitis

Area of pain

Pes Anserine Bursitis

activity as soon as is safely possible. If you return too soon you may worsen your injury, which could lead to prolonged symptoms. Everyone recovers from injury at a different rate. Return to your sport or activity will be determined by how soon your knee recovers, not by how many days or weeks it has been since your injury occurred. In general, the longer you have symptoms before you start treatment, the longer it will take to get better.

You may safely return to your sport or activity when, starting from the top of the list and progressing to the end, each of the following is true:

- Your injured knee can be fully straightened and bent without pain.
- Your knee and leg have regained normal strength compared to the uninjured knee and leg.
- Your knee bursa is not swollen or tender to touch.
- You are able to jog straight ahead without limping.
- You are able to sprint straight ahead without limping.
- You are able to do 45-degree cuts.
- You are able to do 90-degree cuts.
- You are able to do 20-yard figure-of-eight runs.
- You are able to do 10-yard figure-of-eight runs.
- You are able to jump on both legs without pain and jump on the injured leg without pain.
- If you are a swimmer, you need to be able to do the breaststroke kick without pain.

How can I prevent pes anserine bursitis?

Pes anserine bursitis is best prevented by a proper warm-up that includes stretching of the hamstring muscles, the inner thigh muscles, and the top thigh muscles. Gradually increasing your activity level, rather than doing everything at once, will also help prevent its development.

Pes Anserine Bursitis Rehabilitation Exercises

You can stretch your leg right away by doing exercises 1 through 3. Start strengthening your leg by doing exercises 4 through 6.

1. Hamstring stretch: Lie on your back with your buttocks close to a doorway and extend your legs on the floor straight out in front of you through the doorway. Raise your injured leg and rest it against the wall next to the door frame. Hold this position for 30 to 60 seconds, feeling a stretch in the back of your thigh. Repeat 3 times.

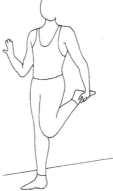

Hamstring stretch

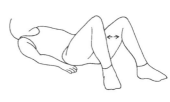

Calf stretch

2. Standing calf stretch: Facing a wall, put your hands against the wall at about eye level. Keep the injured leg back, the uninjured leg forward, and the heel of your injured leg on the floor. Turn your foot on your injured leg slightly inward (as if you were pigeon-toed) as you slowly lean into the wall until you feel a stretch in the back of your calf. Hold for 30 seconds. Do this several times a day.

3. Quadriceps stretch: Stand an arm's length away from a wall, facing straight ahead. Brace yourself by keeping the hand on the uninjured side against the wall. With your other hand, grasp the ankle of the injured leg and pull your heel up toward your buttocks. Don't arch or twist your back. Hold this position for 30 seconds. Repeat 3 times.

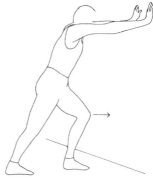

Hip adductor stretch

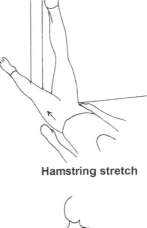

Quadriceps stretch

4. Hip adductor stretch: Lie on your back, bend your knees, and put your feet flat on the floor. Gently spread your knees apart, stretching the muscles on the inside of your thigh. Hold this for 20 seconds. Repeat 3 times.

5. Isometrics:

   A. Quadriceps Isometrics: Sitting on the floor with your injured leg straight and the other leg bent, press the back of your knee down into the floor while tightening the muscles on the top of your thigh. Hold this position for 5 seconds. Repeat 20 times.

   B. Hamstring Isometrics: Sitting on the floor with the injured leg slightly bent, dig the heel of your injured leg into the floor and tighten up the back of your thigh muscles. Hold this position for 5 seconds. Repeat 20 times.

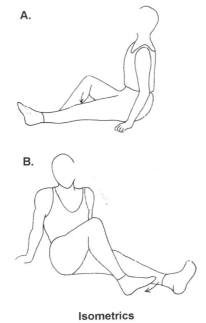

Isometrics

Pes Anserine Bursitis Rehabilitation Exercises

6. Heel slide: Sitting on a firm surface with your legs straight in front of you, slowly slide the heel of your injured leg toward your buttock by pulling your knee to your chest as you slide. Return to the starting position. Repeat 20 times.

Heel slide

Prepatellar (Knee) Bursitis

What is prepatellar bursitis?

Prepatellar bursitis is an irritation or inflammation of a bursa in your knee. A bursa is a fluid-filled sac that acts as a cushion between tendons, bones, and skin.

There are several bursae in the knee. The prepatellar bursa is located just in front of the kneecap near the attachment of the kneecap (patellar) tendon. Prepatellar bursitis is also called housemaid's knee from when maids were injured cleaning floors on their knees. The injury is common in wrestlers, who get it from their knees rubbing on the mats. Volleyball players get it from diving onto their knees for the ball.

How does it occur?

Bursitis can result from:

- overuse
- a direct blow to the area
- chronic friction, such as from frequent kneeling.

What are the symptoms?

Prepatellar bursitis causes pain and swelling over the front of the knee. You may have pain when you bend or straighten your leg.

How is it diagnosed?

Your doctor will examine your knee for tenderness over the bursa.

How is it treated?

Treatment may include:

- using ice packs on your knee for 20 to 30 minutes every 3 to 4 hours for 2 or 3 days or until the pain goes away
- wrapping an elastic bandage around your knee to reduce any swelling or to prevent swelling from occurring
- taking anti-inflammatory medication
- removal by your doctor of some of the fluid within the bursa if it is very swollen
- injection of a corticosteroid medication into the swollen bursa
- leg stretching exercises.

When can I return to my sport or activity?

The goal of rehabilitation is to return you to your sport or

Prepatellar Bursitis

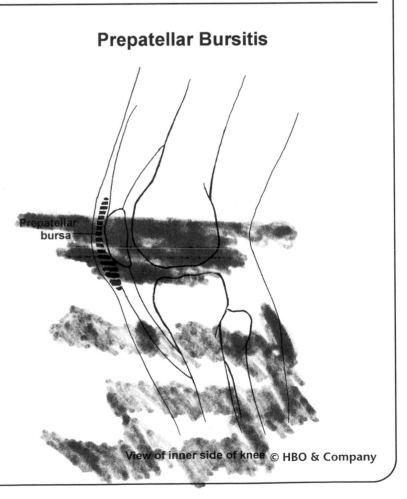

Prepatellar bursa

View of inner side of knee © HBO & Company

Prepatellar (Knee) Bursitis

activity as soon as is safely possible. If you return too soon you may worsen your injury, which could lead to permanent damage. Everyone recovers from injury at a different rate. Return to your sport or activity will be determined by how soon your knee recovers, not by how many days or weeks it has been since your injury occurred. In general, the longer you have symptoms before you start treatment, the longer it will take to get better.

You may safely return to your sport or activity when, starting from the top of the list and progressing to the end, each of the following is true:

- Your injured knee can be fully straightened and bent without pain.
- Your knee and leg have regained normal strength compared to the uninjured knee and leg.
- Your knee bursa is not swollen or tender to touch.
- You are able to put pressure on your bursa (such as kneeling) without pain or swelling.
- You are able to jog straight ahead without limping.
- You are able to sprint straight ahead without limping.
- You are able to do 45-degree cuts.

- You are able to do 90-degree cuts.
- You are able to do 20-yard figure-of-eight runs.
- You are able to do 10-yard figure-of-eight runs.
- You are able to jump on both legs without pain and jump on the injured leg without pain.

How can I prevent prepatellar bursitis?

Prepatellar bursitis is best prevented by avoiding direct blows to the kneecap area and by avoiding prolonged kneeling. Proper protective kneepads will help prevent inflammation of the bursa.

Prepatellar (Knee) Bursitis Rehabilitation Exercises

You can stretch your leg right away by doing exercises 1 through 3. Start strengthening your leg by doing exercises 4 and 5.

1. Hamstring stretch: Lie on your back with your buttocks close to a doorway and extend your legs straight out in front of you along the floor. Raise your injured leg and rest it against the wall next to the door frame. Hold this position for 30 to 60 seconds, feeling a stretch in the back of your thigh. Repeat 3 times.

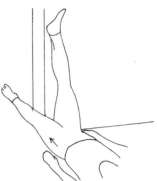

Hamstring stretch

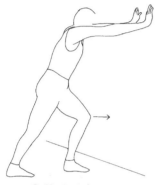

Calf stretch

2. Standing calf stretch: Facing a wall, put your hands against the wall at about eye level. Keep the injured leg back, the uninjured leg forward, and the heel of your injured leg on the floor. Turn your foot on your injured leg slightly inward (as if you were pigeon-toed) as you slowly lean into the wall until you feel a stretch in the back of your calf. Hold for 30 seconds. Do this several times a day.

3. Quadriceps stretch: Stand an arm's length away from a wall, facing straight ahead. Brace yourself by keeping the hand on the uninjured side against the wall. With your other hand, grasp the ankle of the injured leg and pull your heel up toward your buttocks. Don't arch or twist your back. Hold this position for 30 seconds. Repeat 3 times.

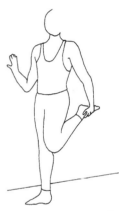

Quadriceps stretch

4. Isometrics:

   A. Quadriceps Isometrics: Sitting on the floor with your injured leg straight and the other leg bent, press the back of your knee down into the floor while tightening the muscles on the top of your thigh. Hold this position for 5 seconds. Repeat 20 times.

   B. Hamstring Isometrics: Sitting on the floor with the injured leg slightly bent, dig the heel of your injured leg into the floor and tighten up the back of your thigh muscles. Hold this position for 5 seconds. Repeat 20 times.

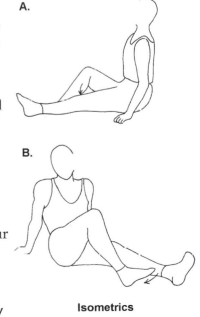

A.

B.

Isometrics

5. Heel slide: Sitting on a firm surface with your legs straight in front of you, slowly slide the heel of your injured leg toward your buttock by pulling your knee to your chest as you slide. Return to the starting position. Repeat 20 times.

Heel slide

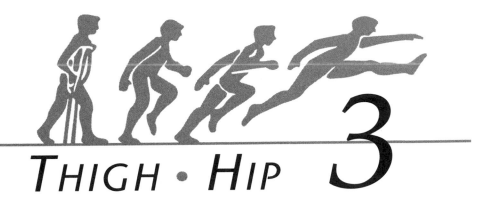

THIGH · HIP 3

Gluteal Strain

What is a gluteal strain?

Your gluteal muscles are the muscles in your buttocks. A strained muscle is when the muscle fibers are stretched or torn.

How does it occur?

A gluteal strain usually occurs with running or jumping. It is often seen in hurdlers or dancers.

What are the symptoms?

A gluteal strain will cause pain in the buttocks. You may have pain when walking up or down stairs and pain when sitting. You will have pain moving your leg backward.

How is it diagnosed?

Your doctor will examine your hips, buttocks, and legs and find that you have tenderness in the gluteal muscles.

How is it treated?

Initially, you should put ice packs on your injury for 20 to 30 minutes every 3 to 4 hours for 2 or 3 days or until the pain goes away. Your doctor may prescribe an anti-inflammatory medication. You will be given a set of rehabilitation exercises.

While you are recovering from your injury, you will need to change your sport or activity to one that does not make your condition worse. For example, if running causes you pain, change to swimming.

When can I return to my sport or activity?

The goal of rehabilitation is to return you to your sport or activity as soon as is safely possible. If you return too soon you may worsen your injury, which could lead to permanent damage. Everyone recovers from injury at a different rate. Return to your sport or activity will be determined by how soon the injured area recovers, not by how many days or weeks it has been since your injury occurred. In general, the

Gluteal Strain

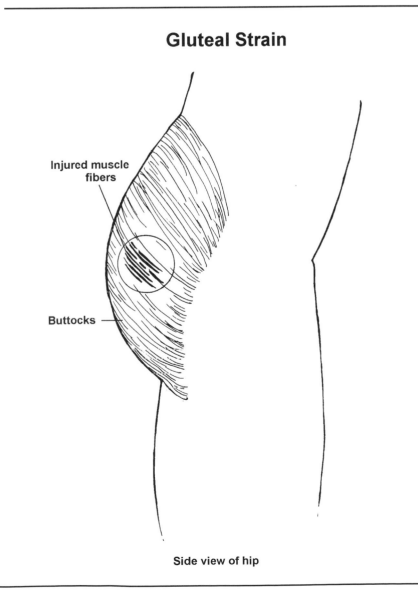

Injured muscle fibers

Buttocks

Side view of hip

Gluteal Strain

longer you have symptoms before you start treatment, the longer it will take to get better.

You may safely return to your sport or activity when, starting from the top of the list and progressing to the end, each of the following is true:

- You have full range of motion on the injured side compared to the uninjured side.
- You have full strength of the injured side compared to the uninjured side.

- You can jog straight ahead without pain or limping.
- You can sprint straight ahead without pain or limping.
- You can do 45-degree cuts, first at half-speed, then at full-speed.
- You can do 20-yard figures-of-eight, first at half-speed, then at full-speed.
- You can do 90-degree cuts, first at half-speed, then at full-speed.

- You can do 10-yard figures-of-eight, first at half-speed, then at full-speed.
- You can jump on both legs without pain and you can jump on the leg on the injured side without pain.

How can a gluteal strain be prevented?

Gluteal strains are best prevented by warming up properly and doing stretching exercises before your activity.

Gluteal Strain Rehabilitation Exercises

You can stretch your gluteal muscles right away. You can begin strengthening your gluteal muscles as soon as the sharp pain goes away and you only have a dull ache using exercise 3, gluteal isometrics. After gluteal isometrics become easier, you can do gluteal strengthening exercises 4, 5, and 6.

After the gluteal strengthening exercises become easy, strengthen your buttock muscles by doing lunges, exercise 7.

1. Single knee to chest stretch: Lie on your back with your legs straight out in front of you. Bring the knee on your injured side up to your chest and grasp the back of your thigh. Pull your knee toward your chest, stretching your buttock muscle. Hold this position for 30 seconds and return to the starting position. Repeat 3 times.

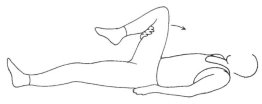

Single knee to chest stretch

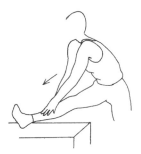

Hamstring stretch

2. Hamstring stretch: With the heel of leg on your injured side resting on a stool about 15 inches high, bend forward at the hips, stretching the back of your thigh muscle. Make sure you don't round your shoulders and bend at the waist. Hold this position for 30 to 60 seconds. Repeat 3 times.

3. Gluteal isometrics: Lie on your stomach with your legs straight out behind you. Squeeze your buttock muscles together and hold for 5 seconds. Release. Repeat 10 times. Do 3 sets of 10.

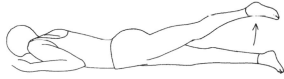

Gluteal isometric

4. Prone hip extension: Lie on your stomach with your legs straight out behind you. Squeeze your buttock muscles and lift the leg on your injured side straight up off the floor about 6 to 8 inches. Keep your knee straight. Hold this for 5 seconds and then slowly lower your leg to the floor. Repeat 10 times. Do 3 sets of 10.

Prone hip extension

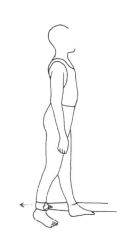

Resisted hip extension

5. Resisted hip extension: Stand facing a door with a Thera-Band tied around your ankle. Knot the other end of the tubing and shut the knot in the door. Pull your leg straight back, keeping your knee straight. Make sure you do not lean forward. Repeat 10 times. Do 3 sets of 10.

To challenge yourself, move farther away from the door and the tubing will provide more resistance.

Gluteal Strain Rehabilitation Exercises

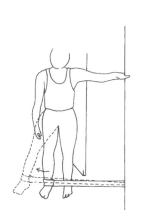

Hip abduction

6. Hip abduction: Stand sideways near a doorway with your uninjured side closest to the door. Tie a Thera-Band around the ankle of your injured leg. Knot the other end of the tubing and close the knot in the door. Extend your leg out to the side, keeping your knee straight. Return to the starting position. Repeat 10 times. Do 3 sets of 10.

To challenge yourself, move farther away from the door.

7. Lunge: Stand and take a large step forward with leg on your injured side. Dip the knee on the uninjured side down toward the floor and bend the leg on your injured side. Return to the starting position. Repeat the exercise, this time stepping forward with the leg on your uninjured side and dipping the leg on the injured side down. Do 10 repetitions on each side.

Lunge

Groin Strain

What is a groin strain?

A strain is a stretch or tear of a muscle or tendon. People commonly call such an injury a "pulled" muscle. The muscles in your groin help bring your legs together. There are two muscles that may commonly get injured in a groin strain: the adductor magnus (the large muscle running down the inner side of the thigh) and the sartorius (a thinner muscle that starts on the outside of your hip, crosses your thigh and attaches near the inside of the knee).

How does it occur?

A groin strain most commonly occurs when you are running or jumping or when there is a forced push-off or cut.

What are the symptoms?

You will have pain or tenderness along the inner side of your thigh or in the groin area. You will have pain when you bring your legs together. You may have pain when lifting your knee up.

How is it diagnosed?

Your doctor will take note of your symptoms and will examine your thigh and hip.

How is it treated?

Treatment may include:

- applying ice to the strained muscle for 20 to 30 minutes every 3 to 4 hours for 2 or 3 days or until the pain goes away
- taking an anti-inflammatory medication prescribed by your doctor
- wearing a supportive bandage called a thigh wrap or taping your thigh or groin
- doing the rehabilitation exercises you are given.

While you are recovering from your injury, you will need to change your sport or activity to one that does not make your condition worse. For example, you may need to swim instead of run.

When can I return to my sport or activity?

The goal of rehabilitation is to return you to your sport or activity as soon as is safely possible. If you return too soon you may worsen your injury, which could lead to permanent damage. Everyone recovers from injury at a different rate. Return to your sport or activity will be determined by how soon your

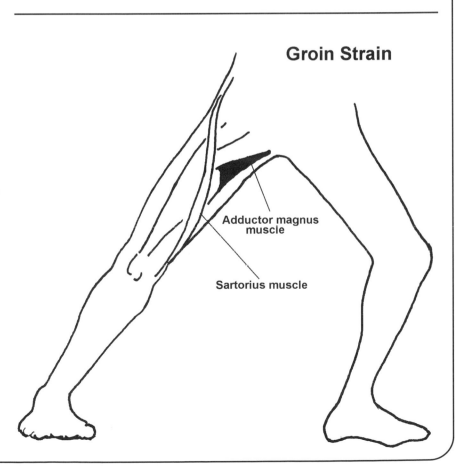

Groin Strain

Adductor magnus muscle

Sartorius muscle

Groin Strain

groin area recovers, not by how many days or weeks it has been since your injury occurred. In general, the longer you have symptoms before you start treatment, the longer it will take to get better.

You may safely return to your sport or activity when, starting from the top of the list and progressing to the end, each of the following is true:

- You have full range of motion in the injured leg compared to the uninjured leg.
- You have full strength of the injured leg compared to the uninjured leg.

- You can jog straight ahead without pain or limping.
- You can sprint straight ahead without pain or limping.
- You can do 45-degree cuts, first at half-speed, then at full-speed.
- You can do 20-yard figures-of-eight, first at half-speed, then at full-speed.
- You can do 90-degree cuts, first at half-speed, then at full-speed.
- You can do 10-yard figures-of-eight, first at half-speed, then at full-speed.

- You can jump on both legs without pain and you can jump on the injured leg without pain.

How can I prevent a groin strain?

A groin strain is best prevented by warming up properly and doing groin muscle stretching exercises prior to your activities. This is especially important in activities such as sprinting or jumping.

Groin Strain Rehabilitation Exercises

Begin stretching your groin muscles as soon as you can tolerate a stretch to that area.

1. Hip adductor stretch: Lie on your back, bend your knees, and put your feet flat on the floor. Gently spread your knees apart, stretching the muscles on the inside of your thigh. Hold this for 20 seconds. Repeat 3 times.

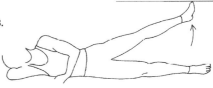

Hip adductor stretch

   You may do exercises 2 and 3 when the pain in the groin muscles decreases.

2. Hamstring stretch: Lie on your back with your buttocks close to a doorway and extend your legs straight out in front of you along the floor. Raise the injured leg up and rest it against the wall next to the door frame. Hold this position for 30 to 60 seconds. You will feel a stretch in the back of your thigh. Repeat 3 times.

3. Sidelying leg raises:

   A. Injured side down: Lie on your injured side. Bend your uninjured leg over your injured leg so that the foot of your uninjured leg is flat on the floor in front of the knee of your injured leg. Tighten the muscles on the front of the thigh of the injured leg and lift that leg 8 to 10 inches off the floor, keeping your knee straight. Slowly lower your leg to the floor. Repeat 10 times. Do 3 sets of 10.

   B. Injured side up: Lying on your uninjured side, tighten the front thigh muscles on your injured leg and lift that leg 8 to 10 inches away from the other leg. Keep the leg straight. Repeat 10 times. Do 3 sets of 10.

Hamstring stretch

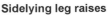

Sidelying leg raises

When the sidelying leg raises become easy, it is time to start strengthening your thigh muscles and groin muscles using the Thera-Band exercises.

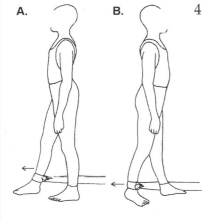

4. Resisted hip strengthening exercises: Tie a loop in one end of the Thera-Band and slip the loop around the ankle of your injured leg. Make a knot in the other end of the tubing and close the knot in a door.

   A. Hip flexion: Stand facing away from the door. Tighten the muscles at the top of your thigh and bring your leg forward away from the door, keeping your knee straight. Return to the starting position. Repeat 10 times. Do 3 sets of 10.

   B. Hip extension: Face the door. Tighten your thigh muscles and pull your leg straight backward. Return to the starting position. Repeat 10 times. Do 3 sets of 10.

Groin Strain Rehabilitation Exercises

C. Hip abduction: Stand sideways to the door, with your injured leg away from the door. Tighten your thigh muscles and extend your leg out to the side. Return to the starting position. Repeat 10 times. Do 3 sets of 10.

D. Hip adduction: Stand sideways to the door, with your uninjured leg away from the door. Bring your injured leg across your body sideways, crossing over your uninjured leg and stretching the Thera-Band. Return to the starting position. Repeat 10 times. Do 3 sets of 10.

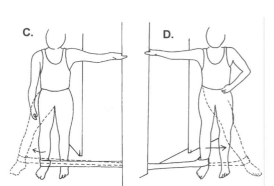

Resisted hip strengthening exercises

© HBO & Company

Hamstring Strain

What is a hamstring strain?

A strain is a stretch or tear of a muscle or tendon. People commonly call such an injury a "pulled" muscle.

Your hamstring muscle group is in the back of your thigh and allows you to bend your knee. It is made up of three large muscles: the biceps, semimembranosus, and semitendinosus.

How does it occur?

A hamstring muscle strain usually occurs when these muscles are contracted forcefully during activities such as running or jumping.

What are the symptoms?

You will often feel a burning or a popping as the injury occurs. You will have pain when walking or when bending or straightening your leg. A few days after the injury, you may have bruising on your leg just below the injury.

How is it diagnosed?

Your doctor will examine your leg and find tenderness at the site of the injury.

How is it treated?

Treatment may include:

- applying ice packs to your hamstrings for 20 to 30 minutes every 3 to 4 hours for 2 to 3 days or until the pain goes away
- elevating your leg by placing a pillow underneath it
- wrapping an elastic bandage around your leg for compression to keep the swelling from getting worse
- taking anti-inflammatory medication according to your doctor's prescription
- using crutches if it is too painful to walk.

As you return to your activity, you may be given an elastic thigh wrap to give extra support to your hamstrings. While

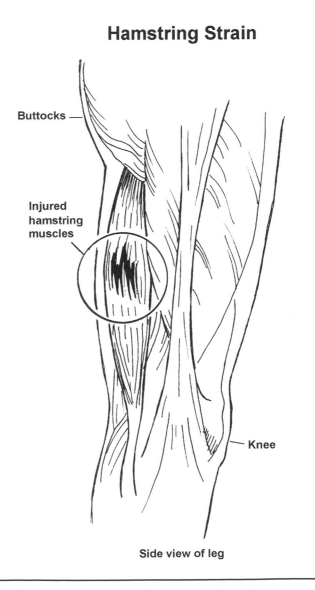

Hamstring Strain

Buttocks

Injured hamstring muscles

Knee

Side view of leg

Hamstring Strain

you are recovering from your injury, you will need to change your sport or activity to one that does not make your condition worse. For example, you may need to swim or bicycle instead of run.

When can I return to my sport or activity?

The goal of rehabilitation is to return you to your sport or activity as soon as is safely possible. If you return too soon you may worsen your injury, which could lead to permanent damage. Everyone recovers from injury at a different rate. Return to your sport or activity will be determined by how soon your leg recovers, not by how many days or weeks it has been since your injury occurred. In

general, the longer you have symptoms before you start treatment, the longer it will take to get better.

You may safely return to your sport or activity when, starting from the top of the list and progressing to the end, each of the following is true:

- You have full range of motion in the injured leg compared to the uninjured leg.
- You have full strength of the injured leg compared to the uninjured leg.
- You can jog straight ahead without pain or limping.
- You can sprint straight ahead without pain or limping.
- You can do 45-degree cuts, first at half-speed, then at full-speed.

- You can do 20-yard figures-of-eight, first at half-speed, then at full-speed.
- You can do 90-degree cuts, first at half-speed, then at full-speed.
- You can do 10-yard figures-of-eight, first at half-speed, then at full-speed.
- You can jump on both legs without pain and you can jump on the injured leg without pain.

How can I prevent a hamstring strain?

A hamstring strain is best prevented by warming up properly and stretching your hamstring muscles prior to your activities. This is especially important in sprinting or jumping.

Hamstring Strain Rehabilitation Exercises

You can begin gently stretching your hamstring right away by doing exercise 1, the standing hamstring stretch. Make sure you do not feel any sharp pain, only a mild discomfort in the back of your thigh when you are doing the stretch.

After the standing hamstring stretch has become easier, you can do exercise 2, the hamstring stretch on a wall. You should also stretch your calf muscle because it attaches near where your hamstring ends. Use exercise 3, the standing calf stretch.

Next, start strengthening your hamstrings using exercises 4, 5, and 6 when the pain is gone.

After your hamstrings have become stronger and you feel your leg is stable, you can begin strengthening the quadriceps (the muscles in the front of the thigh) by doing exercise 7, the wall slide.

1. Standing hamstring stretch: It is generally easiest to begin stretching your hamstring by placing the heel of your injured leg on a stool about 15 inches high. Lean forward, bending at the hips until you feel a mild stretch in the back of your thigh. Make sure you do not roll your shoulders and bend at the waist when doing this or you will stretch your lower back instead. Hold the stretch 30 to 60 seconds. Repeat 3 times.

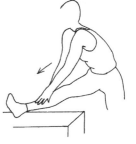

Standing hamstring stretch

2. Hamstring stretch on wall: Lie on your back with your buttocks close to a doorway and your legs extended straight out in front of you and through the doorway. Raise your injured leg and rest the heel against the door frame. Your uninjured leg should still be extended through the doorway. You will feel a very strong stretch in the back of your thigh. Hold this stretch for 60 seconds. Repeat 3 times.

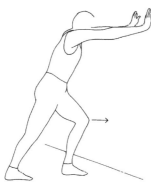

Standing calf stretch

3. Standing calf stretch: Stand facing a wall with your hands on the wall at about chest level. Your injured leg should be about 12 to 18 inches behind your uninjured leg. Keep your injured leg straight with your heel on the floor, and lean into the wall. Bend your front knee until you feel a stretch in the back of the calf muscle of your injured leg. Hold this position for 30 to 60 seconds. Repeat 3 times.

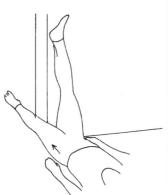

Hamstring stretch on a wall

4. Prone knee bends: You can begin gently strengthening your injured hamstring by lying on your stomach with your legs straight out behind you and bending your knee so that your heel comes toward your buttocks. Bring it back down to the starting position. Repeat 10 times. Do 3 sets of 10.

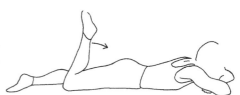

Prone knee bends

As this becomes easier you can wear ankle weights.

Hamstring Strain Rehabilitation Exercises

5. Thera-Band hamstring curls: Sit in a chair facing a door and about 3 feet from the door. Loop and tie one end of the tubing around the ankle of your injured leg. Tie knot in the other end of the Thera-Band and shut the knot in the door. Bend your knee so that your foot slides along the floor and moves back underneath the chair, stretching the tubing. Slowly let your foot slide forward again. Repeat 10 times. Do 3 sets of 10.

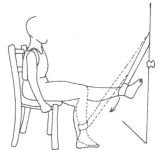

Theraband hamstring curls

You can challenge yourself by moving the chair farther away from the door and increasing the resistance of the Thera-Band.

6. Standing heel raise: Balance yourself while standing behind a chair or other stable object. Raise your body up onto your toes and lift your heels off the floor. Hold this for about 2 seconds and then slowly lower your heels back down to the floor. Repeat 10 times. Do 3 sets of 10.

You can challenge yourself by standing only on your injured leg and lifting your heel off the floor. Do 3 sets of 10.

Standing heel raise

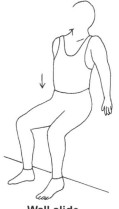

Wall slide

7. Wall slide: Stand with your back, shoulders, and head against a wall and look straight ahead. Keep your shoulders relaxed and your feet 1 foot away from the wall and a shoulder's width apart. Keeping your head against the wall, slide down the wall, lowering your buttocks toward the floor until your thighs are almost parallel to the floor. Hold this position for 20 seconds. Make sure to tighten the thigh muscles as you slowly slide back up to the starting position. Repeat 10 times. Increasing the amount of time you are in the lowered position helps strengthen your quadriceps muscles.

Hip Flexor Strain

What is a hip flexor strain?

A strain is a stretch or tear of a muscle or tendon, a band of tissue that connects muscle to bone. The tendon may be inflamed. Inflammation of a tendon is called tendonitis. The hip flexor muscles allow you to lift your knee and bend at the waist.

How does it occur?

Hip flexor strain occurs from overuse of the muscles that help you flex your knee or do high kicks. This injury occurs in bicyclists, athletes who jump or run with high knee kicks, athletes like soccer players who do forceful kicking activities, and people who practice the martial arts.

What are the symptoms?

You have pain in the upper groin region where the thigh meets the pelvis.

How is it diagnosed?

Your doctor will examine your hip and thigh. You will have tenderness at the muscle and tendon.

How is it treated?

Treatment may include:

- putting ice packs on the injured area for 20 to 30 minutes every 3 to 4 hours

for 2 to 3 days or until the pain goes away

- taking anti-inflammatory medications prescribed by your doctor
- doing rehabilitation exercises to help you return to your activity.

While you are recovering from your injury, you will need to change your sport or activity to one that does not make your condition worse. For example, you may need to swim instead of bicycling or running.

When can I return to my sport or activity?

The goal of rehabilitation is to return you to your sport or activity as soon as is safely possible. If you return too soon you may worsen your injury, which could lead to permanent damage. Everyone recovers from injury at a different rate. Return to your sport or activity will be determined by how soon your hip flexor muscles recover, not by how many days or weeks it

Hip Flexor Strain

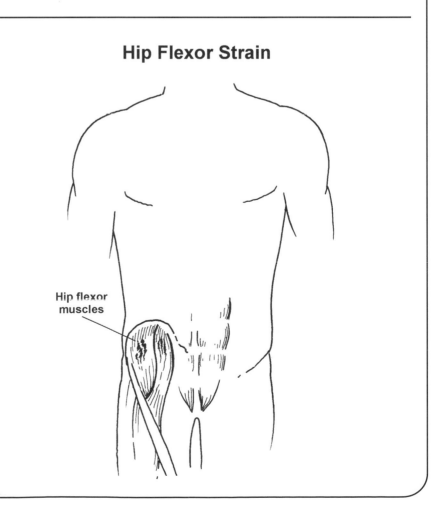

Hip flexor muscles

Hip Flexor Strain

has been since your injury occurred. In general, the longer you have symptoms before you start treatment, the longer it will take to get better.

You may safely return to your sport or activity when, starting from the top of the list and progressing to the end, each of the following is true:

- You have full range of motion in the leg on the injured side compared to the leg on the uninjured side.

- You have full strength of the leg on the injured side compared to the leg on the uninjured side.

- You can jog straight ahead without pain or limping.

- You can sprint straight ahead without pain or limping.

- You can do 45-degree cuts, first at half-speed, then at full-speed.

- You can do 20-yard figures-of-eight, first at half-speed, then at full-speed.

- You can do 90-degree cuts, first at half-speed, then at full-speed.

- You can do 10-yard figures-of-eight, first at half-speed, then at full-speed.

- You can jump on both legs without pain and you can jump on the leg on the injured side without pain.

How can I prevent a hip flexor strain?

Hip flexor strains are best prevented by warming up properly and doing stretching exercises before your activity. If you are a bicyclist make sure your seat is raised to the proper height.

Hip Flexor Strain Rehabilitation Exercises

You can begin stretching your hip muscles right away by doing exercises 1 and 2. Make sure you only feel a mild discomfort when stretching and not a sharp pain. You may do exercises 3, 4, and 5 when the pain is gone.

1. Hip flexor stretch: Kneel on both knees and place your uninjured leg forward, with the foot resting flat on the floor. From this position, lean forward at the hip and attempt to press your pelvis down toward the floor while slightly arching your back until you feel a stretch at the front of your hip. Hold this position for 30 seconds. Repeat 3 times.

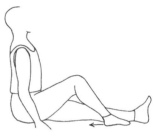

Hip flexor stretch

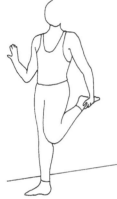

Quadriceps stretch

2. Quadriceps stretch: Stand and hold onto a table or a counter. With the hand on your uninjured side, grasp the top part of the ankle on your injured leg and pull your foot toward your buttock until you feel a stretch on the front of your thigh. Hold this position for 30 seconds. Repeat 3 times.

3. Heel slide: Sit on a firm surface with your legs straight in front of you. Slowly slide the heel of your injured leg toward your buttock by pulling your knee to your chest as you slide. Return to the starting position. Repeat this 20 times.

Heel slide

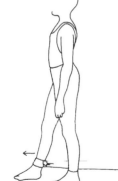

Resisted hip flexion

4. Straight leg raise: Lie on the floor on your back and tighten up the top of the thigh muscles on your injured leg. Point your toes up toward the ceiling and lift your leg up off the floor about 10 inches. Keep your knee straight. Slowly lower your leg back down to the floor. Repeat 10 times. Do 3 sets of 10.

Straight leg raise

5. Resisted hip flexion: Stand facing away from a door. Tie a loop in one end of a Thera-Band and put it around your injured ankle. Tie a knot in the other end of the tubing and shut the knot in the door near the bottom. Tighten up the front of your thigh muscle and bring your leg forward, keeping your knee straight. Repeat 10 times. Do 3 sets of 10.

Hip Pointer

What is a hip pointer?

A hip pointer is a deep bruise on the top portion of your pelvis, called the iliac crest.

How does it occur?

A hip pointer is caused by a direct blow to the iliac crest. This injury most commonly occurs in a contact sport such as football, when a helmet is driven into the iliac crest.

What are the symptoms?

You have tenderness in the top portion of your hip.

How is it diagnosed?

Your doctor will examine your hip and pelvis. Your doctor may get an x-ray if he or she thinks there might be a fracture to that part of the iliac bone.

How is it treated?

At first, treat your injury with ice packs for 20 to 30 minutes every 3 to 4 hours for 2 to 3 days or until the pain goes away. A hip pointer needs time to heal itself. Protect yourself from further injury by placing padding over the injury.

When can I return to my sport or activity?

The goal of rehabilitation is to return you to your sport or activity as soon as is safely possible. If you return too soon you may worsen your injury, which could lead to permanent damage. Everyone recovers from injury at a different rate. Return to your sport or activity will be determined by how soon your hip recovers, not by how many days or weeks it has been since your injury occurred. In general, the longer you have symptoms before you start treatment, the longer it will take to get better.

You may return to your sport or activity after a hip pointer when you have no pain when walking or running. You will usually have pain with contact to the hip pointer for several weeks after the injury. If a pad taped over the hip pointer provides enough protection during contact, you may continue participating in your sport or activity.

How can I prevent a hip pointer?

A hip pointer is usually not preventable. However, if you are playing a con- tact sport it is important to wear proper protective padding over this area of your body.

Hip Pointer

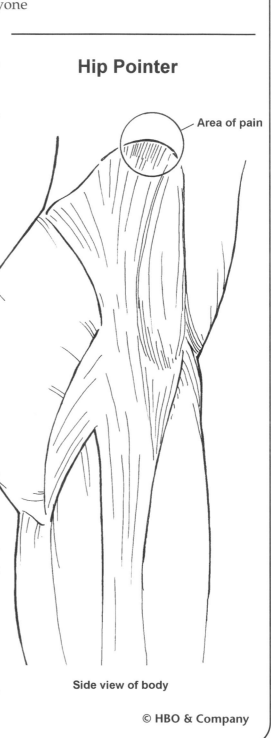

Area of pain

Side view of body

© HBO & Company

Pelvic Avulsion Fractures

What is a pelvic avulsion fracture?

There are several muscles in the thigh that attach to various parts of the pelvis. An avulsion is the tearing away of a body part from its point of attachment. An avulsion fracture occurs when a tendon that attaches a muscle to a bone pulls part of the bone away.

How does it occur?

An avulsion fracture may occur after sudden, forceful contraction of the muscle. It is often seen in athletes with tight muscles. Common sites for avulsion fractures include where the sartorius muscle attaches to the top front of the pelvis; where the rectus femoris muscle attaches to the front of the pelvis; where the hamstring muscle group attaches to the part of the pelvis called the ischial tuberosity (the part of your pelvis that you sit on).

What are the symptoms?

You will feel pain at the attachment site of the muscles. There will be tenderness and swelling.

How is it diagnosed?

Your doctor will review your symptoms and examine the injured area. Since the muscle has been torn away from its attachment site, it is possible that you may not be able to perform a muscle function. Your doctor may order an x-ray that would show a piece of bone pulled away from its muscular attachment site.

How is it treated?

These avulsion fractures require rest. In general, they will heal with 4 to 6 weeks of rest. You may need to use crutches for most of this time. If the bony fragment is large or is torn away from its original site by a significant distance, surgery may be required.

At the time of the initial injury you should apply ice to the area for 20 to 30 minutes every 3 to 4 hours for 2 to 3 days or until the pain goes away. Your doctor may prescribe anti-inflammatory medications.

When can I return to my sport or activity?

The goal of rehabilitation is to return you to your sport or activity as soon as is safely possible. If you return too soon you may worsen your injury, which could lead to permanent damage. Everyone recovers from injury at a different rate. Return to your sport or activity will be determined by how soon the injured area recovers, not by how many days or weeks it has been since your injury occurred. In general, the

Pelvic Avulsion Fractures

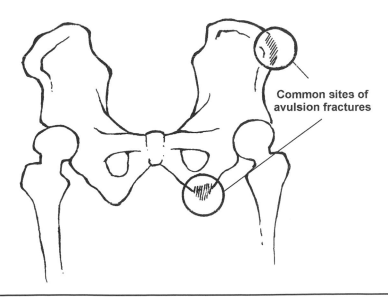

Common sites of avulsion fractures

Pelvic Avulsion Fractures

longer you have symptoms before you start treatment, the longer it will take to get better.

You may safely return to your sport or activity when, starting from the top of the list and progressing to the end, each of the following is true:

- You have full range of motion in the injured leg compared to the uninjured leg.
- You have full strength of the injured leg compared to the uninjured leg.
- You can jog straight ahead without pain or limping.

- You can sprint straight ahead without pain or limping.
- You can do 45-degree cuts, first at half-speed, then at full-speed.
- You can do 20-yard figures-of-eight, first at half-speed, then at full-speed.
- You can do 90-degree cuts, first at half-speed, then at full-speed.
- You can do 10-yard figures-of-eight, first at half-speed, then at full-speed.

- You can jump on both legs without pain and you can jump on the injured leg without pain.

How can pelvic avulsion fractures be prevented?

Since tight muscles are a common cause of avulsion fractures, be sure to do stretching exercises to prevent these injuries from happening again. Warm up properly and stretch your thigh, hamstring, and groin muscles before your activity.

Piriformis Syndrome

What is piriformis syndrome?

Piriformis syndrome refers to irritation of the sciatic nerve as it passes through the piriformis muscle located deep in the buttock. Inflammation of the sciatic nerve, called sciatica, causes pain in the back of the hip that can often travel down into the leg.

How does it occur?

The piriformis muscle is located deep in the buttock and pelvis and allows you to rotate your thigh outward. The sciatic nerve travels from your back into your leg by passing through the piriformis muscle. If the piriformis muscle is unusually tight or if it goes into spasm, the sciatic nerve can become inflamed or irritated. Piriformis syndrome may also be related to intense downhill running.

What are the symptoms?

You have pain deep in your buttock that may feel like a burning pain. The pain usually travels down across your lower thigh. Your pain may increase when you move your thigh outward, such as when you are sitting cross-legged.

How is it diagnosed?

Your doctor will talk to you about when your symptoms began. Since your sciatic nerve begins in the back, it can be irritated from a back injury, such as a herniated disk. Your doctor will ask if you have had any injuries to your back or hip. He or she will examine your back to see if the sciatic nerve is irritated there. He or she will examine your hip and legs and move them to see if movement causes increased pain.

Your doctor may order x-rays, a computed tomography (CT) scan, or a magnetic resonance image (MRI) of your back to see if there is a back injury. There are no x-ray tests that can detect if the nerve is being irritated at the piriformis muscle.

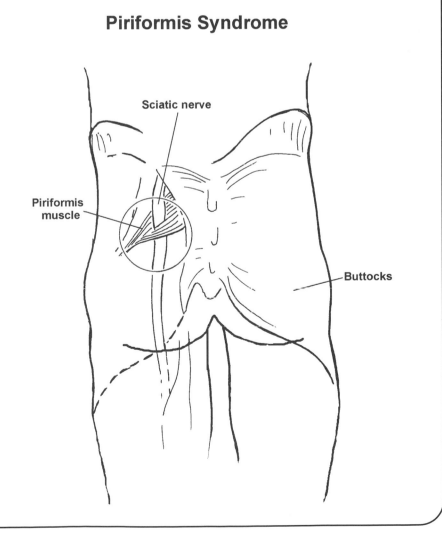

Piriformis Syndrome

Sciatic nerve

Piriformis muscle

Buttocks

Piriformis Syndrome

How is it treated?

Treatment may include:

- placing ice packs on your buttock for 20 to 30 minutes every 3 to 4 hours for the first 2 to 3 days or until the pain goes away
- rest
- taking prescribed anti-inflammatory medications or muscle relaxants
- learning and doing stretching exercises of the piriformis muscle.

When can I return to my sport or activity?

The goal of rehabilitation is to return you to your sport or activity as soon as is safely possible. If you return too soon you may worsen your injury, which could lead to permanent damage. Everyone recovers from injury at a different rate. Return to your sport or activity will be determined by how soon the nerve recovers, not by how many days or weeks it has been since your injury occurred. In general, the longer you have symptoms before you start treatment, the longer it will take to get better.

You may safely return to your sport or activity when, starting from the top of the list and progressing to the end, each of the following is true:

- You have full range of motion in the affected leg compared to the unaffected leg.
- You have full strength of the affected leg compared to the unaffected leg.
- You can jog straight ahead without pain or limping.
- You can sprint straight ahead without pain or limping.

- You can do 45-degree cuts, first at half-speed, then at full-speed.
- You can do 20-yard figures-of-eight, first at half-speed, then at full-speed.
- You can do 90-degree cuts, first at half-speed, then at full-speed.
- You can do 10-yard figures-of-eight, first at half-speed, then at full-speed.
- You can jump on both legs without pain and you can jump on the affected leg without pain.

How I prevent piriformis syndrome?

Piriformis syndrome is best prevented by stretching the muscles that rotate your thigh inward and outward. It is important to have a good warm-up before starting your sport or activity.

Piriformis Syndrome Rehabilitation Exercises

You may do all of these exercises right away.

1. Piriformis stretch: Lie on your back with both knees bent and the foot on your uninjured side flat on the floor. Rest the ankle of your injured leg over the knee of your uninjured leg. Grasp the thigh of your uninjured leg and pull that knee toward your chest. You will feel a stretch along the buttocks and possibly along the outside of your hip on the injured side. Hold this for 30 seconds. Repeat 3 times.

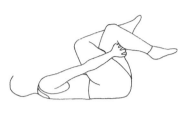

Piriformis stretch

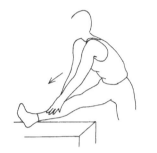

Standing hamstring stretch

2. Standing hamstring stretch: Place the heel of your injured leg on a stool about 15 inches high. Lean forward, bending at the hips until you feel a mild stretch in the back of your thigh. Hold the stretch for 30 to 60 seconds. Repeat 3 times.

3. Pelvic tilt: Lie on your back with your knees bent and you feet flat on the floor. Tighten your abdominal muscles and flatten your spine on the floor. Hold this position for 5 seconds, then relax. Repeat 10 times. Do 3 sets.

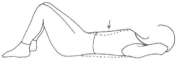

Pelvic tilt

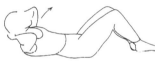

Partial curl

4. Partial curls: Lie on your back with your knees bent and your feet flat on the floor. Clasp your hands behind your head to support it. Keep your elbows out to the side and don't pull with your hands. Slowly raise your shoulders and head off the floor by tightening your abdominal muscles. Hold this position for 3 seconds. Return to the starting position. Repeat 10 times. Build up to 3 sets.

5. Prone hip extension: Lie on your stomach. Tighten up your buttocks muscles and lift your right leg off the floor about 8 inches. Keep your knee straight. Hold for 5 seconds and return to the starting position. Repeat 10 times. Do 3 sets on each side.

Prone hip extension

Quadriceps Contusion (Thigh Bruise) and Strain

What is a thigh bruise (quadriceps contusion) and strain?

A thigh bruise is a bruise (contusion) to the large group of muscles in the front of the thigh that help straighten the leg. These muscles are called the quadriceps. A thigh bruise is also called a charley horse. A strain is a partial tear of a muscle and is often called a pulled muscle.

How does it occur?

A thigh bruise is caused by a direct blow to the muscles of the thigh. A strain may be caused from overuse or from an abrupt movement of the thigh in activities such as sprinting or jumping.

What are the symptoms?

You have pain in the middle of your thigh and have difficulty walking or running. You may have difficulty bending or straightening your leg or lifting your knee. An area of your thigh may be swollen and discolored.

A thigh bruise or strain usually heals without complications. However, a large bruise may bleed a lot into the quadriceps muscle. This bleeding is called a hematoma. The hematoma may become calci-fied and form a hard lump in the quadriceps muscle. This lump is called osteomyositis ossificans and may cause stiffness or a bump in the muscle that may be very long lasting.

How is it diagnosed?

Your doctor will ask about your symptoms and examine your thigh. If your doctor suspects an area of calcification, an x-ray may be ordered.

How is it treated?

Right after your injury your doctor may wrap your leg in a bent-knee position and place ice over your thigh. This will put a maximum stretch on the thigh muscles, keeping them from becoming too tight or stiff during healing.

Other treatment may include:

- putting ice packs on your thigh for 20 to 30 minutes every 3 to 4 hours for 2 or 3 days or until the pain goes away
- lying down and elevating your thigh by putting a pillow under it
- taking an anti-inflammatory medication prescribed by your doctor

- wearing an elastic thigh wrap when you return to sports
- having prescribed physical therapy, which would include rehabilitation exercises and deep tissue

Quadriceps Contusion (Thigh Bruise)

Injured quadriceps muscle

Front view of thigh

Quadriceps Contusion (Thigh Bruise) and Strain

treatments such as ultrasound or electrical stimulation.

While you are recovering from your injury you will need to change your sport or activity to one that does not make your condition worse. For example, you may need to swim instead of run.

When can I return to my sport or activity?

The goal of rehabilitation is to return you to your sport or activity as soon as is safely possible. If you return too soon you may worsen your injury, which could lead to permanent damage. Everyone recovers from injury at a different rate. Return to your sport or activity will be determined by how soon your thigh recovers, not by how many days or weeks it has been since your injury

occurred. In general, the longer you have symptoms before you start treatment, the longer it will take to get better.

You may safely return to your sport or activity when, starting from the top of the list and progressing to the end, each of the following is true:

- You have full range of motion in the injured leg compared to the uninjured leg.
- You have full strength of the injured leg compared to the uninjured leg.
- You can jog straight ahead without pain or limping.
- You can sprint straight ahead without pain or limping.
- You can do 45-degree cuts, first at half-speed, then at full-speed.

- You can do 20-yard figures-of-eight, first at half-speed, then at full-speed.
- You can do 90-degree cuts, first at half-speed, then at full-speed.
- You can do 10-yard figures-of-eight, first at half-speed, then at full-speed.
- You can jump on both legs without pain and you can jump on the injured leg without pain.

How can I prevent a thigh bruise or strain?

A thigh bruise usually occurs from a direct blow to the thigh, which may not be preventable. However, in contact sports such as football be sure to wear the proper protective equipment. Strains are best prevented by warming up and stretching properly before your activity.

Quadriceps Contusion (Thigh Bruise) and Strain Rehabilitation Exercises

You may do all of these exercises right away.

1. Quadriceps stretch: Stand an arm's length away from a wall, facing straight ahead. Brace yourself by keeping your hand on your uninjured side against the wall. With your other hand grasp the ankle of your injured leg and pull your heel up toward your buttocks. Don't arch or twist your back and hold your knees together. Hold this position 30 to 60 seconds. Repeat 3 times. Do this several times a day. Avoid forcing painful movement.

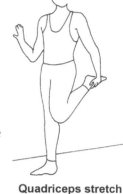

Quadriceps stretch

2. Quadriceps isometrics: Sitting on the floor with your injured leg straight and your other leg bent, press the back of your knee into the floor by tightening the muscles on the top of your thigh. Hold this position 5 seconds. Relax. Repeat 20 to 30 times.

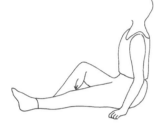

Quadriceps isometrics

3. Straight leg raise: Sit on the floor with your injured leg straight and the other leg bent so your foot is flat on the floor. Tighten the muscles on the top of your thigh and raise your leg off the floor 6 to 8 inches. Hold this position 5 seconds. Repeat 10 times. Do 3 sets.

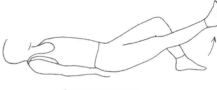

Straight leg raise

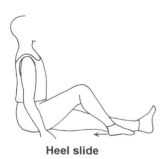

Heel slide

4. Heel slide: Sitting on the floor with your legs straight out in front of you, slowly slide the heel of your injured leg toward your buttocks by pulling your knee toward your chest as you slide. Return to the starting position. Repeat 20 to 30 times.

5. Prone knee bends: Lie on your stomach with your legs straight out behind you. Bend your knee so that your heel comes toward your buttocks. Hold 5 seconds. Relax and return your foot to the floor. Repeat 10 times. Do 3 sets. As this becomes easier you can add weights to your ankle.

Prone knee bends

Snapping Hip Syndrome

What is snapping hip syndrome?

Snapping hip syndrome is a condition in which you feel a snap on the outside portion of your hip as you walk or run. It may happen only occasionally or it may happen all the time.

How does it occur?

Several groups of muscles cross the hip as they pass from the thigh bone to the pelvis. When you bring your knee forward during walking, you may have a feeling of snapping in the hip. The snapping usually occurs because of tightness in a muscle called the iliopsoas or tightness in a muscle called the tensor fascia lata.

What are the symptoms?

You feel snapping in your hip as you walk or run.

How is it diagnosed?

Your doctor will examine your hip and thigh. He or she may be able to feel the muscle group that is snapping as the leg moves forward.

How is it treated?

Since this problem usually occurs because some muscles are too tight and some muscles are too loose, you will be given exercises to both strengthen and stretch your hip and thigh muscles. Your doctor may prescribe an anti-inflammatory medication if this area is painful. If this area becomes inflamed, your doctor may recommend that you put ice packs on the area for 20 to 30 minutes every 3 to 4 hours for 2 to 3 days or until the pain goes away.

When can I return to my sport or activity?

The goal of rehabilitation is to return you to your sport or activity as soon as is safely

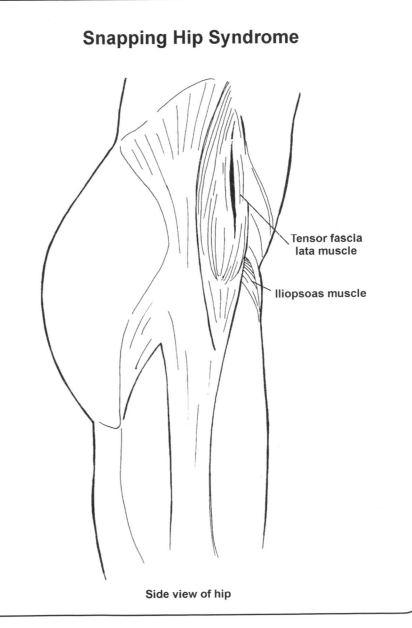

Snapping Hip Syndrome

Tensor fascia lata muscle

Iliopsoas muscle

Side view of hip

Snapping Hip Syndrome

possible. If you return too soon you may worsen your injury, which could lead to permanent damage. Everyone recovers from injury at a different rate. Return to your sport or activity will be determined by how soon your hip recovers, not by how many days or weeks it has been since your injury occurred. In general, the longer you have symptoms before you start treatment, the longer it will take to get better.

You may safely return to your sport or activity when, starting from the top of the list and progressing to the end, each of the following is true:

- You have full range of motion in the affected hip compared to the unaffected hip.
- You have full strength of the affected hip compared to the unaffected hip.
- You can jog straight ahead without pain or limping.
- You can sprint straight ahead without pain or limping.
- You can do 45-degree cuts, first at half-speed, then at full-speed.
- You can do 20-yard figures-of-eight, first at half-speed, then at full-speed.

- You can do 90-degree cuts, first at half-speed, then at full-speed.
- You can do 10-yard figures-of-eight, first at half-speed, then at full-speed.
- You can jump on both legs without pain and you can jump on the affected leg without pain.

How can I prevent snapping hip syndrome?

Snapping hip syndrome may be prevented by stretching the muscles that cross the hip from the pelvis to the thigh bone.

Snapping Hip Syndrome Rehabilitation Exercises

You may do all of these exercises right away.

1. Quadriceps stretch: Stand an arm's length away from the wall, facing straight ahead. Brace yourself by keeping the hand on the uninjured side against the wall. With your other hand, grasp the ankle of the injured leg and pull your heel toward your buttocks. Don't arch or twist your back and keep your knees together. Hold this stretch for 30 to 60 seconds. Repeat 3 times.

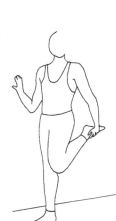

Quadriceps stretch

2. Hamstring stretch: Lie on your back with your buttocks close to a doorway, and extend your legs straight out in front of you along the floor. Raise the injured leg and rest it against the wall next to the door frame. Your other leg should extend through the doorway. You should feel a stretch in the back of your thigh. Hold this position for 30 to 60 seconds. Repeat 3 times.

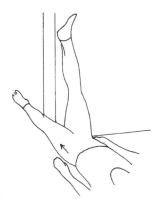

Hamstring stretch

3. Piriformis stretch: Lie on your back with both knees bent and the foot of the uninjured leg flat on the floor. Rest the ankle of your injured leg over the knee of your uninjured leg. Grasp the thigh of the uninjured leg, and pull that knee toward your chest. You will feel a stretch along the buttocks and possibly along the outside of your thigh on the injured side. Hold this stretch for 30 to 60 seconds. Repeat 3 times.

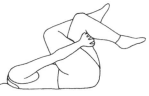

Piriformis stretch

4. Iliotibial band stretch (standing): Cross your uninjured leg in front of your injured leg and bend down and touch your toes. You can move your hands across the floor toward the uninjured side and you will feel more stretch on the outside of your thigh on the injured side. Hold this position for 30 seconds. Return to the starting position. Repeat 3 times.

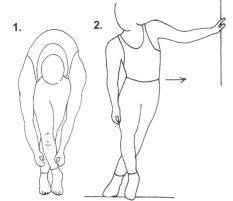

Iliotibial band stretches

5. Iliotibial band stretch (side-leaning): Stand sideways near a wall, your injured leg toward the inside. Place the hand on your injured side on the wall for support. Cross your uninjured leg over the injured leg, keeping the foot the injured leg stable. Lean into the wall. Hold the stretch for 10 seconds and repeat. Do 3 sets of 15.

Snapping Hip Syndrome Rehabilitation Exercises

6. Gluteal strengthening: To strengthen your buttock muscles, lie on your stomach with your legs straight out behind you. Tighten your buttock muscles and lift your injured leg off the floor 8 inches, keeping your knee straight. Hold 5 seconds. Relax and return to the starting position. Repeat 10 times. Do 3 sets.

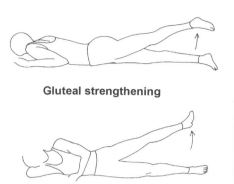

Gluteal strengthening

Hip abduction

7. Hip abduction: Lie on your uninjured side with your legs straight. Lift your injured leg up toward the ceiling, keeping your knee straight. Hold this position for 5 seconds. Repeat 10 times. Do 3 sets.

© HBO & Company

Trochanteric Bursitis

What is trochanteric bursitis?

Trochanteric bursitis is irritation or inflammation of the trochanteric bursa. A bursa is a fluid-filled sac that acts as a cushion between tendons, bones, and skin. The trochanteric bursa is located on the upper, outer area of the thigh. There is a bump on the outer side of the upper part of the thigh bone (femur) called the greater trochanter. The trochanteric bursa is located over the greater trochanter.

How does it occur?

The trochanteric bursa may be inflamed by a group of muscles or tendons rubbing over the bursa and causing friction against the thigh bone. This injury can occur with running, walking, or bicycling, especially when the bicycle seat is too high.

What are the symptoms?

You have pain on the upper outer area of your thigh or in your hip. The pain is worse when you walk, bicycle, or go up or down stairs. You have pain when you move your thigh bone and feel tenderness in the area over the greater trochanter.

How is it diagnosed?

Your doctor will ask about your symptoms and examine your hip and thigh.

How is it treated?

Treatment may include the following:

- putting ice packs on your thigh for 20 to 30 minutes every 3 to 4 hours for 2 to 3 days or until the pain goes away
- taking anti-inflammatory medication prescribed by your doctor
- getting a corticosteroid injection into the bursa to reduce the pain and swelling.

While you are recovering from your injury you will need to change your sport or activity to one that does not make your condition worse. For example, you may need to swim instead of running or bicycling. If you are bicycling, you may need to lower your bicycle seat.

When can I return to my sport or activity?

The goal of rehabilitation is to return you to your sport or activity as soon as is safely possible. If you return too soon you may worsen your injury, which could lead to permanent damage. Everyone

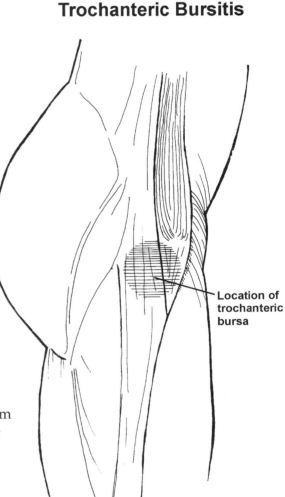

Trochanteric Bursitis

Location of trochanteric bursa

Side view of hip and thigh

Trochanteric Bursitis

recovers from injury at a different rate. Return to your sport or activity will be determined by how soon your leg recovers, not by how many days or weeks it has been since your injury occurred. In general, the longer you have symptoms before you start treatment, the longer it will take to get better.

You may safely return to your sport or activity when, starting from the top of the list and progressing to the end, each of the following is true:

- You have full range of motion in the injured leg compared to the uninjured leg.
- You have full strength of the injured leg compared to the uninjured leg.
- You can jog straight ahead without pain or limping.
- You can sprint straight ahead without pain or limping.
- You can do 45-degree cuts, first at half-speed, then at full-speed.
- You can do 20-yard figures-of-eight, first at half-speed, then at full-speed.

- You can do 90-degree cuts, first at half-speed, then at full-speed.
- You can do 10-yard figures-of-eight, first at half-speed, then at full-speed.
- You can jump on both legs without pain and you can jump on the injured leg without pain.

How can I prevent trochanteric bursitis?

Trochanteric bursitis is best prevented by warming up properly and stretching the muscles on the outer side of your upper thigh.

Trochanteric Bursitis Rehabilitation Exercises

You can begin stretching the muscles that run along the outside of your hip using exercises 1 and 2. You can do strengthening exercises 3 through 5 when the sharp pain lessens.

1. Piriformis stretch: Lying on your back with both knees bent, rest the ankle of your injured leg over the knee of your uninjured leg. Grasp the thigh of your uninjured leg and pull that knee toward your chest. You will feel a stretch along the buttocks and possibly along the outside of your hip on the injured side. Hold this for 30 seconds. Repeat 3 times.

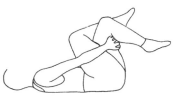

Piriformis stretch

2. Iliotibial band stretch: Standing, cross your uninjured leg in front of your injured leg and bend down and touch your toes. You can move your hands across the floor toward the uninjured side and you will feel more of a stretch on the outside of your injured leg. Hold this position for 30 seconds. Return to the starting position. Repeat 3 times.

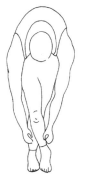

Iliotibial band stretch

3. Straight leg raise: Lie on your back with your legs straight out in front of you. Tighten up the top of your thigh muscle on the injured leg and lift that leg about 8 inches off the floor, keeping the thigh muscle tight throughout. Slowly lower your leg back down to the floor. Do this 10 times. Do 3 sets of 10.

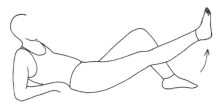

Straight leg raise

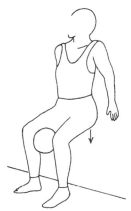

Wall squat with a ball

4. Wall squat with a ball: Stand with your back, shoulders, and head against a wall and look straight ahead. Keep your shoulders relaxed and your feet 1 foot away from the wall and a shoulder's width apart. Place a rolled up pillow or a nerf ball between your thighs. Keeping your head against the wall, slowly squat while squeezing the pillow or ball at the same time. Squat down until you are almost in a sitting position. Your thighs will not yet be parallel to the floor. Hold this position for 10 seconds and then slowly slide back up the wall. Make sure you keep squeezing the pillow or ball throughout this exercise. Do 10 repetitions and build up to 3 sets of 10.

5. Gluteal strengthening: Lie on your stomach with your legs straight out behind you and tighten up your buttock muscles. Lift your injured leg off the floor, keeping the knee straight. Lift your leg about 6 to 8 inches off of the floor, hold for 3 seconds, and slowly return your leg to the floor. Do 3 sets of 10 repetitions.

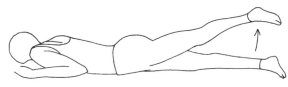

Gluteal strengthening

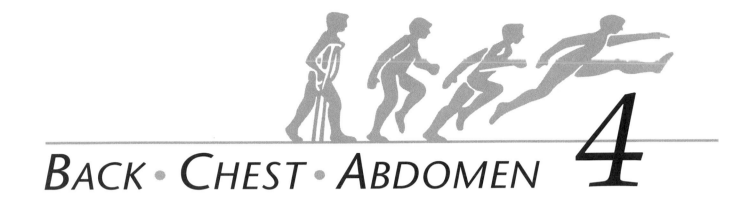

BACK · CHEST · ABDOMEN 4

Abdominal Muscle Strain

What is an abdominal muscle strain?

A strain is a stretch or tear of a muscle or tendon. People commonly call such an injury a "pulled" muscle. Your abdominal muscles may be strained during a forceful activity.

How does it occur?

During a vigorous activity, such as lifting or even hard coughing or sneezing, these muscles may become strained.

What are the symptoms?

There will be pain over the abdominal muscles.

At times these muscles may be torn. A tear all the way through the muscles and the covering of the abdomen (called the fascia) may result in an abdominal wall hernia. In a hernia, some of the contents of the belly (intestines and connective tissue) protrude through the tear and cause a bulge in the abdominal wall.

How is it diagnosed?

Your doctor will examine your abdomen. Your doctor will ask you to do an exercise such as a sit-up or abdominal "crunch," and this will reproduce some of your symptoms. If you have a hernia, your doctor will be able to feel and see a bulge in your abdomen.

How is it treated?

After your initial injury, you should apply ice to the strained muscle for 20 to 30 minutes every 3 to 4 hours for 2 to 3 days or until the pain goes away. Your doctor may prescribe an anti-inflammatory medication. If you have an abdominal hernia you may need surgery to correct this problem.

When can I return to my sport or activity?

The goal of rehabilitation is to return you to your sport or activity as soon as is safely possible. If you return too soon you may worsen your injury, which could lead to permanent damage. Everyone recovers from injury at a different rate. Return to your activity will be determined by

Abdominal Muscle Strain

Injured muscle fibers

Abdominal Muscle Strain

how soon your abdominal muscles recover, not by how many days or weeks it has been since your injury occurred. In general, the longer you have symptoms before you start treatment, the longer it will take to get better.

You may return to your activity when you can bend at the waist to touch your toes and straighten back up without pain. You should be able to do a sit-up or abdominal crunch without pain. If you have a hernia, be cautious about doing strenuous abdominal activities and talk to your doctor about having it repaired.

How can I prevent abdominal muscle strains?

Abdominal muscle strains are best prevented by having well toned abdominal muscles prior to vigorous activities. You can accomplish this by doing sit-ups or abdominal crunches or by using one of the popular abdominal exercise machines. It is important not to overdo it when beginning your exercise program. When lifting heavy objects it is important to lift correctly, with knees bent and your back and abdomen straight.

Abdominal Muscle Strain Rehabilitation Exercises

You may do exercise 1 right away. You may do exercises 2, 3, and 4 when the pain is gone.

1. Pelvic tilt: Lying on your back with your knees bent and your feet flat on the floor, tighten your stomach muscles and gently press the arch of your back into the floor. Hold this position for 5 seconds. Repeat 10 times.

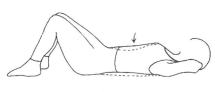

Pelvic tilt

After you have mastered this, tighten your abdominal muscles, press your lower back to the floor and lift one foot off the floor about 3 to 4 inches. Hold it for 5 seconds and then put it down. Repeat with the opposite leg. Make sure you keep your pelvis tilted using your abdominal muscles, not your legs. Repeat this 10 times on each side.

2. Partial curl: Lie on your back on the floor or another firm surface. Clasp your hands behind your neck for support, keeping your elbows pointed out to the side. Look straight up at the ceiling, tighten your stomach muscles, and slowly lift your shoulders off the floor toward the ceiling. Make sure to keep your elbows pointed out to the side and don't use your arms to lift your upper body off the floor. Hold for 3 seconds and slowly lower your shoulders to the floor. Repeat 10 times. Do 3 sets of 10.

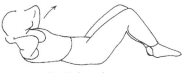

Partial curl

After you have become good at the partial curl you can do a diagonal curl to help strengthen your oblique abdominal muscles.

3. Diagonal curl: Lie on your back with your knees bent and your feet flat on the floor. Clasp your hands behind your neck to support your head. Tighten your stomach muscles and lift your head and shoulders off of the floor while rotating your trunk toward the right. Make sure you don't use your arms to lift your body off the floor. Hold this for 3 seconds. Return to the starting position. Then rotate toward your left side. Do this 10 times on each side. Do 3 sets of 10.

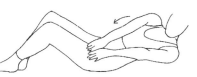

Diagonal curl

4. Lower abdominal exercise: Lie on your back with your knees bent, and hold your feet just off the floor. Next, hold yourself in a pelvic tilt. Your knees should be pointed toward the ceiling. Lower your right foot until it barely touches the floor and then bring it back up to the starting position. Do the same with your left foot. Remember to hold the pelvic tilt while you lower each foot until it just touches the floor. Repeat 10 times on each side.

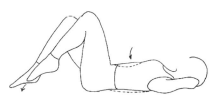

Lower abdominal exercise

Broken Collarbone
(Fractured Clavicle)

What is a broken collarbone?

A broken collarbone is a break in the clavicle, the bone in your upper chest that connects your breastbone (sternum) to part of your shoulder blade (scapula). A broken collarbone is also known as a fractured clavicle.

How does it occur?

A broken collarbone can occur in several ways. You may fall on your outstretched arm and hand, you may fall on your shoulder, or you may be hit directly in the collarbone.

What are the symptoms?

You will have pain and swelling at the area of the break. It will be difficult to move your arm or shoulder. You may have heard a crack at the time of the injury.

How is it diagnosed?

Your doctor will examine your collarbone and find tenderness and swelling. An x-ray will show a fracture.

How is it treated?

To ease your discomfort, your collarbone may be immobilized in a "figure of 8" splint or brace that holds your shoulders back (as if you were standing at attention). Your arm may be placed in a sling. It may take 6 to 12 weeks for your clavicle to heal.

When can I return to my sport or activity?

It is important that the clavicle is fully healed before you return to your sport or activity so your collarbone doesn't break again. You must be able to move your clavicle, shoulder, and arm without pain.

Your doctor may take another x-ray to be sure that the bone has healed.

You can begin rehabilitation exercises after your broken collarbone has healed and after you've seen your doctor.

How can I prevent a broken clavicle?

Clavicle fractures are usually the result of accidents that cannot be prevented.

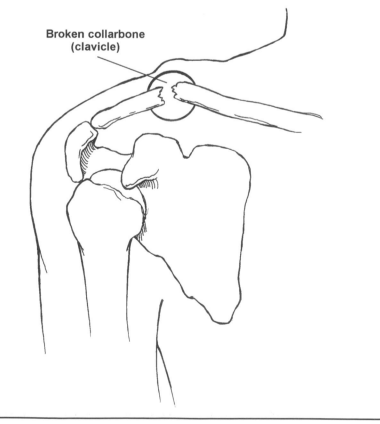

**Broken Collarbone
(Clavicle Fracture)**

Broken collarbone
(clavicle)

— Broken Collarbone Rehabilitation Exercises —

Phase I

1. Wand exercises

A. Shoulder flexion: Stand upright and hold a stick in both hands. Stretch your arms by lifting them over your head, keeping your elbows straight. Hold for 5 seconds and return to the starting position. Repeat 10 times.

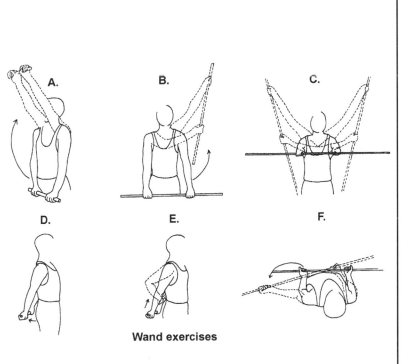

Wand exercises

B. Shoulder abduction and adduction: Stand upright and hold onto a stick with both hands. Rest the stick against the front of your thighs. While keeping your elbows straight, use your uninjured arm to push your injured arm out to the side and up as high as possible. Hold for 5 seconds and return to the starting position. Repeat 10 times.

C. Horizontal abduction and adduction: Stand upright and hold a stick in both hands. Place your arms straight out in front of you at shoulder level. Keep your arms straight and swing the stick to one side, feel the stretch, and hold for 5 seconds. Then swing the stick to the other side, feel the stretch, and hold for 5 seconds. Repeat 10 times.

D. Shoulder extension: Stand upright holding a stick in both hands behind your back. Move the stick away from your back, keeping your elbows straight. Hold the end position for 5 seconds then relax and return to the starting position. Repeat 10 times.

E. Internal rotation: Stand upright holding a stick in both hands behind your back. Move the stick up and down your back by bending your elbows. Hold the bent position for 5 seconds and then return to the starting position. Repeat 10 times.

F. External rotation: Lying on your back, hold a stick with both hands, palms up. Your upper arms should be resting on the floor, your elbows at your sides and bent 90 degrees. Using your good arm, push your injured arm out away from your body while keeping your injured elbow at your side. Hold the stretch for 5 seconds. Return to the starting position. Repeat 10 times.

Broken Collarbone Rehabilitation Exercises

2. Active shoulder range of motion

A. Flexion: Stand with your arms hanging straight down by your side. Lift both arms, thumbs up, over your head. Hold for 5 seconds. Return to the starting position. Repeat 10 times.

B. Shoulder abduction and adduction: Stand with your arms at your sides. Bring your arms up, out to the side, and toward the ceiling. Hold for 5 seconds. Return to the starting position. Repeat 10 times.

Active range of motion

C. Horizontal abduction and adduction: Stand with your arms held straight out in front of you at shoulder level. Pull your arms apart and out to the sides as far as possible. Hold them back for 5 seconds, then bring them back together in front of you. Repeat 10 times. Remember to keep your arms at shoulder level throughout this exercise.

D. Shoulder extension: Standing, move your involved arm back, keeping your elbow straight. Hold this position for 5 seconds. Return to the starting position and repeat 10 times.

E. Scapular range of motion: Shrug your shoulders up. Then squeeze your shoulder blades back and down, making a circle with your shoulders. Return to the starting position. Hold each position 5 seconds and do the entire exercise 10 times.

Phase II

1. Sidelying horizontal abduction: Lie on your uninjured side with your injured arm relaxed across your chest. Slowly bring your injured arm up off the floor, elbow straight, so that your hand is pointing toward the ceiling. Repeat 10 times. Hold a weight in your hand as the exercise becomes easier.

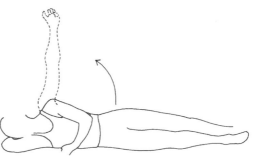

Sidelying horizontal abduction

2. Prone shoulder extension: Lie on your stomach on a table or a bed with your involved arm hanging down over the edge. With your elbow straight, slowly lift your arm straight back and toward the ceiling. Return to the starting position. Repeat 10 times. As this becomes easier, hold a weight in your hand.

Prone shoulder extension

Broken Collarbone Rehabilitation Exercises

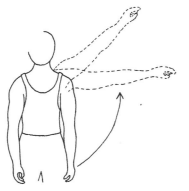

Biceps curls

3. Biceps curls: Standing, hold a weight of some sort (a soup can or hammer) in your hand. Bend the elbow of your involved arm and bring your hand, palm up, toward your shoulder. Slowly return to the starting position and straighten your elbow. Repeat 10 times.

4. Triceps: Lie on your back with your arms toward the ceiling. Bend your involved elbow completely so that the hand on your injured side is resting on the shoulder of that side and your elbow is pointing toward the ceiling. You can use your other hand to help support your upper arm just below the elbow. Then straighten your elbow completely so that your hand is pointing toward the ceiling. Return to the starting position. Repeat 10 times. Hold a weight in your hand when this exercise becomes easy.

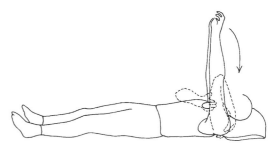

Triceps

5. Abduction: Stand with your injured arm at your side, palm resting against your side. With your elbow straight, lift your hand arm out to the side and toward the ceiling. Hold this position for 5 seconds. Repeat 10 times. Add a weight to your hand as this exercise becomes easier.

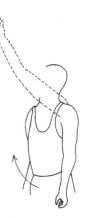

Shoulder flexion

6. Shoulder flexion: Stand with your injured arm hanging down at your side. Keeping your elbow straight, bring your arm forward and up toward the ceiling. Hold this position for 5 seconds. Repeat 10 times. As this exercise becomes easier, add a weight.

Abduction

© HBO & Company

Herniated Disk

What is a herniated disk?

Disks are small, circular cushions between vertebrae (the bones of the spine). Normally, disks act as shock absorbers to cushion your vertebrae from each other as you move. A herniated disk is a disk that has bulged out from its proper place. It may press on nearby nerves and cause severe pain.

How does it occur?

When a disk is damaged, the soft rubbery center of the disk squeezes out through a weak point in the hard outer layer. A disk may be damaged by:

- a fall or accident
- repeated straining of your back
- a sudden strenuous action such as lifting a heavy weight or twisting violently.

A herniated disk may also happen spontaneously without any specific injury.

What are the symptoms?

Symptoms of a herniated disk in your neck may begin suddenly or gradually. You may wake up and feel a sudden aching. Or you may have a twisted neck that you cannot straighten without extreme pain. You may also have numbness, tingling, or weakness in one or both arms. If your herniated disk is below

your neck, your symptoms may develop gradually or begin suddenly. Symptoms include:

- back pain
- pain down one or both legs
- numbness, tingling, or weakness in one or both legs
- changes in bladder and bowel habits.

How is it diagnosed?

Your health care provider will review your symptoms and ask about the history of your pain. Then he or she will examine your spine and test

the movement and reflexes in your arms and legs. Finally, your provider may want you to have one or more of the following tests:

- x-rays of your spine
- CT scan (computerized x-ray images of your spine)
- magnetic resonance imaging, also called MRI (an image of your spine and herniated disk generated by sound waves)
- electromyography (tests of electrical activity in your muscles)
- myelography (injection of dye into the fluid around the

Herniated Disk

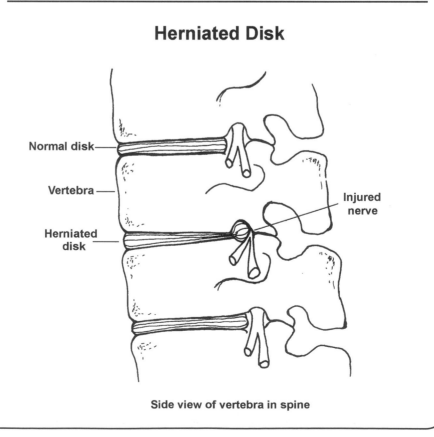

Side view of vertebra in spine

Herniated Disk

spinal cord that can be seen on x-rays)

- diskography (injection of dye into a disk and x-rays taken).

How is it treated?

In most cases, treatment without surgery will relieve your pain.

Treatment for a herniated disk in your neck may include:

- hot or cold packs
- anti-inflammatory drugs
- muscle relaxants
- prescription pain relievers
- a neck collar or neck brace to relieve muscle spasms
- neck and shoulder massage
- traction, which is the process of putting bones or muscles under tension with a system of weights and pulleys to keep them from moving or to relieve pressure on them.

For a herniated disk in your back, treatment may include:

- several days or more of lying flat on your back on a firm mattress or on an ordinary bed with a stiff board under the mattress, or lying on your belly with a pillow under your chest, whichever is more comfortable
- muscle relaxants
- anti-inflammatory drugs
- prescription pain relievers

- hot or cold packs, depending on your health care provider's preference
- traction
- back massage or physical therapy
- steroid injections into the space near the herniated disk to control pain and inflammation.

As your pain lessens, your health care provider will want you to begin a physical therapy program in which you will do exercises to strengthen your back muscles and joints. Recently, stabilizing exercises have been used successfully to treat herniated disks. This therapy involves learning how to control the movement of your spine in all recreation and work activities.

If you continue to have symptoms, you may need to have surgery. However, most people who have herniated disks do not need surgery.

How long will the effects of a herniated disk last?

The initial intense pain should go away within a few weeks, but some pain may remain for a few months. You may be prone to backaches throughout your life and therefore must remember to protect your spine when lifting or being physically active.

If the weakness and numbness in your legs continue or if you

lose control of your bowel or bladder function, contact your health care provider immediately.

How can I take care of myself?

Practice correct posture when you are walking, sitting, standing, lying down, or working.

- When lifting heavy objects, don't bend over from your waist. Kneel or squat down by the object, while keeping your back as straight as possible. Use your thigh muscles to do the lifting. Avoid twisting.
- When you stand, always stand up straight with your shoulders back, abdomen in, and the small of the back flat. When standing for long periods, move around frequently and shift your weight from one foot to another while standing as straight as possible.
- When you sit, have your feet flat on the floor or elevated. Get up every 20 minutes or so and stretch. Sit in a chair that has good back support.
- Sleep on a firm mattress or one with a bed board under it. Lie on your side (never on your stomach) with your knees bent or on your back with a small pillow under your head and another pillow under your knees.

Herniated Disk

When can I return to my sport or activity?

The goal of rehabilitation is to return you to your sport or activity as soon as is safely possible. If you return too soon you may worsen your injury, which could lead to permanent damage. Everyone recovers from injury at a different rate. Return to your sport will be determined by how soon your herniated disk recovers, not by how many days or weeks it has been since your injury occurred. In general, the longer you have symptoms before you start treatment, the longer it will take to get better.

It is important that your herniated disk has fully recovered before you return to any strenuous activity and that you have been seen by your health care provider. You must be able to perform all of your rehabilitation exercises without pain. You must have full range of motion of your back and neck and have no shooting pain into your legs or arms. You must be able to run, jump, and twist without any pain.

What can be done to help prevent a herniated disk?

Herniated disks can often be prevented by keeping your weight down, eating a proper diet, and exercising to keep your muscles firm. Strong, flexible muscles can stabilize your spine and protect it from injury. This includes keeping your stomach muscles strong. Walking and swimming are two good exercises for strengthening and protecting your spine.

Herniated Disk Rehabilitation Exercises

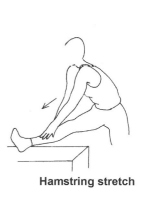

Hamstring stretch

1. Hamstring stretch: Place the heel of your injured leg on a stool about 15 inches high. Lean forward, bending at the hips until you feel a mild stretch in the back of your thigh. Make sure you do not roll your shoulders and bend at the waist when doing this or you will stretch your lower back instead. Hold the stretch 30 to 60 seconds. Repeat 3 times.

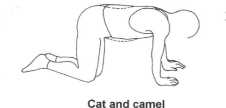

Cat and camel

2. Cat and camel: Get down on your hands and knees. Let your stomach sag, allowing your back to curve downward. Hold this position for 5 seconds, then arch your back. Repeat 10 times. Do 2 sets.

Pelvic tilt

3. Pelvic tilt: Lie on your back with your knees bent and your feet flat on the floor. Tighten your stomach muscles to flatten your lower back against the floor. Hold for 5 seconds, then relax. Repeat 10 times. Do 3 sets.

4. Prone hip extension: Lie on your stomach with your legs straight out behind you. Tighten your buttock muscles and lift your right leg off the floor, keeping your knee straight. Hold this position for 5 seconds. Then lower your leg and relax. Repeat the same with your left leg. Hold 5 seconds and then lower the leg and relax. Repeat 10 times on each side. Build up to 3 sets of 10.

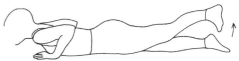

Prone hip extension

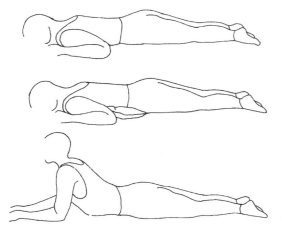

Prone-lying exercises

5. Prone-lying exercises: Lie face down on the floor for 5 minutes. If this hurts too much, lie face down with a pillow under your stomach. This should relieve your leg pain. When you can lie on your stomach for 5 minutes without pillows, then you can move to the next step. Lie on your stomach and prop yourself up on your elbows for 10 seconds at a time. You should have no pain in your legs when you do this, but it is normal to feel pain in your lower back. Repeat 10 times and do this several times a day.

Herniated Disk Rehabilitation Exercises

6. Partial curl: Do this exercise only when you no longer have pain in your buttocks or legs. Lie on your back with your knees bent and your feet flat on the floor. Tighten your stomach muscles and flatten your back against the floor. Tuck your chin to your chest. With your hands stretched out in front of you, curl your upper body forward until your shoulders clear the floor. Hold this position for 3 seconds. Don't hold your breath. It helps to breathe out as you lift your shoulders up. Relax. Repeat 10 times. Build to 3 sets of 10. To challenge yourself, clasp your hands behind your head and keep your elbows out to the side.

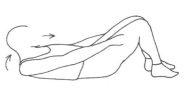

Partial curl

If you have a herniated disk, you should limit driving and other sitting activities to no more than 30 minutes at a time. Walking is also good exercise for you.

Low Back Pain

What is low back pain?

Low back pain is pain and stiffness in the lower back. It is one of the most common reasons people miss work.

How does it occur?

Low back pain is usually caused when a ligament or muscle holding a vertebra in its proper position is strained. Vertebrae are bones that make up the spinal column through which the spinal cord passes. When these muscles or ligaments become weak, the spine loses its stability, resulting in pain. Because nerves reach all parts of the body from the spinal cord, back problems can lead to pain or weakness in almost any part of the body.

Low back pain can occur if your job involves lifting and carrying heavy objects, or if you spend a lot of time sitting or standing in one position or bending over. It can be caused by a fall or by unusually strenuous exercise. It can be brought on by the tension and stress that cause headaches in some people. It can even be brought on by violent sneezing or coughing.

People who are overweight may have low back pain because of the added stress on their back.

Back pain may occur when the muscles, joints, bones, and connective tissues of the back become inflamed as a result of an infection or an immune system problem. Arthritic disorders as well as some congenital and degenerative conditions may cause back pain.

Back pain accompanied by loss of bladder or bowel control, difficulty in moving your legs, or numbness or tingling in your arms or legs may indicate an injury to your spine and nerves, which requires immediate medical treatment.

What are the symptoms?

Symptoms include:
- pain in the back or legs
- stiffness and limited motion.

The pain may be continuous or may occur only in certain positions. It may be aggravated by coughing, sneezing, bending, twisting, or straining during a bowel movement. The pain may occur in only one spot or may spread to other areas, most commonly down the buttocks and into the back of the thigh.

A low back strain typically does not produce pain past the knee into the calf or foot. Tingling or numbness in the calf or foot may indicate a herniated disk or pinched nerve. Be sure to see your doctor if you have weakness in your leg, especially if you cannot lift your foot, because this is a sign of nerve damage. New bowel or bladder problems related to your back pain may indicate severe injury to your spinal cord, and you should see your doctor. Pain that increases

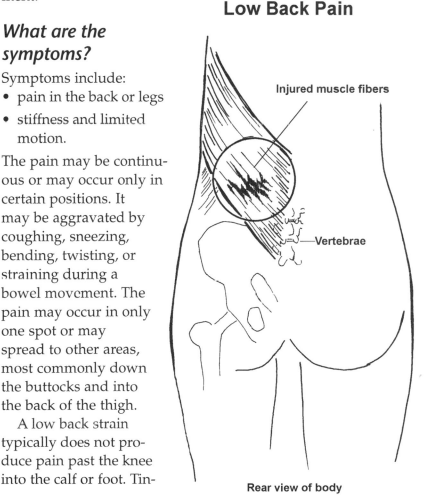

Low Back Pain

Injured muscle fibers

Vertebrae

Rear view of body

Low Back Pain

despite treatment indicates a more severe problem, which should be evaluated.

How is it diagnosed?

Your doctor will review your medical history and examine you. He or she may order x-rays. In certain situations a myelogram, CT scan, or MRI may be ordered.

How is it treated?

The early stages of back pain with muscle spasms should be treated with ice packs for 20 to 30 minutes every 4 to 6 hours for the first 2 to 3 days. You may lie on a frozen gel pack, crushed ice, or a bag of frozen peas.

The following are ways to treat low back pain:

- After the initial injury, applying heat from a heating pad or hot water bottle.
- Resting in bed on a firm mattress. Often it helps to lie on your back with your knees raised. However, some people prefer to lie on their side with their knees bent.
- Taking aspirin, ibuprofen, or other anti-inflammatory medications; muscle relaxants; or other pain medications if recommended by your doctor.
- Having your back massaged by a trained person.

- Having traction, if recommended by your doctor.
- Wearing a belt or corset to support your back.
- Talking with a counselor, if your back pain is related to tension caused by emotional problems.
- Beginning a program of physical therapy, or exercising on your own. Begin a regular exercise program to gently stretch and strengthen your muscles as soon as you can. Your doctor or physical therapist can recommend exercises that will not only help you feel better but will strengthen your muscles and help avoid back trouble later.

When the pain subsides, ask your doctor about starting an exercise program such as the following:

- Exercise moderately every day, using stretching and warm-up exercises suggested by your doctor or physical therapist.
- Exercise vigorously for about 30 minutes two or three times a week by walking, swimming, using a stationary bicycle, or doing low-impact aerobics.

Participating regularly in an exercise program will not only help your back, it will also help keep you healthier overall.

How long will the effects last?

The effects of back pain last as long as the cause exists or until your body recovers from the strain, usually a day or two but sometimes weeks.

How can I take care of myself?

In addition to the treatment described above, keep in mind these suggestions:

- Use an electric heating pad on a low setting (or a hot water bottle wrapped in a towel to avoid burning yourself) for 20 to 30 minutes. Don't let the heating pad get too hot, and don't fall asleep with it. You could get a burn.
- Try putting an ice pack wrapped in a towel on your back for 20 minutes, one to four times a day. Set an alarm to avoid frostbite from using the ice pack too long.
- Put a pillow under your knees when you are lying down.
- Sleep without a pillow under your head.
- Lose weight if you are overweight.
- Practice good posture. Stand with your head up, shoulders straight, chest forward, weight balanced evenly on both feet, and pelvis tucked in.

Low Back Pain

Pain is the best way to judge the pace you should set in increasing your activity and exercise. Minor discomfort, stiffness, soreness, and mild aches need not interfere with activity. However, limit your activities temporarily if:

- Your symptoms return.
- The pain increases when you are more active.
- The pain increases within 24 hours after a new or higher level of activity.

When can I return to my sport or activity?

The goal of rehabilitation is to return you to your sport or activity as soon as is safely possible. If you return too soon you may worsen your injury, which could lead to permanent damage. Everyone recovers from injury at a different rate. Return to your sport will be determined by how soon your back recovers, not by how many days or weeks it has been since your injury occurred. In general, the longer you have symptoms before you start treatment, the longer it will take to get better.

It is important that you have fully recovered from your low back pain before you return to your sport or any strenuous activity. You must

be able to have the same range of motion that you had before your injury. You must be able to run, jump and twist without pain.

What can I do to help prevent low back pain?

You can reduce the strain on your back by doing the following:

- Don't push with your arms when you move a heavy object. Turn around and push backwards so the strain is taken by your legs.
- Whenever you sit, sit in a straight-backed chair and hold your spine against the back of the chair.
- Bend your knees and hips and keep your back straight when you lift a heavy object.
- Avoid lifting heavy objects higher than your waist.
- Hold packages you carry close to your body, with your arms bent.
- Use a footrest for one foot when you stand or sit in one spot for a long time. This keeps your back straight.
- Bend your knees when you bend over.
- Sit close to the pedals when you drive and use your seat belt and a hard backrest or pillow.

- Lie on your side with your knees bent when you sleep or rest. It may help to put a pillow between your knees.
- Put a pillow under your knees when you sleep on your back.
- Raise the foot of the bed 8 inches to discourage sleeping on your stomach unless you have other problems that require that you keep your head elevated.

To rest your back, hold each of these positions for 5 minutes or longer:

- Lie on your back, bend your knees, and put pillows under your knees.
- Lie on your back, put a pillow under your neck, bend your knees to a 90-degree angle, and put your lower legs and feet on a chair.
- Lie on your back, bend your knees, and bring one knee up to your chest and hold it there. Repeat with the other knee, then bring both knees to your chest. When holding your knee to your chest, grab your thigh rather than your lower leg to avoid overflexing your knee.

Low Back Pain Rehabilitation Exercises

The goal of these exercises is to strengthen your abdominal muscles, stretch your lower back, hip flexors, and hamstrings. These exercises may help reduce lower back pain by correcting muscle imbalances in strength and flexibility of the trunk and hips.

1. Hamstring stretch: Place the heel of one leg on a stool about 15 inches high. Lean forward, bending at the hips until you feel a mild stretch in the back of your thigh. Make sure you do not roll your shoulders and bend at the waist when doing this or you will stretch your lower back instead. Hold the stretch 30 to 60 seconds. Do the same exercise with the other leg. Repeat 3 times.

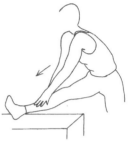

Hamstring stretch

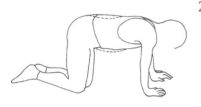

Cat and camel

2. Cat and camel: Get down on your hands and knees. Let your stomach sag, allowing your back to curve downward. Hold this position for 5 seconds, then arch your back. Repeat 10 times. Do 2 sets.

3. Pelvic tilt: Lie on your back with your knees bent and your feet flat on the floor. Tighten your stomach muscles to flatten your lower back against the floor. Hold for 5 seconds, then relax. Repeat 10 times. Do 3 sets.

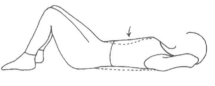

Pelvic tilt

4. Partial curl: Lie on your back with your knees bent and your feet flat on the floor. Tighten your stomach muscles and flatten your back against the floor. Tuck your chin to your chest. With your hands stretched out in front of you, curl your upper body forward until your shoulders clear the floor. Hold this position for 3 seconds. Don't hold your breath. It helps to breathe out as you lift your shoulders up. Relax. Repeat 10 times. Build to 3 sets of 10. To challenge yourself, clasp your hands behind your head and keep your elbows out to the side.

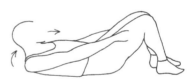

Partial curl

5. Prone hip extension: Lie on your stomach with your legs straight out behind you. Tighten your buttock muscles and lift your right leg off the floor, keeping your knee straight. Hold this position for 5 seconds. Then lower your leg and relax. Repeat the same with your left leg. Hold 5 seconds and then lower the leg and relax. Repeat 10 times on each side. Build up to 3 sets of 10.

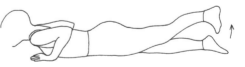

Prone hip extension

6. Single knee to chest: Now do a pelvic tilt and pull one knee up to your chest. Hold for 5 seconds and return to the starting position. Alternate sides, and repeat it 10–20 times.

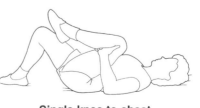

Single knee to chest

Low Back Pain Rehabilitation Exercises

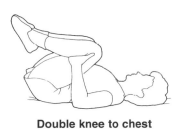

Double knee to chest

7. Double knee to chest: Again, do a pelvic tilt and now pull both knees up to your chest. Hold for 5 seconds and repeat it 10–20 times. You may need to lift one leg at a time until your stomach muscles get stronger.

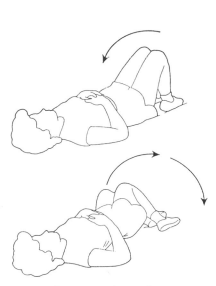

Lower trunk rotation

8. Lower trunk rotation: Do a pelvic tilt. Keeping shoulders down flat, gently rotate the knees to one side, then the other, as far as you can. Repeat 10–20 times.

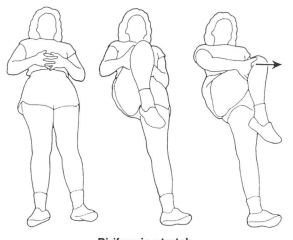

Piriformis stretch

9. Piriformis stretch: Lie on your back as shown. Pull one knee up and across your trunk so you feel a comfortable stretch in the top buttocks and back. Hold for 5-15 seconds and repeat 5-10 times on each side.

You can modify this exercise by reaching for your knee with the opposite hand and keeping your shoulders flat on the floor. Pull your knee over as far as you can allowing your trunk to rotate.

Rib Injury

What is a rib injury?

There are 12 ribs on each side of the chest that protect the heart, lungs, and the upper abdominal contents. All of the ribs are attached to the vertebrae (backbone) in the rear. In the front, 10 of them are attached to the sternum (breastbone) by pieces of cartilage. Direct blows to the ribs may bruise or break the ribs or injure to the rib cartilage. The ribs may tear away from the cartilage that attaches them to the breastbone. This tearing away from the cartilage is called a costochondral separation.

How does it occur?

Rib injuries usually result from a direct blow to the chest wall. Breaks usually occur in the curved portion of the outer part of the rib cage. A costochondral separation may occur when you land hard on your feet or even when you cough or sneeze violently.

What are the symptoms?

A rib injury causes pain and tenderness over the place of injury. You may have pain when you breathe, move, laugh, or cough.

How is it diagnosed?

Your doctor will review your symptoms, examine your rib cage, and listen to your lungs.

Your doctor may order a chest x-ray to look for any rib damage, lung damage, or bleeding around the lungs.

How is it treated?

Treatment may include:

- rest
- putting an ice pack over the injured rib for 20 to 30 minutes every 3 to 4 hours for 2 to 3 days or until the pain goes away
- taking an anti-inflammatory or other pain medication.

When can I return to my sport or activity?

The goal of rehabilitation is to return you to your sport or activity as soon as is safely possible. If you return too soon you may worsen your injury, which could lead to permanent damage. Everyone recovers from injury at a different rate. Return to your sport or activity will be determined by how soon your ribs recover, not by how many days or weeks it has been since your injury occurred. In general, the longer you have symptoms before you start treatment, the longer it will take to get better.

If you broke a rib it may take 4 to 6 weeks to heal. Your doctor may take an x-ray to see that the bone has healed before he or she allows you to return to your activity, especially if it is a contact sport. You may

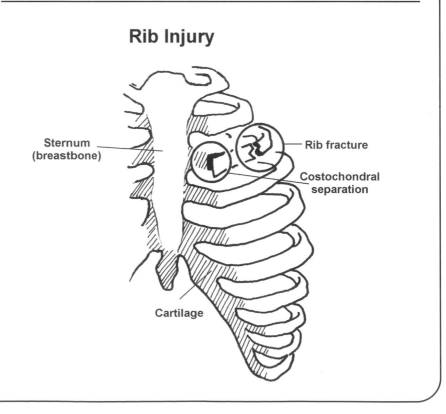

Rib Injury

Sternum (breastbone)

Rib fracture

Costochondral separation

Cartilage

Rib Injury

participate in noncontact activities sooner if you can do so without pain in your ribs and without pain when you breathe. If you have bruised your ribs or separated the cartilage from the ribs, you may return to your activity when you can do so without pain.

How can I prevent a rib injury?

Ribs are often injured in accidents that are not preventable. However, in contact sports such as football it is important to wear appropriate protective equipment.

Spondylolysis and Spondylolisthesis

What are spondylolysis and spondylolisthesis?

Your lower back is called your lumbar spine. It is made up of five bones called lumbar vertebrae. The vertebrae have two major parts, a solid part called the body and a bony ring through which the lower part of the spinal cord and nerves travel. Between the bodies of the vertebrae is shock absorbing material called disks. Part of the ring of each vertebra, called the pars, touches the vertebra above it and the vertebra below it.

Spondylolysis is a condition where there is a break in one or both sides of the ring of a vertebra. Spondylolisthesis is a condition in which a break in both sides of the ring allows the body of the vertebra to slip forward. Spondylolysis and spondylolisthesis most commonly occur at the fourth or fifth lumbar vertebrae. These conditions are also call pars defects, pars stress fractures, or stress fractures.

How does it occur?

Spondylolysis and spondylolisthesis result from repetitive extension of the back (bending backward). This causes weakness in the rings of the lumbar vertebrae, even-tually leading to a break (fracture) in a ring. Less commonly, these conditions may result from an injury to the back. Some doctors feel that certain people are born with weak vertebral rings.

Athletes most commonly troubled by spondylolysis or spondylolisthesis are gymnasts, dancers, and football players.

How is it diagnosed?

Your doctor will examine your back and look for tenderness along your vertebrae or spasm in the muscles next to your vertebrae. Your doctor will order an x-ray, which will show a break in the ring of a vertebra or slippage of a vertebra. Your doctor may order a bone scan to look for a break that has just recently occurred.

Spondylolysis

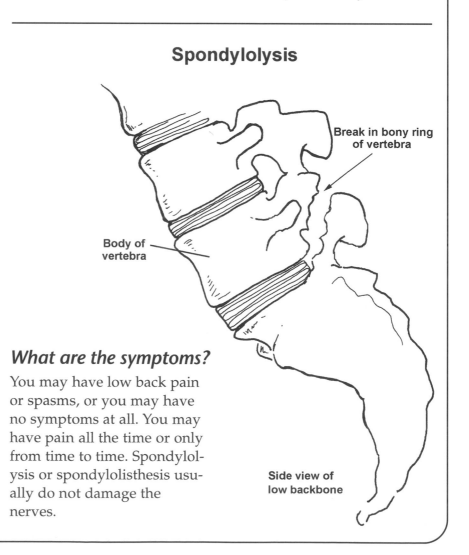

Break in bony ring of vertebra

Body of vertebra

Side view of low backbone

What are the symptoms?

You may have low back pain or spasms, or you may have no symptoms at all. You may have pain all the time or only from time to time. Spondylolysis or spondylolisthesis usually do not damage the nerves.

Spondylolysis and Spondylolisthesis

How is it treated?

For periods of acute pain your doctor may prescribe anti-inflammatory medication or other pain medications. You should place ice packs on your back for 20 to 30 minutes every 3 to 4 hours for 2 to 3 days or until the pain goes away.

You can participate in your sport or activity as long as you do not have pain. You may need to change your sport or activity to one that does not involve hyperextending the back.

If your doctor thinks the break is new and that the bones could heal, he or she may recommend wearing a brace for one to three months. Severe cases of spondylolisthesis may require surgery. Spondylolysis and spondylolisthesis are chronic problems. It is very important to keep your back in the best possible physical condition. Do not become overweight.

How can I prevent spondylolysis and spondylolisthesis?

You can best prevent these conditions by having strong back and abdominal muscles and by avoiding being overweight. If you have spondylolysis you may be able to prevent progression to spondylolisthesis by doing back exercises and by avoiding forced back extension activities, such as might occur during tackling in football.

It is important to have strong abdominal muscles when the structures of your spine are weakened. These exercises help build strong stomach muscles.

When can I return to my sport or activity?

The goal of rehabilitation is to return you to your sport or activity as soon as is safely possible. If you return too soon you may worsen your injury, which could lead to permanent damage. Everyone recovers from injury at a different rate. Return to your sport will be determined by how soon your back recovers, not by how many days or weeks it has been since your injury occurred. In general, the longer you have symptoms before you start treatment, the longer it will take to get better.

It is important that you have fully recovered from your low back pain before you return to your sport or any strenuous activity. You must be able to have the same range of motion that you had before your injury. You must be able to run, jump and twist without pain.

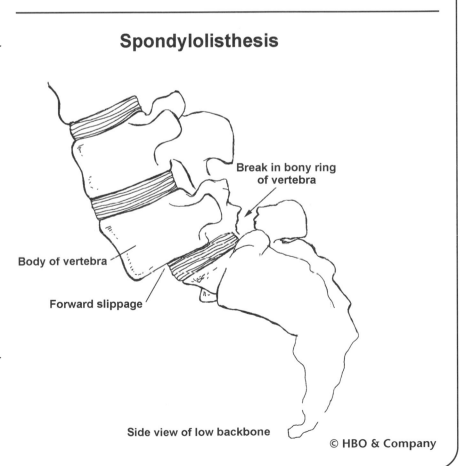

Spondylolisthesis

Break in bony ring of vertebra

Body of vertebra

Forward slippage

Side view of low backbone

© HBO & Company

Spondylolysis and Spondylolisthesis —
Rehabilitation Exercises

1. Pelvic tilt: Lying on your back with your knees bent and your feet flat on the floor, tighten your stomach muscles and push your lower back into the floor. Hold 5 seconds and relax. Repeat 10 times. Do 3 sets of 10.

   As the pelvic tilt becomes easier, you can progress to an exercise called the dead bug.

2. Dead bug: Tighten your stomach muscles and press your lower back into the floor. Lift up one leg several inches off the floor, hold for 5 seconds, then lower it. Lift the other leg off the floor, hold for 5 seconds, then lower it. Alternate legs, doing 5 repetitions with each leg and then relaxing the pelvic tilt. Do 3 sets of 10.

3. Partial curl: Lie on your back on the floor or another firm surface. Clasp your hands behind your neck for support, keeping your elbows pointed out to the side. Look straight up at the ceiling and tighten your stomach muscles by doing a pelvic tilt. Lift your shoulders off the floor toward the ceiling. Make sure to keep your elbows pointed out to the side and don't use your arms to lift your upper body off the floor. Hold for 3 seconds and then slowly lower your shoulders to the floor. Repeat 10 times. Do 3 sets of 10.

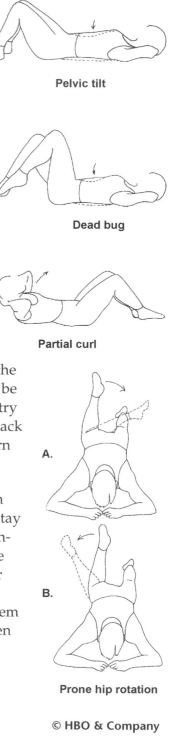

Pelvic tilt

Dead bug

Partial curl

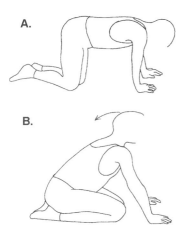

A.

B.

All-fours-to-heels sit

4. All-fours-to-heels sit: Kneel on the floor on all fours. Your palms should be flat on the floor in front of you and your back should be kept flat. Shift your weight backward and try to sit on your heels. Be sure to keep your back flat. Hold this position for 6 seconds. Return to the starting position. Do this 10 times.

5. Prone hip rotation: Lie on your stomach on the floor. Bend your knees so your thighs stay on the floor and your lower legs are perpendicular to the floor. Keep your knees on the floor and shoulder width apart. Cross your legs over each other as far as you can. Keeping your knees on the floor, uncross your lower legs and move them as far apart as possible. Hold for 2 seconds. Repeat 10 to 20 times. When you can do this exercise easily, add ankle weights.

A.

B.

Prone hip rotation

© HBO & Company

Sternoclavicular Joint Separation

What is a sternoclavicular joint separation?

The sternoclavicular joint is located where the collarbone (clavicle) attaches to the breastbone (sternum). These bones are held together by a piece of connective tissue called a ligament. A sternoclavicular separation occurs when the ligament tears.

How does it occur?

A sternoclavicular joint separation most commonly occurs when there is a direct blow to the sternum or a fall onto the shoulder or outstretched hands that causes a force along the length of the collarbone. It may occur in a contact sport when a player's shoulder hits the ground and another player lands on top of the other shoulder.

What are the symptoms?

You will have pain, swelling, and tenderness over the sternoclavicular joint. There may be movement between the breastbone and the collarbone. Your collarbone may be displaced either in front of your breastbone or behind your breastbone.

How is it diagnosed?

Your doctor will review your symptoms and examine your sternoclavicular joint. An x-ray or CT (computed tomography) scan may be ordered to see if there is a gap between your collarbone and breastbone.

How is it treated?

Treatment may include:

- putting ice packs on the injury for 20 to 30 minutes every 3 to 4 hours for 2 to 3 days or until the pain goes away
- taking anti-inflammatory medication or pain medications prescribed by your doctor
- wearing a sling
- resting your shoulder and arm on the side of the separation until the pain goes away.

In cases where the collarbone is forced behind the breastbone, there may be a risk of damage to the heart or the blood vessels in the chest and surgery may be required to repair the separation.

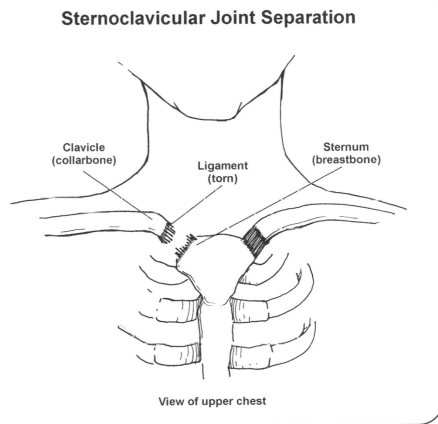

Sternoclavicular Joint Separation

Clavicle (collarbone)   Ligament (torn)   Sternum (breastbone)

View of upper chest

Sternoclavicular Joint Separation

In some cases, the sternoclavicular joint heals but may have some instability, or movement, when you move your arm or shoulder. If this instability causes pain, your doctor may recommend surgery.

When can I return to my sport or activity?

The goal of rehabilitation is to return you to your sport or activity as soon as is safely possible. If you return too soon you may worsen your injury, which could lead to permanent damage. Everyone recovers from injury at a different rate. Return to your sport or activity will be determined by how soon the injured area recovers, not by how many days or weeks it has been since your injury occurred.

You may safely return to your sport or activity when:

- You no longer have pain at the sternoclavicular joint.

- You have full range of motion and strength of your shoulder.

How can I prevent a sternoclavicular joint separation?

A sternoclavicular joint separation is usually caused by an accident that cannot be prevented.

Sternoclavicular Joint Separation Rehabilitation Exercises

You may do exercises 1 and 2 right away. You may do exercises 3 through 6 when the first two exercises are nearly painless.

1. Chest stretch: Grasp hands behind your back and lift your arms away from your body. Hold 10 seconds. Repeat 5 times.

2. Shoulder range of motion:

   A. Flexion and extension: Standing with your elbows straight, slowly lift your arm in front of you and over your head. Return to the starting position, with your elbow straight and bring your arm back behind you. Repeat 10 times.

   B. Abduction: Standing with your elbow straight, slowly bring your arm out to your side and over your head. Return to the starting position with your elbow straight. Repeat 10 times.

   C. External rotation: Standing with your elbow at your side and bent 90 degrees, slowly rotate your forearm and hand out to the side. Return to the starting position. Repeat 10 times.

   D. Horizontal motion: Standing with your arm out in front of you, elbow straight and at shoulder level, move your arm in a horizontal direction out to the side. Return to the starting position. Repeat 10 times.

Chest stretch

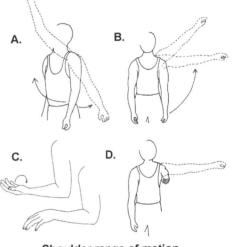

Shoulder range of motion

3. Sitting shoulder flexion: Using a small weight of some kind (soup can, hammer), lift your arm up in front of you with the elbow straight and try to reach over your head. Return to the starting position with your elbow straight. Repeat 10 times.

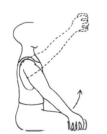

Sitting shoulder flexion

4. Supine horizontal motion: Lie on your back, hold your arm out straight, and move your arm up until your hand is toward the ceiling. Return your arm to the starting position. Repeat 10 times. As you get stronger, hold a weight in your hand as you do this exercise.

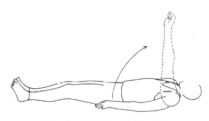

Supine horizontal motion

5. Prone extension: Lie on your stomach with your arm hanging over a table or bed. Lift your arm straight back behind you toward the ceiling. Keep your elbow straight. Repeat 10 times. As you get stronger, add a weight to your hand.

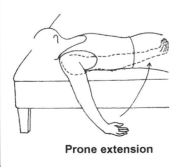

Prone extension

Sternoclavicular Joint Separation
Rehabilitation Exercises

6. Prone horizontal motion: Lying on your stomach with your face facing the floor, raise your arms straight out from the side and squeeze your shoulder blades together. Keep your elbows straight and your thumbs up. Repeat 10 times. As you get stronger, add a weight.

Prone horizontal motion

© HBO & Company

Tailbone Injuries

What is a tailbone injury?

Your tailbone (coccyx) is actually made up of several bones that are located at the end of your lower back. Tailbones can be bruised or broken.

How does it occur?

A tailbone injury usually occurs from a direct fall onto the coccyx.

What are the symptoms?

Your tailbone is very tender. You have pain when you are sitting. You may also have pain when you walk and when you have a bowel movement.

How is it diagnosed?

Your doctor will review your symptoms and examine your back and tailbone. Your doctor may order an x-ray to see if your tailbone is broken.

How is it treated?

An injured tailbone needs time to heal. A bruised tailbone may take several days to several weeks to completely heal. A fractured tailbone takes 4 to 6 weeks to heal. In either case, people sometimes have pain for a long time.

While your tailbone injury is healing it is very important to use a doughnut cushion when you are sitting. A doughnut cushion may be purchased at a medical supply house or you may use a child's swimming inner tube.

You should place an ice pack on your tailbone for 20 to 30 minutes every 3 to 4 hours for 2 to 3 days or until the pain goes away. Your doctor may prescribe an anti-inflammatory or pain medications.

It is important to avoid constipation while your tailbone is healing. Drink plenty of fluids and increase the amount of fiber in your diet.

How can I prevent tailbone injuries?

Most tailbone injuries are caused by accidents that cannot be prevented. In some contact sports such as football or hockey, it is important to wear protective equipment.

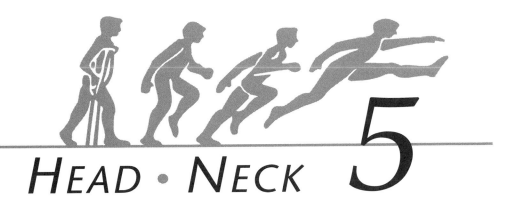

HEAD · NECK 5

Brachial Plexus Injury
(Stinger/Burner)

What is a stinger?

A stinger or burner is an injury to the nerves that travel from your neck and down your arm.

There are seven bones in your neck called vertebrae. The vertebrae are held together by ligaments. Your spinal cord goes from the bottom of your brain through a canal in your vertebrae down to your lower back. Nerves come off the spinal cord that make your limbs and body move and have sensation. These are called peripheral nerves. A group of peripheral nerves called the brachial plexus leaves the spinal cord and travels between the vertebrae and into the shoulder, giving your arm its ability to function. These are the nerves that are injured when you have a stinger.

How does it occur?

A stinger is almost always seen in contact sports when the head and neck are forcibly moved or hit to one side, stretching the brachial plexus on the opposite side. Sometimes when the head and neck are forcibly pushed to one side there is compression of the nerves in the brachial plexus on the same side. The nerves become irritated as a result of being stretched or compressed.

What are the symptoms?

A stinger usually causes intense pain from the neck down to the arm. You may feel like your arm is on fire. You may have a "pins and needles" sensation. Your arm or hand may be weak. It is possible that you may not have any symptoms after a period of rest following your injury.

How is it diagnosed?

Your doctor will ask about your symptoms and examine your head, neck, shoulder, arm, and hand. You may have a sensation of burning or tingling if your doctor pushes down on your head or pushes your head to the side.

Your doctor may do neck x-rays to be sure there is no damage to the vertebrae. If the injury is serious, your doctor may do a CT (computerized tomography) scan or MRI (magnetic resonance imaging). Your doctor may send you to a specialist for tests such as an electromyogram (EMG) or nerve conduction studies (NCS).

How is it treated?

Treatment may include:

- resting your neck and arms until the pain and symptoms are gone

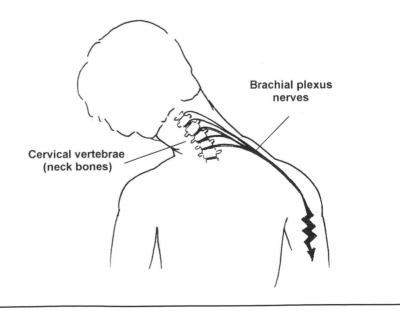

Stinger/Burner (Brachial Plexus Injury)

Brachial plexus nerves

Cervical vertebrae (neck bones)

Brachial Plexus Injury (Stinger/Burner)

- putting an ice pack on your neck and shoulders for 20 to 30 minutes every 3 to 4 hours for 2 to 3 days or until the pain goes away
- taking an anti-inflammatory medication
- doing exercises to strengthen your neck.

Chronic stiff neck muscles may be treated with heat, massage, or muscle stimulation.

When can I return to my sport or activity?

The goal of rehabilitation is to return you to your sport or activity as soon as is safely possible. If you return too soon you may worsen your injury, which could lead to permanent damage. Everyone recovers from injury at a different rate. Return to your sport or activity will be determined by how soon your nerves recover, not by how many days or weeks it has been since your injury occurred. In general, the longer you have symptoms before you start treatment, the longer it will take to get better. Before you return to competition in contact sports, it is important that your neck and shoulders be healed and strong. You must have full range of motion of your neck. This means you must be able to turn your head fully to look over both shoulders, extend your head backward as far as possible, flex your neck forward until your chin touches your chest, and move your head in each direction so that your ear touches your shoulder. If any of these actions causes burning in your neck or shoulder, you are not yet able to return.

How can I prevent a stinger?

A stinger is best prevented by keeping the muscles in your neck strong. It is important to use good technique in contact sports such as football and not to strike with your head when blocking or tackling.

© HBO & Company

Brachial Plexus Injury (Stinger/Burner) Rehabilitation Exercises

A.

B.

C.

Cervical isometrics

You can begin these exercises when moving your neck in all directions (up, down, right, left) does not cause numbness or tingling down your arm or into your hand.

1. Cervical isometrics
    A. Neck flexion: Sit tall, eyes straight ahead, and chin level. Place your palm against your forehead and gently push your forehead into your palm. Hold for 5 seconds and release. Repeat 5 times.
    B. Neck extension: Clasp your hands together and place them behind your head. Press the back of your head into your palm. Hold 5 seconds and repeat 5 times.
    C. Neck side bend: Place the palm of your hand at the side of your temple and press your temple into the palm of your hand. Hold 5 seconds, repeat 5 times, and then do it to the other side.

2. Cervical strengthening exercises
    A. Neck curl: Lie on your back with your knees bent and feet flat on the floor. Tuck your chin in and slowly lift your head off the floor. Roll your neck so that your eyes are facing your knees. Slowly return to the starting position and repeat 10 times.

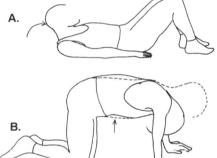

A.

B.

Cervical strengthening exercises

    B. Hands and knees neck extension: Get on your hands and knees on the floor. Let your head hang down so that the top of your head is facing the floor and your eyes are facing your thighs. Lift your head up so that your eyes are now facing straight down into the floor and the top of your head is straight out in front of you. Repeat 10 times.

3. Neck side bend: Lie on your right side, right arm held straight over your head, and your head resting on that arm. Lift your head up so that your left ear goes toward your left shoulder. Return to the starting position. Repeat 10 times. Lie on your left side and bring your right ear toward your right shoulder, lifting your head off the floor. Repeat 10 times.

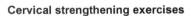

Neck side bend

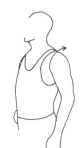

Shoulder shrugs

4. Shoulder shrugs: Stand with your head directly over your shoulders, with your spine straight. Shrug your shoulders up and then relax. Repeat 10 times. Do 3 sets of 10.

© HBO & Company

Concussion

What is a concussion?

A concussion is an injury to the brain that is caused by a blow to the head. Concussions are the most common head injuries in sports. A concussion may cause a person to become temporarily confused, disoriented, have memory loss (amnesia), or become unconscious.

How does it occur?

A concussion occurs when you are hit in the head, jarring your brain. The most common sports for concussions are football, gymnastics, ice hockey, and wrestling. However, concussions can occur in any sport or activity where you may get hit in the head.

What are the symptoms?

If you have had a concussion you may have any of the following symptoms:

- confusion
- disorientation
- memory loss (amnesia)
- loss of consciousness
- nausea
- dizziness
- headache
- loss of balance.

You may have these symptoms, called post-concussive syndrome, for several days or weeks after the injury.

Concussions are graded as I, II, or III, depending upon the severity of the confusion, amnesia, or loss of consciousness.

How is it diagnosed?

Your doctor will examine you and find out what happened. If you have amnesia, the doctor may need to get this information from other people who were there. The doctor will do a neurologic examination, testing your strength, sensation, balance, reflexes, and memory. He or she will also examine your eyes with a flashlight to see if your pupils are of equal size. Your doctor may choose to do a special x-ray called a computed tomography (CT) scan or a magnetic resonance image (MRI) of your head to be sure there is no damage to your brain.

How is it treated?

The treatment for a concussion is rest. The headache may be treated with a mild pain reliever and the nausea may be treated with a medication for nausea.

To avoid complications from the concussion, it is very important that you do not return to your sport or activity too soon. In a very mild concussion, you may be allowed to return to your sport or activity after 20 to 30 minutes. If there has been a loss of memory or loss of consciousness, the you may not be able to return for 1 week. After a severe concussion, you may not be able to return to sports for up to 1 month.

If you have had repeated concussions, your doctor may talk to you about limiting your participation in certain sports.

What symptoms should be watched for?

If you have had a concussion, you need to be watched by a relative or a friend for 8 to 12 hours. You should be awakened and checked every 2 to 4 hours while sleeping. Symptoms to report to a doctor include:

- confusion
- convulsions or seizures
- unequal pupil sizes
- restlessness or irritability
- trouble using your legs or arms
- repeated vomiting
- headache that will not go away after being treated with acetaminophen (Tylenol)
- stiff neck
- garbled speech
- bleeding from the ears or nose

Concussion

- bleeding from the ears or nose
- decreasing alertness
- unusual sleepiness.

How can I prevent a concussion?

A concussion is caused by a blow to the head. It is important in contact sports that you wear proper protective head gear that fits well. In sports such as football, it is important to use proper blocking and tackling techniques and not to use your head for initial contact. In sports such as bicycling and rollerblading, wear a helmet.

Corneal Abrasion

What is corneal abrasion?

The cornea is the transparent covering on the front part of the eye. It covers the pupil and the colored part of the eye. A corneal abrasion is a scratch on the cornea.

How does it occur?

A corneal abrasion commonly occurs when an object scratches your eye. This can happen in sports such as basketball or football when a player gets poked in the eye, or in tennis or racquetball when a player gets hit in the eye with the ball.

What are the symptoms?

You have pain in your eye. Your eye may become red and be teary. Your vision may be blurred.

How is it diagnosed?

Your health care provider will examine your eye. He or she will check your vision and look at the surface of your eye. Your health care provider may put a painless dye in your eye to help make the scratch easier to see. The stain will temporarily make your vision yellow. The yellowness will go away in a few minutes.

How is it treated?

If you have gotten something in your eye, after a drop of anesthetic your health care provider can remove it quickly and painlessly.

The covering of the eye has a great ability to heal itself. This healing will be aided by the use of antibiotic drops or ointment. Your health care provider may patch your eye and may recommend a follow-up eye exam in the next 24 to 48 hours.

How long will the effects last?

Most corneal abrasions heal within a day or two. Once the cornea has healed, you can usually resume your normal activities right away.

How can I prevent corneal abrasions?

Corneal abrasions from sports injuries or occupational hazards are best prevented by wearing protective eyeglasses, sports goggles, or eye shields that attach to the facemasks of helmets.

Nose Injury

What is a nose injury?

A nose injury may be a:

- nosebleed
- bruised nose (contusion)
- broken nose (fracture)
- damaged nasal septum (the nasal septum is the tissue that separates the nasal passages).

How does it occur?

Nose injuries are almost always caused by a direct hit to the nose.

What are the symptoms?

Symptoms may include:

- pain
- bleeding
- swelling
- sometimes deformity or crookedness
- difficulty breathing through the nose
- grating or grinding noise with movement of broken nose bones.

How is it diagnosed?

Your health care provider will examine your nose. He or she will look for swelling, tenderness, bleeding, and movement of bones. Your provider will look in your nostrils to see if the septum is swollen or bent to the side (deviated). You may have:

- an x-ray to see if the nose is broken
- a CT scan to look at the nasal septum and the sinuses.

How is it treated?

If your nose is bleeding:

- Pinch your nostrils firmly together just below the nasal bones for 10 minutes or until the bleeding stops.
- It may help to put ice on your nose.
- Sit up and lean forward.
- Breathe through your mouth.

If the bleeding doesn't stop with pressure, your health care provider may need to put gauze packing in your nose to stop the bleeding.

After the nosebleed stops, try not to blow your nose because the bleeding may start again. Avoid taking aspirin or other anti-inflammatory medicines because they may make bleeding worse. Take acetaminophen instead.

Many broken noses heal normally with no special treatment. If you have broken your nose and it is crooked:

- Your health care provider may straighten it right after the injury.

- You may be sent to a specialist to have it straightened.
- You may need surgery.

If the septum has become deviated and you have trouble breathing, you may need to have surgery in the future.

When can I return to my sport or activity?

- Do not start any activities until the nosebleed has completely stopped.
- If you have broken your nose and you play a contact sport, wear a special nose and face shield for 4 to 6 weeks after the injury. Shields may be purchased at a sporting goods store or may be custom-made for you.

How can I prevent a nose injury?

Nose injuries are usually caused by an accident that cannot be prevented. If you play a sport for which preventive face gear is available, such as hockey or lacrosse, make sure you wear the shield.

Neck Spasms

What are neck spasms?

Neck spasms are involuntary contractions of the muscles in your neck. The muscles become tight, hard, and painful.

How do they occur?

Neck spasms may occur from an injury, overuse, poor posture, or stress. For example, it is common for a person doing a lot of computer work to feel his or her neck stiffen. Spasms may even occur from an uncomfortable night's sleep.

What are the symptoms?

The muscles in your neck feel hard, tight, and painful. When the muscles that extend from your shoulders to your head go into spasm, the spasms may even cause headaches. You may have tender spots in your neck, sometimes called trigger points, that cause pain elsewhere.

How are they diagnosed?

Your doctor will review your medical history and examine your neck.

How are they treated?

- Stretching: Spasms are best treated with stretching exercises.

- Massage: You may be able to massage your neck yourself by finding the tight muscles and putting deep pressure on these muscles. You might also get a massage from a friend or therapist.

- Medication: Your doctor may recommend an anti-inflammatory medication such as ibuprofen or naproxen or may prescribe a muscle relaxant.

- Ice: If your neck spasm has just occurred, put ice packs on your neck for 20 to 30 minutes three to four times a day.

- Moist heat: Sometimes, especially with recurrent spasms, moist heat can help. Put warm, moist towels on your neck for 20 minutes, or take hot showers or baths.

- Physical therapy: Your doctor may recommend physical therapy for an exercise program and other treatments.

- Injection: If the above treatments do not help the spasm get better, your doctor may recommend a shot of an anesthetic or a medicine like cortisone into the muscle.

- Stress management: Neck spasms are a common physical symptom caused by stress or depression.

Neck Strain and Neck Spasm

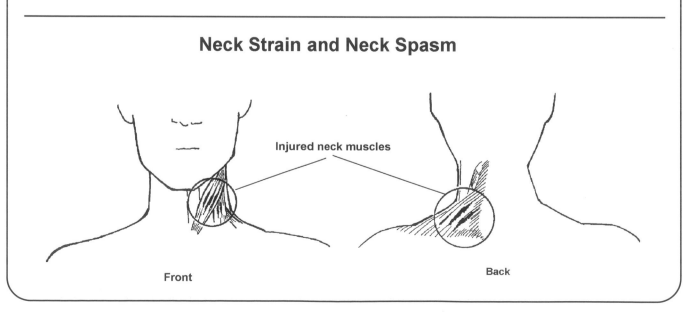

Injured neck muscles

Front

Back

Neck Spasms

Identification of these problems and treatment of them may help considerably with neck spasms.

When can I return to my sport or activity?

You may return to your sport or activity when:

- You no longer have neck pain.

- You can move your neck fully and comfortably.

How can I help prevent neck spasms?

Know what you can do about the common causes of neck spasm: overuse, stress, and poor posture. For example, use good posture at your computer terminal, take frequent breaks, and do stretching exercises.

When you first feel tightness or pain in your neck, start the treatment that has helped you the most. Treating early, mild symptoms right away can often stop the symptoms from becoming worse.
You may do these exercises right away.

© HBO & Company

Neck Spasm Rehabilitation Exercises

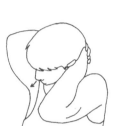

Forward

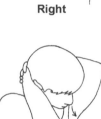

Right

Left

Neck flexion

1. Neck flexion forward: Clasp your hands behind your head and let the weight of your arms pull your chin to your chest. Relax. Hold for a count of 10. Do this 3 times.

2. Neck flexion, right side: Turn your head to the right and clasp your hands behind your head. Let the weight of your arms pull your chin to the right side of your chest. Relax. Hold for a count of 10. Do this 3 times.

3. Neck flexion, left side: Turn your head to the left and clasp your hands behind your head. Let the weight of your arms pull your chin to the left side of your chest. Relax relax. Hold for a count of 10. Do this 3 times.

4. Ear to shoulder, right side: Lean your right ear toward your right shoulder. Reach your right arm over your head and place your fingers over your left ear. Gently pull your head toward your right shoulder. Hold for a count of 10. Do this 3 times.

5. Ear to shoulder, left side: Lean your left ear toward your right shoulder. Reach your left arm over your head and place your fingers over your right ear. Gently pull your head toward your left shoulder. Hold for a count of 10. Do this 3 times.

6. Neck rotation, right side: Rotate your neck by looking over your right shoulder. Lift your right hand and place your palm on the left side of your chin. Push your chin with your palm toward your right shoulder. Hold for a count of 10. Do this 3 times.

7. Neck rotation, left side: Rotate your neck by looking over your left shoulder. Lift your left hand and place your palm on the right side of your chin. Push your chin with your palm toward your left shoulder. Hold for a count of 10. Do this 3 times.

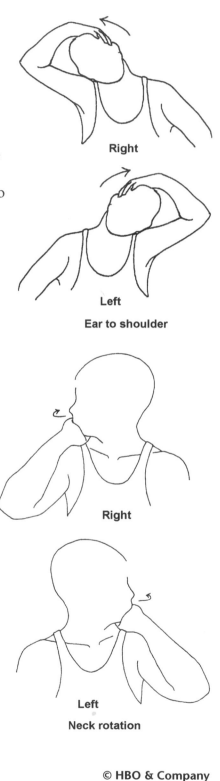

Right

Left

Ear to shoulder

Right

Left

Neck rotation

Neck Strain

What is neck strain?

A strain is a tear of a muscle or tendon. Your neck is surrounded by small muscles running close to the vertebrae and larger muscles that make up the visible muscles of the neck.

How does it occur?

Neck strains most commonly occur when the head and neck are forcibly moved, such as in a whiplash injury or from contact in sports.

What are the symptoms?

You literally have a pain in the neck. When these muscles go into spasm you feel hard, tight muscles in your neck that are very tender to the touch. You have pain when you move your head to either side or when you try to move your head up or down. The spas-ming muscles can cause headaches.

How is it diagnosed?

Your health care provider will examine your neck. Your neck muscles will be tender and tight, and you may have pain over the bones in your neck. Your health care provider may order x-rays to make sure the vertebrae are not injured.

How is it treated?

Right after the injury you should place an ice pack on your neck for 20 to 30 minutes every 3 or 4 hours for 2 to 3 days or until the pain goes away.

Your health care provider may prescribe an anti-inflammatory medication and a neck collar to support your neck and prevent further injury.

If you still have neck pain several days after the injury and after using ice, your health care provider may recommend using moist heat on your neck. You can buy a moist-heat pad or make your own by soaking towels in hot water. You should apply moist heat to the neck for 20 to 30 minutes every 3 or 4 hours until the pain goes away. You may find that it helps to alternate putting heat and ice on your neck.

How long will the effects last?

Most people recover from neck strains in a few days to a few weeks, but some people take longer to get better.

When can I return to my sport or activity?

The goal of rehabilitation is to return you to your sport or

Neck Strain and Neck Spasm

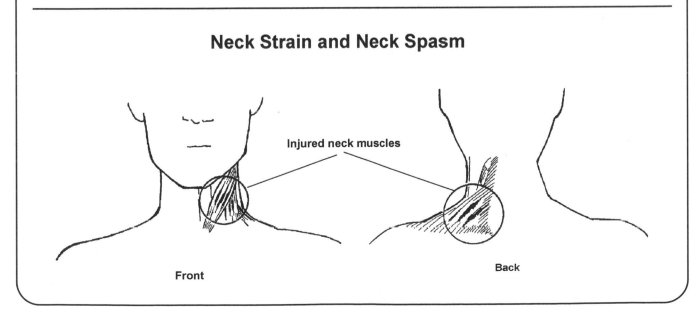

Injured neck muscles

Front   Back

Neck Strain

activity as soon as is safely possible. If you return too soon you may worsen your injury, which could lead to permanent damage. Everyone recovers from injury at a different rate. Return to your sport or activity will be determined by how soon your neck recovers, not by how many days or weeks it has been since your injury occurred. In general, the longer you have symptoms before you start treatment, the longer it will take to get better.

If you participate in contact sports, it is important to rehabilitate your neck and shoulders before going back to competition. You must have full range of motion of your neck. This means you must be able to:

- turn your head fully to look over both shoulders
- extend your head backward as far as possible
- flex your neck forward until your chin touches your chest
- move your head in each direction so that your ear touches your shoulder.

If any of these actions cause burning in your neck or shoulder or pain or spasm in your neck or shoulder muscles, you are not yet able to return.

How can I prevent neck strain?

Neck strain is best prevented by having strong and supple neck muscles. If you have a job that requires you to be in one position all day (for example, work at a computer all day), it is very important to take breaks and relax your neck muscles.

In many cases an injury to the neck occurs during an accident that is not preventable.

Neck Strain Rehabilitation Exercises

Do these exercises only if you do not have pain or numbness running down your arm or into your hand. Exercises 1 through 4 are meant to help your neck remain flexible. Exercise 5 will help you maintain or regain your range of motion.

1. Neck range of motion exercises

    A. Neck rotation: Sit in a chair, keeping your neck, shoulders, and trunk straight. First, turn your head slowly to the right. Move it gently to the point of pain. Move it back to the forward position. Relax. Then move it to the left. Repeat 10 times.

    B. Neck side bend: Tilt your head so that your right ear moves toward your right shoulder. Move it to the point of pain. Then tilt your head so your left ear moves toward your left shoulder. Make sure you do not rotate your head while tilting or raise your shoulder toward your head. Repeat this exercise 10 times in each direction.

    C. Neck flexion: Bend your head forward, reaching your chin toward your chest. Hold for 5 seconds. Repeat 10 times.

    D. Neck extension: Bring your head back so that your chin is pointing toward the ceiling. Repeat 10 times.

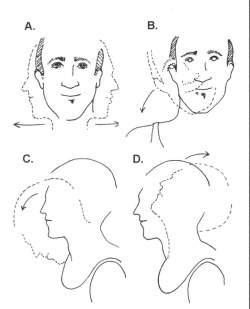

Neck range of motion exercises

2. Upper trapezius stretch: The upper trapezius muscle connects your shoulder to your head. Sitting in an upright position, put your right arm behind your back and gently grasp the right side of your head with your left hand to help tilt your head toward the left. You will feel a gentle stretch on your right side. Hold for 20 seconds. Repeat 3 times on each side.

Upper trapezius stretch

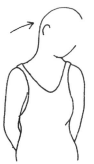

Scalene stretch

3. Scalene stretch: This stretches the neck muscles that attach to your ribs. Sitting in an upright position, clasp both hands behind your back, lower your left shoulder, and tilt your head toward the right. Hold this position for 20 seconds and then come back to the starting position. Lower your right shoulder and tilt your head toward the left until you feel a stretch. Hold for 20 seconds. Repeat 3 times on each side.

Neck Strain Rehabilitation Exercises

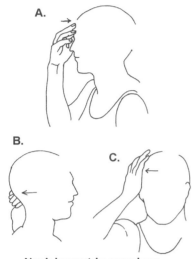

Neck isometric exercises

4. Neck isometric exercises

A. Neck flexion: Sit upright, look straight ahead, and keep your chin level. Apply light pressure with your fingertips to your forehead, resisting bending your head forward. Hold for 5 seconds. Repeat 5 times.

B. Neck extension: Sitting upright, apply light pressure with your fingertips to the back of your head, resisting the bending backward of your head. Hold for 5 seconds. Repeat 5 times.

C. Neck side bend: Sitting upright, place your right palm on the right side of your head and press your head into your palm. Hold this for 5 seconds and then relax. Repeat the same resistance using your left hand on the left side of your head. Repeat on each side 5 times.

5. Head lifts

A. Neck curl: Lie on your back with your knees bent and your feet flat on the floor. Tuck your chin and lift your head toward your chest, keeping your shoulders on the floor. Hold for 5 seconds. Repeat 10 times.

B. Neck side bend: Turn onto your right side. With your right forearm underneath your head, lift your head slowly toward your left shoulder. Hold for 5 seconds. Repeat 10 times. Switch to your left side and repeat the exercise lifting your head toward your right shoulder.

C. Hands and knees neck extension: Get on your hands and knees and look down at the floor. Keep your back straight and let your head slowly drop toward your chest. Then tuck your chin and lift your head up until your neck is level with your back. Hold this position for 5 seconds. Repeat 10 times.

Head lifts

Outer Ear Infection
(Otitis Externa)

What is otitis externa?

Otitis externa is an infection of the outer ear caused by bacteria, fungi, or allergies. Otitis externa is also called swimmer's ear.

How does it occur?

Otitis externa can occur from an injury or from contaminated water in your ear canal. Frequent showering or swimming can increase the risk of getting an infection. It often occurs in the summer from swimming in polluted water. Hair spray or hair dye may irritate the ear canal skin as well. Some people get otitis externa repeatedly.

What are the symptoms?

Symptoms include:

- itching (often the first symptom; eczema develops in the ear canal and often the skin is broken)
- redness
- extreme pain and swelling in ear canal
- foul discharge from the ear
- crusting around the ear canal opening.

In some cases, swelling or pus may affect your hearing.

How is it diagnosed?

The doctor will examine your ears with a viewing instrument. He or she may take a sample of pus and culture it to look for bacteria or fungi.

How is it treated?

Your doctor will carefully clean and dry your ear. If your ear is very swollen, he or she may insert a wick soaked in an antibiotic into the ear to apply the medicine to the infected area. You may need to put drops in your ear several times a day to keep the wick moist.

Your doctor may prescribe an antibiotic in pill form if you have a severe infection. In addition, he or she may suggest a topical medication, such as cream or ointment, for some types of infection.

How long will the effects last?

The pain and swelling will go away gradually as the antibiotics or other medications take effect. Most cases of otitis externa clear up completely in 5 to 7 days.

How can I take care of myself?

The doctor will tell you how to take care of your ear and how to remove the wick.

Follow the treatment plan prescribed by the doctor. Also:

- Keep water out of your ears until the infection is completely gone.
- Take baths instead of showers. If you need to wash your hair several times a week, consider washing your hair in a sink instead of in the shower.
- Don't put anything in your ears, including Q-tips, that should not be inserted into the ear canal.

How can I help prevent otitis externa?

- Wear earplugs or use something such as lamb's wool to keep your ears dry when you swim and shower.
- Dry your ears carefully if you get water in them. You may want to use a hair dryer.
- Avoid any substance that may cause an allergic reaction of the ear canal skin. Read product labels carefully and ask your doctor before you use chemicals or medications in the area of your ear.

© HBO & Company

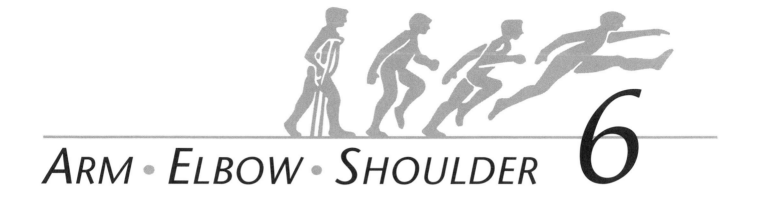

ARM · ELBOW · SHOULDER 6

Biceps Tendonitis

What is biceps tendonitis?

Tendons are connective tissue bands that attach muscles to bones. The biceps muscle is located in the front part of the upper arm and attaches at the elbow and in two places at the shoulder. Biceps tendonitis, also called bicipital tendonitis, is inflammation that causes pain in the front part of the shoulder or upper arm.

How does it occur?

Biceps tendonitis occurs from overuse of the arm and shoulder or from an injury to the biceps tendon.

What are the symptoms?

You feel pain when you move your arm and shoulder, especially when you move your arm forward over shoulder height. You feel pain when you touch the front of your shoulder.

How is it diagnosed?

Your doctor will examine your arm and shoulder for tenderness along the biceps muscle and biceps tendons.

How is it treated?

Treatment may include:
• placing ice packs on your shoulder for 20 to 30 minutes every 3 to 4 hours

for 2 or 3 days or until the pain goes away
• taking anti-inflammatory medication
• getting an injection of a corticosteroid medication to reduce the inflammation and pain
• doing rehabilitation exercises.

When can I return to my sport or activity?

The goal of rehabilitation is to return you to your sport or activity as soon as is safely possible. If you return too soon you may worsen your injury, which could lead to permanent damage. Everyone recovers from injury at a different rate. Return to your activity will be determined by how soon your shoulder recovers, not by how many days or weeks it has been since your injury occurred. In general, the longer you have symptoms before you start treatment, the longer it will take to get better.

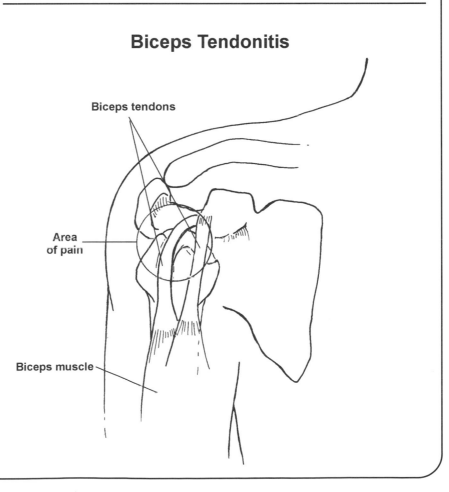

Biceps Tendonitis

Biceps tendons

Area of pain

Biceps muscle

Biceps Tendonitis

You may safely return to your sport or activity when:

- Your injured shoulder has full range of motion without pain.
- Your injured shoulder has regained normal strength compared to the uninjured shoulder.

In throwing sports, you must gradually rebuild your tolerance to throwing. This means you should start with gentle tossing and gradually throw harder. In contact sports, your shoulder must not be tender to touch and contact should progress from minimal contact to harder contact.

How can I prevent biceps tendonitis?

You can best prevent biceps tendonitis by doing a proper warm-up and stretching exercises for your arm and shoulder before your activity.

Biceps Tendonitis Rehabilitation Exercises

1. Active range of motion
   A. Flexion: Gently try to bend your elbow, bringing your hand toward your shoulder, palm up. Hold for 5 seconds. Repeat 10 times. Do 3 sets.
   B. Extension: Gently relax your arm out straight. Hold 5 seconds. Repeat 10 times. Do 3 sets.
   C. Pronation and supination: With your elbow bent at a 90-degree angle, move your forearm so your palm faces up and then faces down. Hold each position for 5 seconds. Repeat palm up and palm down 10 times each. Do 3 sets.

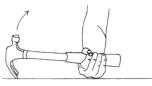

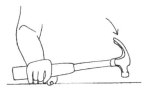

Active range of motion

2. Biceps strengthening: Begin by holding a soup can or similar object in your hand. Bend your elbow by bringing your hand toward your shoulder. Hold 5 seconds. Repeat 10 times. Do 3 sets.

3. Pronation and supination strengthening: Hold a hammer in your hand. With your elbow bent at a 90-degree angle, move your forearm so your palm faces up and then faces down. Hold each position 10 seconds. Repeat palm up and palm down 10 times each. Do 3 sets.

Biceps strengthening

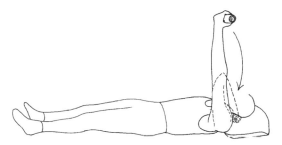

Pronation and supination strengthening

4. Triceps strengthening: Lie on your back with your injured arm pointing toward the ceiling. Hold a light weight in your hand. Bend your elbow completely, so that your hand is resting on the same shoulder and your elbow is pointing toward the ceiling. Straighten the elbow completely so that your hand is pointing toward the ceiling. Return to the starting position. Repeat 10 times. Do 3 sets. Increase the amount of weight when this becomes too easy.

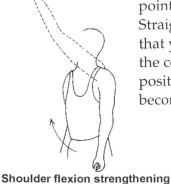

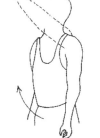

Shoulder flexion strengthening

Triceps strengthening

5. Shoulder flexion strengthening: Stand with your injured arm hanging down at your side. Keeping your elbow straight, bring your arm forward and up toward the ceiling. Hold this position for 5 seconds. Repeat 10 times. Do three sets. When this becomes too easy, hold a weight.

Frozen Shoulder

(Adhesive Capsulitis)

What is a frozen shoulder?

A frozen shoulder is stiffness and pain in the shoulder.

How does it occur?

A frozen shoulder develops after a shoulder injury that causes pain and does not allow you to move your shoulder enough. If you have limited movement of your shoulder for weeks, months, or years because of the injury, the capsule surrounding the shoulder joint may become very stiff. Your shoulder may develop scar tissue, or adhesions, in the joint.

What are the symptoms?

Your shoulder will lose its normal ability to move in all directions. You may not be able to lift your arm above your head or be able to scratch your back. Movement of the shoulder may be very painful. You may feel grinding when moving your shoulder.

How is it diagnosed?

Your doctor will examine your shoulder and may take x-rays. In some cases, he or she may want to do an arthrogram (an x-ray of your shoulder after dye is injected into your shoulder joint) or an MRI (magnetic resonance imaging) scan.

How is it treated?

Your doctor will probably send you to physical therapy for a supervised exercise program. You will also be given exercises to do at home. Your doctor may prescribe an anti-inflammatory medication and may choose to do an injection of a corticosteroid medication into your shoulder joint. When your shoulder is painful it is important to use ice packs on your shoulder for 20 to 30 minutes 3 or 4 times a day.

In cases that do not respond to therapy, your doctor may talk to you about doing a "manipulation under anesthesia." In this procedure, you are put to sleep with a general anesthetic and your doctor moves your shoulder in various directions to break up the adhesions, bands of scar tissue, in your shoulder capsule.

When can I return to my sport or activity?

The goal of rehabilitation is to return you to your sport or activity as soon as is safely possible. If you return too soon you may worsen your injury, which could lead to permanent damage. Everyone recovers from injury at a different rate. Return to your activity will be determined by how soon your shoulder recovers, not by how many days or weeks it has been since your injury occurred. In general, the longer you have symptoms before you start treatment, the longer it will take to get better.

You may safely return to your sport or activity when:

- Your injured shoulder has full range of motion without pain.
- Your injured shoulder has regained normal strength compared to the uninjured shoulder.

In throwing sports, you must gradually rebuild your tolerance to throwing. This means you should start with gentle tossing and gradually throw harder. In contact sports, your shoulder must not be tender to touch and contact should progress from minimal contact to harder contact.

How can I prevent a frozen shoulder?

After you have had an injury to your shoulder it is important that you do not limit your shoulder motion for a prolonged period of time. It is important to do your shoulder rehabilitation exercises as they have been prescribed. If you feel that you are losing range of motion in your shoulder you should see your doctor.

© HBO & Company

Frozen Shoulder Rehabilitation Exercises

1. Wand exercises

   A. Shoulder flexion: Stand upright and hold a stick in both hands, palms down. Stretch your arms by lifting them over your head, keeping your elbows straight. Hold for 5 seconds and return to the starting position. Repeat 10 times.

   B. Shoulder abduction: Stand upright and hold a stick with both hands, palms down. Rest the stick against the front of your thighs. While keeping your elbows straight, use your good arm to push your injured arm out to the side and up as high as possible. Hold for 5 seconds. Repeat 10 times.

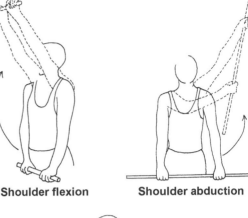

Shoulder flexion   **Shoulder abduction**

   C. Shoulder extension: Stand upright and hold a stick in both hands behind your back. Move the stick away from your back. Hold the end position for 5 seconds. Relax and return to the starting position. Repeat 10 times.

   D. Internal rotation: Stand upright holding a stick with both hands behind your back. Place the hand on your uninjured side behind your head grasping the stick, and the hand on your injured side behind your back at your waist. Move the stick up and down your back by bending your elbows. Hold the bent position for 5 seconds and then return to the starting position. Repeat 10 times.

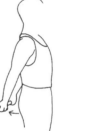
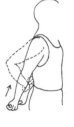

Shoulder extension   **Internal rotation**

   E. External rotation: Lie on your back and hold a stick in both hands, palms up. Your upper arms should be resting on the floor, your elbows at your sides and bent 90 degrees. Using your good arm, push your injured arm out away from your body while keeping the elbow of the injured arm at your side. Hold the stretch for 5 seconds. Repeat 10 times.

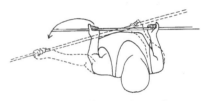

External rotation

2. Scapular range of motion: Shrug your shoulders up. Squeeze your shoulder blades together, then push your shoulder blades down. Relax and return to the starting position. Hold each position for 5 seconds. Repeat 10 times.

3. Active shoulder flexion: Stand with your arm hanging down at your side. Keep your elbow straight and lift your arm up over your head as far as you can reach. Hold the end position for 5 seconds. Repeat 10 times. Do 3 sets.

Scapular range of motion

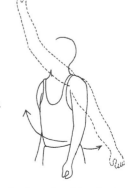

Active shoulder flexion

© HBO & Company

Labral Tear

What is a labral tear of the shoulder?

The shoulder joint is a ball and socket joint. The labrum is a lip of connective tissue where the shoulder ligaments connect to the edge of the socket that holds the ball of the upper arm bone into the socket of the shoulder blade.

How does it occur?

The labrum can be torn by:

- dislocating your shoulder
- falling onto your arm
- having your arm jerked away from your body
- using your arm to break a fall
- lifting a heavy object
- use of your shoulder in sports with a repetitive, high velocity overhead movement, such as throwing or tennis serving.

What are the symptoms?

The symptoms of a labral tear are:

- arm and shoulder pain
- shoulder weakness
- arm weakness
- painful overhead movements of the shoulder
- clicking or grinding when moving your shoulder

How is it diagnosed?

Your doctor will perform a physical exam and check your shoulder for pain, tenderness, loss of motion or laxity as you move your arm in all directions. Your doctor will ask you whether your shoulder pain began suddenly or gradually. An x-ray may be ordered to see if there are any fractures in the shoulder.

Your doctor may recommend that you get an MRI (magnetic resonance imaging) of your shoulder, a special test that can see bone, ligaments, cartilage and muscle. The MRI may be done with an arthrogram. A special dye is injected into the shoulder to outline the structures within the joint, and allows a better look at the labrum.

Your doctor may perform an arthroscopy, a surgical procedure in which a small fiberoptic instrument is inserted into your shoulder joint so your doctor can see all the structures in your shoulder. Many times labral tears are finally diagnosed when arthroscopy is performed to look inside the persistently painful or symptomatic shoulder.

What is the treatment?

Large labral tears usually need to be fixed in surgery. The tear in the labrum may be reattached or trimmed away. If there is scar tissue, it may be removed. Torn ligaments may be re-attached.

Small labral tears may become painless by avoiding uncomfortable activities. Initially you will be treated by:

- applying ice packs to your shoulder for 20-30 minutes 3 to 4 times a day
- taking anti-inflammatory medications such as ibuprofen
- doing shoulder rehabilitation exercises

When can I return to my sport or activity?

The goal of rehabilitation is to return you to your sport or

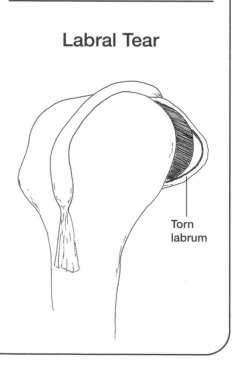

Labral Tear

Torn labrum

Labral Tear

activity as soon as is safely possible. If you return too soon, you may worsen your injury, which could lead to permanent damage. Everyone recovers from injury at a different rate. Return to your sport or activity is determined by how soon your shoulder recovers, not by how many days or weeks it has been since your injury occurred.

You may safely return to your sport or activity when:

your injured shoulder has full range of motion without pain your injured shoulder has regained normal strength compared to the uninjured shoulder.

In throwing sports, you must gradually build your tolerance to throwing. This means you should start with gently tossing and gradually throw harder. In contact sports, your shoulder must not be tender to touch and contact should progress from minimal contact to harder contact.

How can I prevent a labral tear?

Many labral tears are caused by accidents that cannot be prevented. However, it is important to use good form while throwing, playing racquet sports or lifting heavy objects.

Lateral Epicondylitis
(Tennis Elbow)

What is lateral epicondylitis (tennis elbow)?

Lateral epicondylitis (tennis elbow) is the name for a condition in which the bony bump at the outer side of the elbow is painful and tender.

The elbow joint is made up of the bone in the upper arm (humerus) and one of the bones in the lower arm (ulna). The bony bumps at the bottom of the humerus are called epicondyles. The bump on the outer side of the elbow, to which certain forearm muscles are attached by tendons, is called the lateral epicondyle.

Lateral epicondylitis is also referred to as wrist extensor tendonitis.

How does it occur?

Tennis elbow results from overusing the muscles in your forearm that straighten and raise your hand and wrist. When these muscles are overused, the tendons are repeatedly tugged at the point of attachment (the lateral epicondyle). As a result, the tendons become inflamed. Repeated, tiny tears in the tendon tissue cause pain. Among the activities that can cause tennis elbow are tennis and other racquet sports, carpen-

try, machine work, typing, and knitting.

What are the symptoms?

The symptoms of tennis elbow are:

- pain or tenderness on the outer side of the elbow
- pain when you straighten or raise your wrist and hand
- pain made worse by lifting a heavy object
- pain when you make a fist, grip an object, shake hands, or turn door handles
- pain that shoots from the elbow down into the forearm or up into the upper arm.

How is it diagnosed?

Your doctor will ask you about your daily and recreational activities. He or she will examine your elbow and arm and will have you do movements that may cause pain in the outer part of your elbow. Your doctor may order x-rays of the elbow.

How is it treated?

Treatment includes the following:

- Put an ice pack on your elbow for 20 to 30 minutes every 3 to 4 hours for 2 to 3 days or until the pain goes away.

Lateral Epicondylitis (Tennis Elbow)

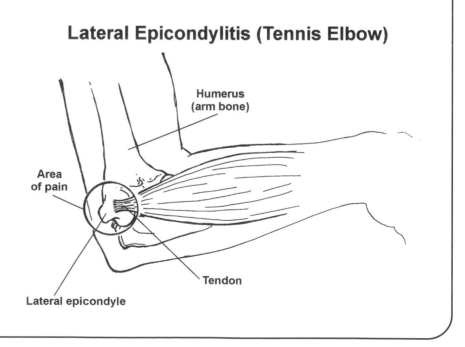

Humerus (arm bone)

Area of pain

Tendon

Lateral epicondyle

Lateral Epicondylitis (Tennis Elbow)

- You can also do ice massage. Massage your elbow with ice by freezing water in a Styrofoam cup. Peel the top of the cup away to expose the ice and hold onto the bottom of the cup while you rub the ice over your elbow for 5 to 10 minutes.
- Do the exercises recommended by your doctor.

Your doctor may recommend that you:

- Take anti-inflammatory medication, such as ibuprofen, for 4 to 6 weeks.
- Wear a tennis elbow strap. This strap wraps around the forearm below the elbow, acting as a new attachment site for the forearm muscles and keeping them from pulling on the painful epicondyle.

While you are recovering from your injury you will need to avoid repetitive motion of the elbow and to change your sport or activity to one that does not make your condition worse. For example, you may need to run instead of play tennis. If you play tennis, your doctor may advise you to use a tennis racquet with a larger grip. He or she may suggest improvements in the way you hold or swing your racquet.

If ice, rest, anti-inflammatory medication, and an elbow strap do not relieve your symptoms, you may need physical therapy. Also, your doctor may recommend an injection of a corticosteroid medication around the lateral epicondyle to reduce the inflammation. In severe cases, surgery may be recommended.

When can I return to my sport or activity?

The goal of rehabilitation is to return you to your sport or activity as soon as is safely possible. If you return too soon you may worsen your injury, which could lead to permanent damage. Everyone recovers from injury at a different rate. Return to your sport or activity will be determined by how soon your elbow recovers, not by how many days or weeks it has been since your injury occurred. In general, the longer you have symptoms before you start treatment, the longer it will take to get better.

You may return to your sport or activity when your are able to forcefully grip your tennis racquet, bat, or golf club, or do activities such as working at a keyboard without pain in your elbow. In sports such as gymnastics, it is important that you are able to bear weight on your elbow painlessly. It is important that there is no swelling around your injured elbow and that it has regained its normal strength compared to your uninjured elbow. You must have full range of motion of your elbow.

How can I prevent tennis elbow?

To prevent tennis elbow:

- Use proper form during your activities, whether they are sports or job-related. For instance, be sure your tennis stroke is correct and that your tennis racquet has the proper grip size.
- Warm up before playing tennis or doing other activities that involve your elbow or arm muscles. Gently stretch your elbow and arm muscles before and after exercise.
- Ice your elbow after exercise or work.
- In job-related activities, be sure your posture is correct and that the position of your arms during your work doesn't cause overuse of your elbow or arm muscles.

Lateral Epicondylitis (Tennis Elbow) Rehabilitation Exercises

You may do stretching exercises 1 through 3 right away. You may do strengthening exercises 4 through 6 when stretching is nearly painless.

1. Wrist range of motion: Bend your wrist forward and backward as far as you can. Repeat 10 times. Do 3 sets.

2. Forearm range of motion: With your elbow at your side and bent 90 degrees, bring your palm facing up and hold for 5 seconds then slowly turn your palm facing down and hold for 5 seconds. Repeat 10 times. Do 3 sets. Make sure you keep your elbow bent at 90 degrees throughout this exercise.

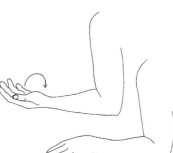

Wrist range of motion

3. Elbow range of motion: Gently bring your palm up toward your shoulder and bend your elbow as far as you can. Then straighten your elbow out as far as you can. Repeat 10 times. Do 3 sets.

4. Wrist strengthening:

   A. Wrist flexion: Holding a soup can or hammer handle with your palm up, slowly bend your wrist up. Slowly lower the weight and return to the starting position. Repeat 10 times. Do 3 sets. Gradually increase the weight of the can you are holding.

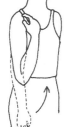

Elbow range of motion

Forearm range of motion

B. Wrist extension: Holding a soup can or hammer handle with your palm down, gently bend your wrist up. Slowly lower the weight and return to the starting position. Repeat 10 times. Do 3 sets. Gradually increase the weight of the can you are holding.

C. Wrist radial deviation: Hold your wrist in the sideways position with your thumb up. Holding a can of soup or hammer handle, gently bend your wrist up with your thumb reaching towards the ceiling. Slowly lower to the starting position. Do not move your forearm throughout this exercise. Repeat 10 times. Do 3 sets.

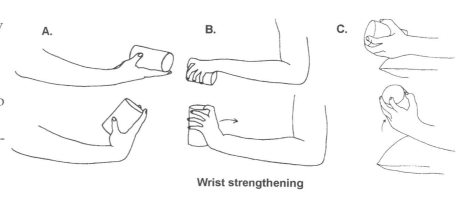

Wrist strengthening

Lateral Epicondylitis (Tennis Elbow) Rehabilitation Exercises

5. Pronation and supination: Hold a soup can or hammer handle in your hand, with your elbow bent 90 degrees. Slowly rotate your hand with palm upward and then palm down. Repeat 10 times. Do 3 sets.

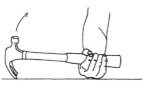

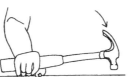

Pronation and supination

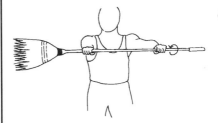

Wrist extension

6. Wrist extension: Stand up and hold a broom handle in both hands. With your arms at shoulder level, elbows straight and palms down, roll the broom handle backward in your hand as if you are reeling something in using the broom handle. Repeat for 1 minute and then rest. Do 3 sets.

Medial Apophysitis
(Little Leaguer's Elbow)

What is medial apophysitis (Little Leaguer's elbow)?

Little Leaguer's elbow is pain on the side of the elbow that is closest to the body.

The elbow joint is made up of the bone in the upper arm (humerus) and one of the bones in the lower arm (ulna). The bony bumps at the end of the humerus are called epicondyles. The bump closest to the body is called the medial epicondyle, and the bump on the outer side of the elbow is called the lateral epicondyle.

The muscles that work to bend the wrist attach at the medial epicondyle, and the muscles that work to straighten the wrist attach at the lateral epicondyle. Too much bending of the wrist will irritate the muscles that attach to the medial epicondyle.

In a child, the bones grow from areas called growth plates. There is a growth plate at the medial epicondyle called the medial apophysis. In Little Leaguer's elbow this growth plate is irritated or inflamed.

How does it occur?

Little Leaguer's elbow is caused by too much throwing. Too much throwing puts stress on the muscles that bend the wrist where they attach to the inner side of the elbow. The growth plate becomes inflamed. In severe cases, the growth plate may actually break way from the upper arm.

What are the symptoms?

Little Leaguer's elbow causes pain at the inner side of the elbow. There may be swelling and tenderness.

How is it diagnosed?

Your doctor will examine your child's arm and elbow. There will be tenderness along the medial epicondyle. Your child will feel pain when he or she throws a ball for the doctor. X-rays may show irritation or a break in the growth plate.

How is it treated?

The most important treatment for Little Leaguer's elbow is to not throw if the growth plate is inflamed. Ice packs should be placed on the elbow for 20 to 30 minutes every 3 to 4

Medial Apophysitis (Little Leaguer's Elbow)

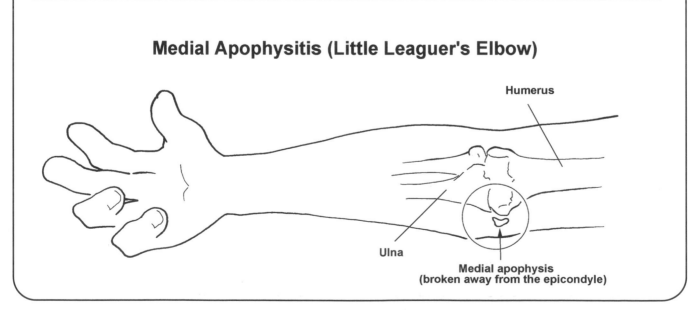

Humerus

Ulna

Medial apophysis
(broken away from the epicondyle)

Medial Apophysitis (Little Leaguer's Elbow)

hours for 2 to 3 days or until the pain goes away. An elastic elbow wrap may be placed on the inflamed elbow to give it more support. The doctor may give your child an anti-inflammatory medication. Your child will be given rehabilitation exercises. In severe cases of Little Leaguer's elbow where there is a break in the bone, surgery may be needed.

When can my child return to his or her sport or activity?

The goal of rehabilitation is to return your child to his or her sport or activity as soon as is safely possible. If your child returns too soon the injury may be worsened, which could lead to permanent dam-

age. Everyone recovers from injury at a different rate. Return to your child's sport or activity will be determined by how soon the elbow recovers, not by how many days or weeks it has been since your child's injury occurred. In general, the longer your child has symptoms before starting treatment, the longer it takes to get better.

Your child may begin throwing when there is no swelling around the injured elbow and it has regained its normal strength compared to the uninjured elbow. Your child must have full range of motion of the elbow. Throwing should be gradually increased but stopped if the elbow becomes painful.

How can Little Leaguer's elbow be prevented?

The best way to prevent Little Leaguer's elbow is to limit the amount of throwing a child does. Since this problem occurs the most in pitchers, there are guidelines for how many pitches or innings a child can throw in a week. In general, a child ages 9 through 12 years old should pitch a maximum of 6 innings per week (and no more than 250 pitches). A youngster ages 13 through 15 should pitch a maximum of 9 innings per week (and no more than 350 pitches).

Medial Apophysitis (Little Leaguer's Elbow)
Rehabilitation Exercises

You may do stretching exercises 1 through 3 right away. You may do strengthening exercises 4 through 6 when stretching is painless.

1. Wrist range of motion: Bend your wrist forward and backward as far as you can. Repeat 10 times. Do 3 sets.

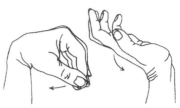

Wrist range of motion

2. Forearm range of motion: With your elbow at your side and bent 90 degrees, bring your palm face up and hold for 5 seconds, then slowly turn your palm face down and hold for 5 seconds. Repeat 10 times. Do 3 sets. Make sure you keep your elbow bent at 90 degrees throughout this exercise.

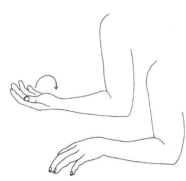

Forearm range of motion

3. Elbow range of motion: Gently bring your palm up toward your shoulder and bend your elbow as far as you can. Then straighten your elbow as far as you can 10 times. Do 3 sets.

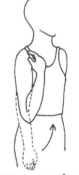

Elbow range of motion

4. Wrist strengthening:

   A. Wrist flexion: Hold a soup can or hammer handle with your palm up. Slowly bend your wrist up. Slowly lower the weight and return to the starting position. Repeat 10 times. Do 3 sets. Gradually increase the weight of the can you are holding.

   B. Wrist extension: Hold a soup can or hammer handle with your palm down. Gently bend your wrist up. Slowly lower the weight and return to the starting position. Repeat 10 times. Do 3 sets. Gradually increase the weight of the can you are holding.

   C. Wrist radial deviation strengthening: Put your wrist in the sideways position with your thumb up. Hold a can of soup or hammer handle and gently bend your wrist up with the thumb reaching toward the ceiling. Slowly lower to the starting position. Do not move your forearm throughout this exercise. Repeat 10 times. Do 3 sets.

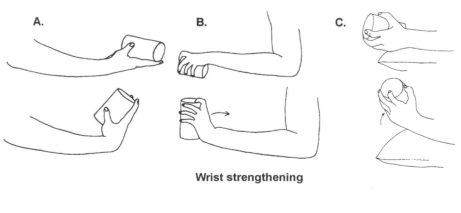

Wrist strengthening

Medial Apophysitis (Little Leaguer's Elbow) Rehabilitation Exercises

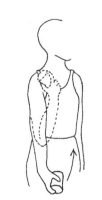

Elbow flexion and extension

5. Pronation and supination strengthening: Hold a soup can or hammer handle in your hand and bend your elbow 90 degrees. Slowly rotate your hand with palm upward and then palm down. Repeat 10 times. Do 3 sets.

6. Elbow flexion and extension: Hold a can of soup with your palm face up. Slowly bend your elbow so that your hand is approaching your shoulder. Then lower it slowly so your elbow is completely straight. Repeat 10 times. Do 3 sets. Slowly increase the weight you are using.

Pronation and supination

Medial Epicondylitis
(Golfer's Elbow)

What is medial epicondylitis (golfer's elbow)?

Medial epicondylitis (golfer's elbow) is a painful inflammation of the bony bump on the inner side of the elbow. The elbow joint is made up of the bone in the upper arm (humerus) and one of the bones in the lower arm (ulna). The bony bumps at the bottom of the humerus are called the epicondyles. The bump on the side closest to the body is called the medial epicondyle, and the bump on the outer side of the elbow is called the lateral epicondyle.

The tendons of the muscles that work to bend your wrist attach at the medial epi-condyle. Medial epicondylitis is also referred to as wrist flex-or tendonitis.

How does it occur?

Medial epicondylitis occurs from overuse of the muscles that enable you to bend your fingers and wrist. When these muscles are overused, the tendons are repeatedly tugged at their point of attachment (the medial epicondyle). As a result, the tendons become inflamed (tendonitis), and repeated, tiny tears in the tendon tissue cause pain. This commonly happens in sports such as golf, in throwing sports, and in racquet sports. It also may happen in occupational activities like carpentry or typing.

What are the symptoms?

Medial epicondylitis causes pain in the elbow at the side closest to the body. You may also have pain along the entire inner side of the forearm when the wrist is bent. You may have pain when you make a fist.

How is it diagnosed?

Your doctor will examine your elbow and find tenderness at the medial epicondyle.

How is it treated?

You should apply ice packs to your elbow for 20 to 30 minutes every 3 to 4 hours for 2 or 3 days or until the pain goes away.

Medial Epicondylitis (Golfer's Elbow)

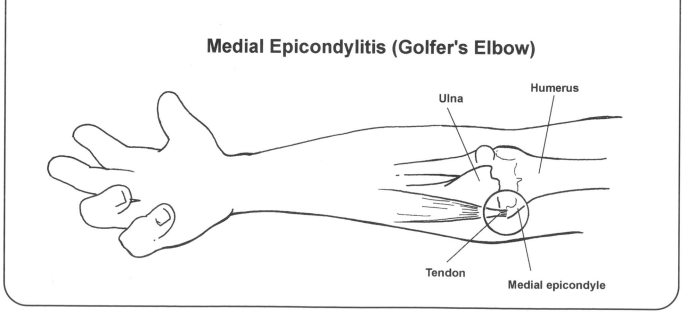

Medial Epicondylitis (Golfer's Elbow)

If your elbow is swollen, you should elevate it by placing a pillow underneath it when you are lying down and by elevating it on the back of a chair or couch while sitting. You may be given an elastic bandage to wrap around your elbow to keep it from swelling.

While you are recovering from your injury, you will need to change your sport or activity to one that does not make your condition worse. For example, instead of playing golf you should walk or write things out by hand instead of typing.

Your doctor may prescribe a tennis elbow strap for you to wear just below the tender spot on your elbow. This will allow the forearm muscles to pull against the strap instead of against the painful epicondyle. Your doctor may prescribe an anti-inflammatory medication. Your doctor may give you an injection of an corticosteroid medication around the medial epicondyle to reduce the inflammation. You will be given elbow exercises. In severe cases of medial epicondylitis surgery may need to be done.

When can I return to my sport or activity?

The goal of rehabilitation is to return you to your sport or activity as soon as is safely possible. If you return too soon you may worsen your injury, which could lead to permanent damage. Everyone recovers from injury at a different rate. Return to your sport or activity will be determined by how soon your elbow recovers, not by how many days or weeks it has been since your injury occurred. In general, the longer you have symptoms before you start treatment, the longer it will take to get better.

You may return when your are able to forcefully grip your tennis racquet, bat, or golf club, or do activities such as working at a keyboard without pain in your elbow. In sports such as gymnastics, it is important that you are able to bear weight on your elbow painlessly. It is important that there is no swelling around your injured elbow and that it has regained its normal strength compared to the uninjured elbow. You must have full range of motion of your elbow.

How can I prevent medial epicondylitis?

Since medial epicondylitis occurs because of overuse to the muscles that bend your wrist, it is important that you do not allow this overactivity to occur. At the earliest signs of pain on the inner side of your elbow, you should slow your activity down and seek treatment. Wearing a tennis elbow strap and doing elbow stretching exercises will help prevent medial epicondylitis.

Medial Epicondylitis (Golfer's Elbow) ─── *Rehabilitation Exercises*

You may do stretching exercises 1 through 3 right away. You may do strengthening exercises 4 through 6 when stretching is nearly painless.

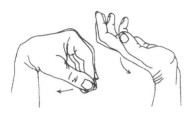

Wrist range of motion

1. Wrist range of motion: Bend your wrist forward and backward as far as you can. Do this 10 times. Do 3 sets.

2. Forearm range of motion: With your elbow at your side and bent 90 degrees, bring your palm facing up and hold for 5 seconds. Slowly turn your palm facing down and hold for 5 seconds. Repeat this 10 times. Do 3 sets. Make sure you keep your elbow bent at 90 degrees throughout this exercise.

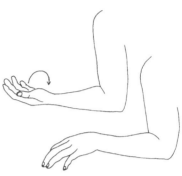

Forearm range of motion

3. Elbow range of motion: Gently bring your palm up toward your shoulder and bend your elbow as far as you can and then straighten your elbow out as far as you can 10 times. Do 3 sets.

4. Wrist strengthening:

   A. Wrist flexion: Hold a soup can or hammer handle with your palm up. Slowly bend your wrist up. Slowly lower the weight and return to the starting position. Repeat this 10 times. Do 3 sets. Gradually increase the weight of the can you are holding.

   B. Wrist extension: Hold a soup can or hammer handle with the palm down. Gently bend your wrist up. Slowly lower the weight and return to the starting position. Repeat this 10 times. Do 3 sets. Gradually increase the weight of the can you are holding.

   C. Wrist radial deviation strengthening: With your wrist in the sideways position and your thumb up, hold a can of soup or hammer handle. Gently bend your wrist up with your thumb reaching towards the ceiling. Slowly lower to the starting position. Do not move your forearm throughout this exercise. Repeat 10 times. Do 3 sets.

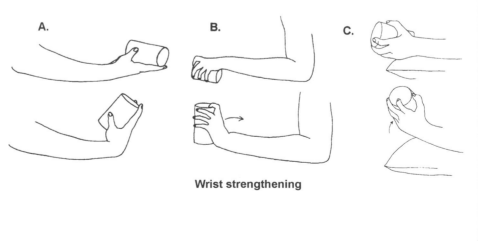

Wrist strengthening

Medial Epicondylitis (Golfer's Elbow) — Rehabilitation Exercises

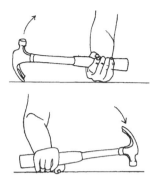

Pronation and supination

5. Pronation and supination strengthening: Hold a soup can or hammer handle, with your elbow bent 90 degrees. Slowly rotate your hand with palm upward and then palm down. Repeat this 10 times. Do 3 sets.

6. Elbow flexion and extension: Hold a can of soup with your palm face up. Slowly bend your elbow so that your hand is approaching your shoulder and then lower it down slowly so your elbow is completely straight. Repeat this 10 times. Do 3 sets. Slowly increase the weight are using.

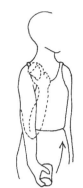

Elbow flexion and extension

— Elbow (Olecranon) Bursitis —

What is elbow (olecranon) bursitis?

A bursa is a fluid-filled sac that acts as a cushion between tendons, bones, and skin. Irritation or inflammation of a bursa is called bursitis. Olecranon bursitis causes pain at the point of the elbow.

How does it occur?

Repeated injury, such as falling onto the elbow or rubbing the elbow against a hard surface, causes irritation to the bursa.

What are the symptoms?

The bursa at the point of the elbow will be swollen. This swelling may or may not be painful. It may hurt to bend and straighten your elbow. There may be warmth and redness. Sometimes the fluid inside the bursa can become infected.

How is it diagnosed?

The doctor will examine your elbow.

How is it treated?

Treatment may include:

- putting ice packs on your elbow for 20 to 30 minutes every 3 to 4 hours for 2 to 3 days or until the pain and swelling go away

- wrapping an elastic bandage around your elbow to keep the bursa from swelling more
- removal of some of the bursa fluid by your doctor with a needle and syringe
- taking anti-inflammatory medication
- protecting your elbow with a pad.

In some cases, problems with longstanding (chronic) olecranon bursitis may require surgical removal of the bursa.

When can I return to my sport or activity?

The goal of rehabilitation is to return you to your sport or activity as soon as is safely possible. If you return too soon you may worsen your injury, which could lead to permanent damage. Everyone recovers from injury at a different rate. Return to your sport will be determined by how soon your elbow recovers, not by how many days or weeks it has been since your injury occurred. In general, the longer you have symptoms before you start treatment, the longer it will take to get better.

You may return to your sport or activity when your are able to forcefully grip your tennis racquet, bat, or golf club, or do activities such as working at a keyboard without pain at your elbow. In sports such as gymnastics, you

Elbow (Olecranon) Bursitis

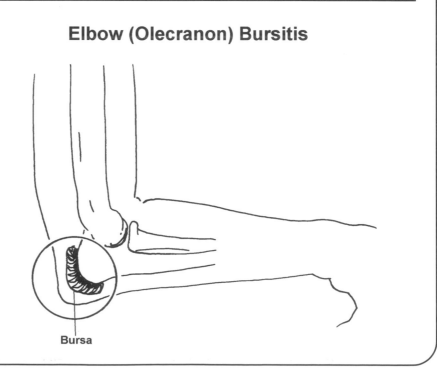

Bursa

Elbow (Olecranon) Bursitis

should be able to bear weight on your elbow painlessly. You should have no swelling around your injured elbow and it should have regained its normal strength compared to your uninjured elbow. You must have full range of motion of your elbow.

How can I prevent olecranon bursitis?

Olecranon bursitis can be best prevented by avoiding direct contact to the point of your elbow. It is important not to irritate the bursa by leaning your elbow onto a surface such as a table or a desk.

Osteochondritis Dissecans (Bone Chips) of the Elbow

What is osteochondritis dissecans of the elbow?

Osteochondritis dissecans of the elbow is a disorder in which fragments of bone or cartilage come loose and float around in the elbow joint. Cartilage is tough, smooth tissue that lines and cushions the surface of the joints. These chips usually come from the upper arm bone (humerus).

How does it occur?

The chips usually result from a forceful injury to the elbow joint. It is also seen in the elbows of throwing athletes and gymnasts.

What are the symptoms?

It hurts when you move your elbow. Your elbow may click or lock or you may feel a bone chip inside the joint. Your elbow may be swollen and you may not be able to completely straighten your arm.

How is it diagnosed?

Your doctor will review your symptoms and examine your elbow. Your doctor may do an x-ray, which may show a bone chip or an abnormal joint surface.

How is it treated?

The treatment for osteochondritis dissecans is to rest your elbow until the symptoms are gone. This may take up to a few weeks. You should apply ice to the elbow for 20 to 30 minutes every 3 to 4 hours for 2 to 3 days or until the pain and swelling go away. Your doctor may prescribe an anti-inflammatory medication or other pain medication. Small bone chips that do not affect elbow motion and do not cause further pain do not need to be removed. Surgery may be needed to remove a large bone chip.

When can I return to my sport or activity?

The goal of rehabilitation is to return you to your sport or activity as soon as is safely possible. If you return too soon you may worsen your injury, which could lead to permanent damage. Everyone recovers from injury at a different rate. Return to your sport or activity will be determined by how soon your elbow recovers, not by how

Osteochondritis Dissecans of the Elbow

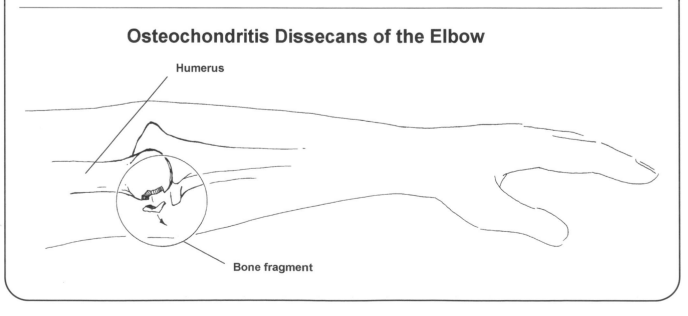

Humerus

Bone fragment

Osteochondritis Dissecans (Bone Chips) of the Elbow

many days or weeks it has been since your injury occurred. In general, the longer you have symptoms before you start treatment, the longer it will take to get better.

You may return to your sport or activity when your are able to forcefully grip your tennis racquet, bat, or golf club, or do activities such as working at a keyboard without pain at your elbow. In sports such as gymnastics, you should be able to bear weight on your elbow painlessly. There should be no swelling around your injured elbow and it should have regained its normal strength compared to your uninjured elbow. You must have full range of motion of your elbow.

How can I prevent osteochondritis dissecans of the elbow?

Osteochondritis dissecans is usually caused by trauma to the elbow and is not preventable.

Rhomboid Muscle Strain or Spasm

What is a rhomboid muscle strain or spasm?

Your rhomboid muscles are in your upper back, connecting the inner edges of your shoulder blades to your spine. A strain is an injury in which muscle fibers or tendons are stretched or torn. A muscle spasm is an involuntary contraction of the muscle.

How does it occur?

A rhomboid muscle strain or spasm usually occurs as a result of overusing your shoulder and arm, especially during overhead activities like serving a tennis ball or reaching to put objects on a high shelf. It can also occur from activities such as rowing.

What are the symptoms?

A rhomboid strain causes pain in your upper back between your shoulder blades and your spine. A spasm feels like a knot or tightness in the muscle. You may have pain when you move your shoulders or when you breathe.

How is it diagnosed?

Your doctor will examine your back and shoulder and will find that these muscles are tender or tight.

How is it treated?

The injury should initially be treated with ice packs for 20 to 30 minutes every 3 to 4 hours for 2 to 3 days or until the pain goes away. You can place crushed ice (in a plastic bag) or a frozen gel pack on the floor, put a towel over the bag or gel pack, and then lie down with your rhomboid muscles against the ice. Your doctor may prescribe an anti-inflammatory medication.

Massage is also very helpful. You can do a form of self-massage by putting a tennis ball on the floor, lying down with your rhomboid muscles against the ball, and gently rolling the ball against your rhomboid muscles.

You will be given a set of rehabilitation exercises to help you return to your sport or activity. While you are recovering from your injury you will need to change your sport or activity to one that does not make your condition worse. For example, you may need to run or bicycle instead of playing tennis or rowing.

When can I return to my sport or activity?

The goal of rehabilitation is to return you to your sport or

Rhomboid Muscle Strain/Spasm

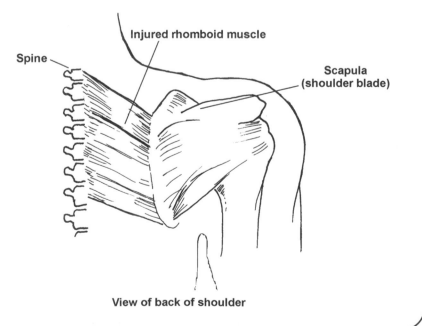

Injured rhomboid muscle

Spine

Scapula (shoulder blade)

View of back of shoulder

Rhomboid Muscle Strain or Spasm

activity as soon as is safely possible. If you return too soon you may worsen your injury, which could lead to permanent damage. Everyone recovers from injury at a different rate. Return to your sport or activity will be determined by how soon your back recovers, not by how many days or weeks it has been since your injury occurred. In general, the longer you have symptoms before you start treatment, the longer it will take to get better.

You may safely return to your sport or activity when the muscles are no longer in spasm and you can move your shoulders and arms without pain.

How can I prevent a rhomboid muscle strain or spasm?

Rhomboid strains and spasms are best prevented by warming up properly and doing stretching exercises before activities such as tennis, rowing, or overhead movements.

Rhomboid Muscle Strain or Spasm
Rehabilitation Exercises

You may do all of these exercises right away.

1. Reach and pull stretch: Stand and clasp your hands in front of you at chest height. Drop your head down, stretching the back of your neck. Reach forward with your arms, stretching your upper back. Hold this position for 10 seconds. Repeat 5 times.

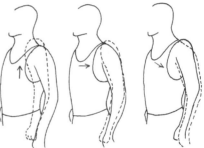

Reach and pull stretch

2. Pec stretch: Stand in a corner about 3 feet away from the corner. Place one hand on each wall at about shoulder height. Lean your chest forward, stretching the front of your chest. Hold this position for 30 seconds. Repeat 3 times.

3. Scapular box: Stand and shrug your shoulders up and hold 5 seconds. Then squeeze your shoulder blades back and together and hold 5 seconds. Next, pull your shoulder blades downward as if putting them in your back pocket. Relax. Repeat this sequence 10 times.

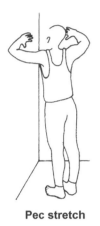

Pec stretch

Scapular box

4. Scapular retraction using Thera-Band: Take a 5-foot section of tubing and tie a knot in the center of it. Shut the knot in a door at about shoulder height. Standing about 3 feet away from the door, take one end of the tubing in each hand. Move your hands up to shoulder level, with your elbows, hands, and shoulders at the same height and parallel to the floor. Squeeze your shoulder blades back and together, and pull your elbows straight back, stretching the tubing for resistance. Hold 5 seconds. Return to the starting position and relax. Repeat 10 times. Do 3 sets.

Scapular retraction using tubing

5. Rhomboid stretch: Stand near a door frame. Lift the arm of your injured rhomboid straight out in front of you and grasp the door frame. Lean back, letting the pull of your body weight stretch your rhomboid muscle. Hold for a count of 10, repeat 5 times.

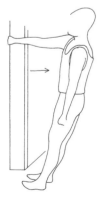

Rhomboid stretch

Rotator Cuff Injury

What is a rotator cuff injury?

A rotator cuff injury is a strain or tear in the group of tendons and muscles that hold your shoulder joint together and help move your shoulder.

How does it occur?

A rotator cuff injury may result from:

- using your arm to break a fall
- falling onto your arm
- lifting a heavy object
- use of your shoulder in sports with a repetitive overhead movement, such as swimming, baseball (mainly pitchers), football, and tennis, which gradually strains the tendon
- manual labor such as painting, plastering, raking leaves, or housework.

What are the symptoms?

The symptoms of a torn rotator cuff are:
- arm and shoulder pain
- shoulder weakness
- shoulder tenderness
- loss of shoulder movement, especially overhead.

How is it diagnosed?

Your doctor will perform a physical exam and check your shoulder for pain, tenderness, and loss of motion as you move your arm in all directions. Your doctor also will ask whether your shoulder pain began suddenly or gradually. An x-ray may be done to rule out fractures and bone spurs. Based on these results, your doctor may order other tests and procedures either right away or later, including:

- an arthrogram, which is an x-ray that is taken after a special dye has been injected into your shoulder joint to outline its soft structures
- magnetic resonance imaging (MRI), which creates images of your shoulder and surrounding structures with sound waves
- arthroscopy, a surgical procedure in which a small instrument is inserted into your shoulder joint so your doctor can look directly at your rotator cuff.

What is the treatment?

A tendon in your shoulder can be inflamed, partially torn, or completely torn. What is done about it depends on how torn it is and how much it hurts.

If your tear is a minor one, it can be left to heal by itself if

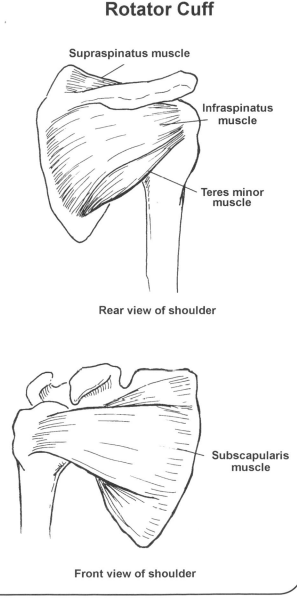

Rotator Cuff

Supraspinatus muscle

Infraspinatus muscle

Teres minor muscle

Rear view of shoulder

Subscapularis muscle

Front view of shoulder

Rotator Cuff Injury

it doesn't interfere with your everyday activities. Your treatment plan should include:

- proper sitting posture, in which your head and shoulders are balanced
- rest for your shoulder, which means avoiding strenuous activity and any overhead motion that causes pain
- ice packs at least once a day, and preferably two or three times a day
- doing the exercises your doctor gives you
- anti-inflammatory drugs
- physical therapy to strengthen your shoulder as it heals.

If you have a bad tear, you may need to have it repaired by arthroscopy. Arthroscopy is also used to perform surgery on a joint, not only for seeing its interior. The rough edges of a torn tendon can be trimmed and left to heal. Larger tears can be stitched back together. After surgery, your treatment

plan will include physical therapy to strengthen your shoulder as it heals.

How long will the effects of a torn rotator cuff last?

Full recovery depends on what is torn and how it is treated.

When can I return to my sport or activity?

The goal of rehabilitation is to return you to your sport or activity as soon as is safely possible. If you return too soon you may worsen your injury, which could lead to permanent damage. Everyone recovers from injury at a different rate. Return to your sport or activity will be determined by how soon your shoulder recovers, not by how many days or weeks it has been since your injury occurred. In general, the longer you have symptoms before you start treatment, the

longer it takes to get better.
You may safely return to your sport or activity when:

- Your injured shoulder has full range of motion without pain.
- Your injured shoulder has regained normal strength compared to the uninjured shoulder.

In throwing sports, you must gradually build your tolerance to throwing. This means you should start with gentle tossing and gradually throw harder. In contact sports, your shoulder must not be tender to touch and contact should progress from minimal contact to harder contact.

What can be done to help prevent this from recurring?

The best way to prevent a recurrence is to strengthen your shoulder muscles and keep them in peak condition with shoulder exercises.

Rotator Cuff Strain Rehabilitation Exercises

You may do all of these exercises right away.

1. Scapular range of motion: Shrug your shoulders up. Then squeeze your shoulder blades together. Then relax your shoulder blades down. Hold each position 5 seconds. Repeat 10 times. Do 3 sets.

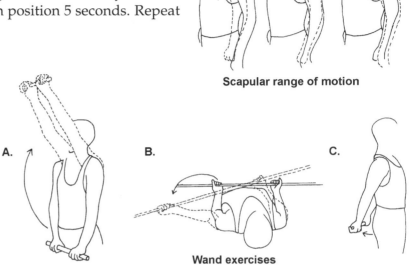

Scapular range of motion

2. Wand exercises
   A. Shoulder flexion: Stand upright and hold a stick in both hands. Stretch your arms by lifting them over your head, keeping your elbows straight. Do not raise them past the point of pain. Hold that position for 5 seconds. Return to the starting position. Repeat 10 times.

Wand exercises

   B. Shoulder external rotation: Lie on your back and hold a stick in both hands with palms up. Your upper arms should be resting on the floor and your elbows at your sides, bent 90 degrees. Using your good arm, push your injured arm out away from your body while keeping the elbow of your injured side at your side. Hold this stretch for 5 seconds. Return to the starting position. Repeat 10 times.

   C. Shoulder extension: Stand upright holding a stick in both hands behind your back. Move the stick away from your back. Hold the end position for 5 seconds and then relax and return to the starting position. Repeat 10 times.

3. Isometrics
   A. External rotation: Standing in a doorway with your elbow bent 90 degrees and the back of your hand pressing against the door frame, attempt to press your hand outward into the door frame. Hold for 5 seconds. Repeat 10 times.

   B. Internal rotation: Standing in a doorway with your elbow bent 90 degrees and the front of your hand pressing against the door frame, attempt to press your palm into the door frame. Hold for 5 seconds. Rest. Repeat 10 times.

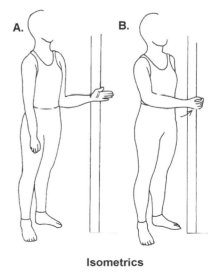

Isometrics

Rotator Cuff Strain Rehabilitation Exercises

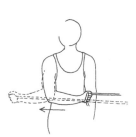

Tubing exercise for external rotation

4. Tubing exercise for external rotation: Stand resting the hand of your injured side against your stomach. With that hand grasp tubing that is connected to a doorknob or other object at waist level. Keeping your elbow in at your side, rotate your arm outward and away from your waist. Make sure you keep your elbow bent 90 degrees and your forearm parallel to the floor. Repeat 10 times. Build up to 3 sets of 10.

5. Supraspinatus exercise: Standing with your arms at your sides and your thumbs pointed toward the floor, lean your trunk forward slightly. Lift your arms up and out from your sides, keeping your elbows straight. Lift your hands only to shoulder level. Hold 5 seconds. Repeat 10 times. Do 3 sets. Gradually add weight to your hands to increase your strength.

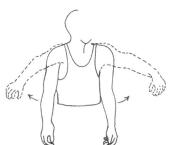

Supraspinatus exercise

Shoulder Bursitis

What is shoulder bursitis?

Shoulder bursitis is an irritation or inflammation of the bursa in your shoulder. A bursa is a fluid-filled sac that acts as a cushion between tendons, bones, and skin.

How does it occur?

The shoulder bursa can become inflamed from repetitive motion of the shoulder. It frequently occurs in sports with overhead activities such as swimming, tennis, or throwing. It may also occur in occupational activities like painting or carpentry.

What are the symptoms?

You have pain on the outer front side of your shoulder. Your shoulder may hurt when you lift your arm above your head. The outer side of your shoulder may become swollen and may at times be warm.

How is it diagnosed?

Your doctor will review your symptoms and examine your shoulder.

How is it treated?

Treatment may include:

- ice packs on your shoulder for 20 to 30 minutes every 3 to 4 hours for 2 to 3 days or until the pain goes away

- anti-inflammatory medication or other pain medications

- an injection of a corticosteroid medication into the bursa to reduce the inflammation and pain

- exercises to help in your recovery.

When can I return to my sport or activity?

The goal of rehabilitation is to return you to your sport or activity as soon as is safely possible. If you return too soon you may worsen your injury, which could lead to permanent damage. Everyone recovers from injury at a different rate. Return to your sport or activity will be determined by how soon your shoulder recovers, not by how many days or weeks it has been since your injury occurred. In general, the longer you have symptoms before you start treatment, the

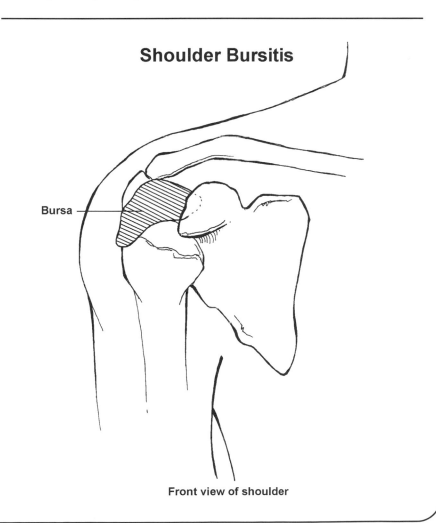

Shoulder Bursitis

Bursa

Front view of shoulder

Shoulder Bursitis

longer it will take to get better. You may safely return to your sport or activity when:

- Your injured shoulder has full range of motion without pain.
- Your injured shoulder has regained normal strength

compared to the uninjured shoulder.

In throwing sports, you must gradually rebuild your tolerance to throwing. This means you should start with gentle tossing and gradually throw harder. In contact sports, your shoulder must not be tender to touch and contact should progress from minimal contact to harder contact.

How can I prevent shoulder bursitis?

Be sure to warm up properly and stretch your shoulder before such activities as throwing, tennis, or swimming. If your shoulder begins to hurt during these activities, you may need to slow down until the pain goes away.

© HBO & Company

Shoulder Bursitis Rehabilitation Exercises

You may do these exercises when your pain has improved.

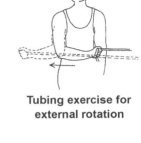

Tubing exercise for external rotation

1. Scapular range of motion: Shrug your shoulders up. Then squeeze your shoulder blades together. Then relax your shoulder blades down. Hold each position 5 seconds. Repeat 10 times. Do 3 sets.

2. Wand exercises

   A. Shoulder flexion: Stand upright and hold a stick in both hands. Stretch your arms by lifting them over your head, keeping your elbows straight. Do not raise them past the point of pain. Hold that position for 5 seconds. Return to the starting position. Repeat 10 times.

   A. **B.** **C.**

   Wand exercises

   B. Shoulder external rotation: Lie on your back and hold a stick in both hands with palms up. Your upper arms should be resting on the floor and your elbows at your sides, bent 90 degrees. Using your good arm, push your injured arm out away from your body while keeping the elbow of your injured side at your side. Hold this stretch for 5 seconds. Return to the starting position. Repeat 10 times.

   C. Shoulder extension: Stand upright holding a stick in both hands behind your back. Move the stick away from your back. Hold the end position for 5 seconds and then relax and return to the starting position. Repeat 10 times.

3. Isometrics

   A. External rotation: Standing in a doorway with your elbow bent 90 degrees and the back of your hand pressing against the door frame, attempt to press your hand outward into the door frame. Hold for 5 seconds. Repeat 10 times.

   B. Internal rotation: Standing in a doorway with your elbow bent 90 degrees and the front of your hand pressing against the door frame, attempt to press your palm into the door frame. Hold for 5 seconds. Repeat 10 times.

   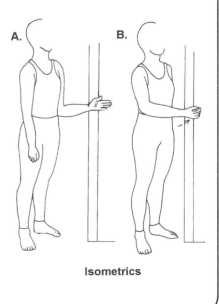

   A. **B.**

   4. Tubing exercise for external rotation: Stand resting the hand of your injured side against your stomach. With that hand grasp tubing that is connected to a doorknob or other object at waist level. Keeping your elbow in at your side, rotate your arm outward and away from your waist. Make sure you keep your elbow bent 90 degrees and your forearm parallel to the floor. Repeat 10 times. Build up to 3 sets of 10.

   Isometrics

Shoulder Bursitis Rehabilitation Exercises

5. Supraspinatus exercise: Standing with your arms at your sides and your thumbs pointed toward the floor, lean your trunk forward slightly. Lift your arms up and out from your sides, keeping your elbows straight. Lift your hands only to shoulder level. Hold 5 seconds. Repeat 10 times. Do 3 sets. Gradually add weight to your hands to increase your strength.

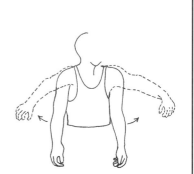

Supraspinatus exercise

Dislocated Shoulder

What is a dislocated shoulder?

A dislocation of the shoulder joint happens when the bones making up your shoulder joint are moved apart so that the joint no longer functions.

Your shoulder is made up of two bones: the ball (the end of the arm bone, or humerus) and the socket (part of your shoulder blade, or scapula). When the ball part of the joint is dislocated in front of the socket, it is called an anterior dislocation. When it is dislocated behind the socket, it is called a posterior dislocation. In severe cases, ligaments, tendons, and nerves also can be stretched and injured.

How does it occur?

The most common type of dislocation is an anterior dislocation. It can be caused by a fall onto your outstretched hand or onto the shoulder itself.

A posterior dislocation may occur as a result of a powerful direct blow to the front of your shoulder. It may also be caused by a violent twisting of your upper arm, such as that caused by an electric shock or seizure.

Dislocated shoulders are common in contact sports such as football, rugby, hockey, and lacrosse. Other sports that may cause the injury include downhill skiing, volleyball, and soccer.

You also may be genetically susceptible to a dislocation, particularly if your shoulder goes out often or easily. Other members of your family may have the same problem.

What are the symptoms?

The main symptom is pain in your shoulder and upper arm that is made worse by movement.

If you have an anterior dislocation, you will find yourself holding your arm on the dislocated side slightly away from your body with your opposite hand. This will keep your dislocated shoulder in the least uncomfortable position. Your shoulder will have a large bump rising up under the skin in front of your shoulder. Your shoulder will look square instead of round.

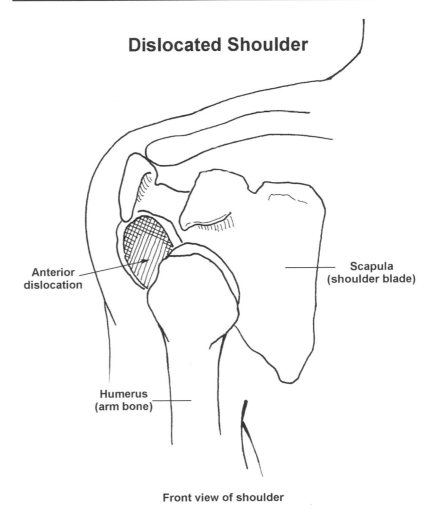

Dislocated Shoulder

Anterior dislocation

Scapula (shoulder blade)

Humerus (arm bone)

Front view of shoulder

Dislocated Shoulder

If you have a posterior dislocation, you will hold your arm on the dislocated side tight against your body. You will have a large bump on the back of your shoulder.

How is it diagnosed?

Your doctor will ask about your medical history, including your symptoms, previous treatment, and family history. During your physical exam, your doctor will check for:

- shoulder tenderness and weakness
- numbness in the shoulder area, arm, or hand
- pain when you move your shoulder or loss of normal shoulder motion
- shoulder instability and deformity.

Your doctor will arrange for an x-ray of the joint and surrounding areas to confirm the dislocation and check for broken bones.

What is the treatment?

You should go to your doctor's office or the hospital emergency room immediately when your shoulder becomes dislocated. Put ice on your shoulder. Cold reduces swelling by controlling internal bleeding and the buildup of fluids in and around the injured area.

Your doctor will reposition the head or ball of the joint back into the joint socket. This can sometimes be done without an anesthetic if it is done within a few minutes after the dislocation occurs. If you have recurrent dislocations, you may be able to learn how to put your shoulder back into place by yourself. However, even in such cases you should see a doctor promptly to make sure the repositioning has been done properly.

Fifteen to thirty minutes after the injury, your dislocated shoulder will probably be quite swollen and painful. You may then need to be given an intravenous (IV) pain medication and muscle relaxant or general anesthesia before the doctor repositions your shoulder. Sometimes local anesthetic can be injected into the joint to help the doctor reposition the bones. After the repositioning, your doctor will have your shoulder x-rayed to make sure it is in the correct position.

Your doctor will place your shoulder and arm in a type of sling called a shoulder immobilizer. It will aid healing by keeping your arm next to your body and stopping you from moving your shoulder. You will keep your shoulder and arm in the immobilizer for 2 to 3 weeks. You may begin shoulder rehabilitation exercises during this time or after you are no longer wearing the immobilizer.

Your doctor may prescribe an anti-inflammatory medication or other pain medicine. You should continue to place ice packs on your shoulder for 20 to 30 minutes every 3 to 4 hours until the pain and swelling are gone.

In some cases, surgery may be needed to get the shoulder repositioned correctly or if it continues to dislocate. If your shoulder joint becomes weak because of repeated dislocations, your doctor may recommend an operation to tighten the ligaments that hold the joint together.

How long will the effects of shoulder dislocation last?

The healing process may take 4 to 12 weeks, depending on the extent of your injury. With proper healing, you should regain full movement of your shoulder.

How can I take care of myself?

Follow your doctor's instructions when you begin to use your arm and shoulder again, or you may reinjure it. Do the rehabilitation exercises that are given to you by your doctor or therapist. Avoid participation in sports until the shoulder has had time to heal.

Dislocated Shoulder

When can I return to my sport or activity?

The goal of rehabilitation is to return you to your sport or activity as soon as is safely possible. If you return too soon you may worsen your injury, which could lead to permanent damage. Everyone recovers from injury at a different rate. Return to your sport will be determined by how soon your shoulder recovers, not by how many days or weeks it has been since your injury occurred.

You may safely return to your sport or activity when:

- Your injured shoulder has full range of motion without pain.
- Your injured shoulder has regained normal strength compared to the uninjured shoulder.

In throwing sports, you must gradually build your tolerance to throwing. This means you should start with gentle tossing and gradually throw harder. In contact sports, your shoulder must not be tender to touch and contact should progress from minimal contact to harder contact.

If you feel your arm popping out of the shoulder joint, contact your doctor.

What can be done to help prevent a dislocated shoulder?

- Avoid situations in which you could suffer another dislocation.
- Wear layers of clothing or padding to help cushion any fall that may be likely.
- Do not return to sports until you have full recovery of motion and strength in the arm.

Dislocated Shoulder Rehabilitation Exercises

Do these exercises as soon as your doctor says you can.

PART I

1. Isometrics:

   A. Adduction: With a pillow between your chest and your arms, squeeze the pillow with your arms and hold 5 seconds. Release and repeat 10 times.

   B. Flexion: Stand facing a wall with your elbow bent at a right angle and held close to your body. Press your fist forward against the wall, hold this for 5 seconds, then rest. Repeat this 10 times.

   C. Extension: Standing facing away from the wall with your elbow touching the wall, press the back of your elbow into the wall and hold for 5 seconds. Rest. Repeat 10 times.

   D. Abduction: Standing with your injured side towards the wall and your elbow bent at a 90-degree angle, press the side of your arm into the wall as if attempting to lift it. Hold for 5 seconds. Rest. Repeat 10 times.

   E. Internal rotation: Standing in a doorway with your elbow bent at a 90-degree angle and your palm resting on the door frame, attempt to press your palms into the door frame and hold 5 seconds. Rest. Repeat 10 times.

   F. External rotation: Standing in a doorway with your elbow bent at a 90-degree angle and the back of your hand pressing against the door frame, attempt to press your hand outward into the door frame. Hold 5 seconds. Rest. Repeat 10 times.

2. Careful range of motion:

   A. Flexion: Standing with your arms straight, raise your arm forward and up over your head. Hold this position for 5 seconds. Return to the starting position and repeat 10 times.

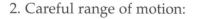

Isometrics

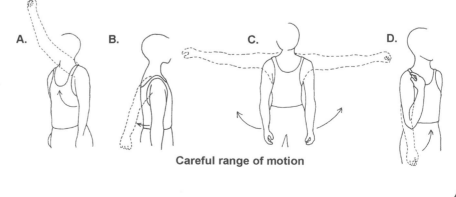

Careful range of motion

Dislocated Shoulder Rehabilitation Exercises

B. Extension: Standing with your arms straight, move your arm backward while keeping your elbow straight. Hold this position for 5 seconds. Repeat 10 times.

C. Abduction: Standing with your arms at your side, slowly raise your arms out away from your body and hold in position for 5 seconds. Return to the starting position. Repeat 10 times.

D. Elbow flexion: Standing, bend your elbow, bring your hand toward your shoulder. Return to starting position. Repeat 10 times. As this becomes easier, add a weight to your hand to give you some resistance.

PART II

3. Tubing exercises:

A. Internal rotation: Using tubing connected to a door knob or other object at waist level, keep your elbow in at your side and rotate your arm inward across your body. Make sure you keep your forearm parallel to the floor. Repeat 10 times. Do 2 sets of 10.

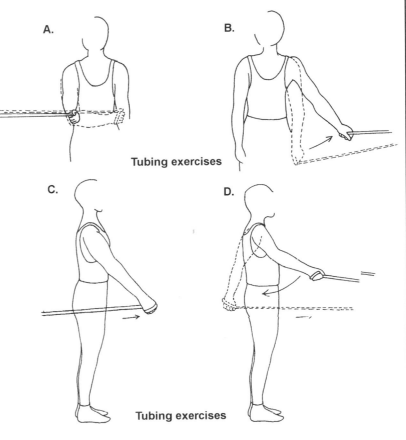

Tubing exercises

Tubing exercises

B. Adduction: Stand sideways with your injured side toward the door and out approximately 8 to 10 inches. Slowly bring your arm next to your body holding onto the tubing for resistance. Repeat 10 times. Do 2 sets of 10.

C. Flexion: Facing away from the door with the tubing connected to the door knob, keep your elbow straight and pull your arm forward. Repeat 10 times. Do 2 sets of 10.

D. Extension: Using the tubing, pull your arm back. Be sure to keep your elbow straight. Repeat 10 times. Do 2 sets of 10.

4. Latissimus dorsi strengthening: Sit on a firm chair. Place your hands on the seat on either side of you. Lift your buttocks off the chair. Hold this position for 5 seconds and then relax. Repeat 10 times. Do 2 sets of 10.

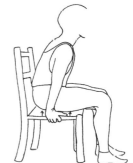

Latissimus dorsi strengthening

© HBO & Company

Shoulder Separation

What is a shoulder separation?

A shoulder separation occurs when you tear the ligaments that hold your collarbone (clavicle) to the joint where it meets the shoulder blade. Your collarbone may move out of its normal place and push up the skin on the top of your shoulder. Another term for shoulder separation is acromioclavicular (AC) separation or sprain.

Shoulder separations, or sprains, are graded I, II, or III, depending on how far the collarbone is separated from the shoulder. A grade I sprain has tenderness but no actual separation. A grade II sprain has slight separation of the clavicle from the shoulder, and grade III has a greater separation.

How does it occur?

A shoulder separation can result from a blow to your shoulder or a fall on your shoulder. It also can result from a fall on your outstretched hand or arm. It is a common injury in contact sports such as football, rugby, hockey, or lacrosse. It may occur from falling onto a hard surface, such as might happen during downhill skiing, volleyball, rock climbing, and soccer.

What are the symptoms?

Symptoms include the following:
- severe pain at the moment the injury occurs
- limited shoulder movement and tenderness on top of your shoulder at the end of your collarbone
- swelling and bruising of your shoulder area
- a misshapen shoulder.

How is it diagnosed?

Your doctor will examine your shoulder for tenderness and a bump over the tip of your collarbone.

To make sure it is an AC separation and not a fracture, x-rays are necessary.

How is it treated?

Immediately after your injury put an ice pack on your shoulder for 20 to 30 minutes. Con-

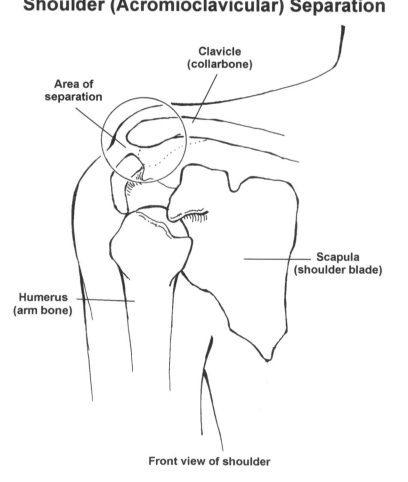

Shoulder (Acromioclavicular) Separation

Clavicle (collarbone)

Area of separation

Scapula (shoulder blade)

Humerus (arm bone)

Front view of shoulder

Shoulder Separation

tinue to put ice on your shoulder every 3 to 4 hours for the first 2 to 3 days, then as needed for the next several weeks. Cold helps reduce the pain, swelling, and inflammation.

The treatment of your separated shoulder depends on the severity. Grade I separations and some grade II and grade III separations may be placed in a sling or shoulder immobilizer. The sling or immobilizer will keep you from lifting your arm away from your chest and help healing of the ligaments. Your shoulder will be immobilized until you are pain free. Then you will begin rehabilitation exercises. Your doctor may prescribe an anti-inflammatory medication or other pain medication.

For most grade II and grade III separations treatment is the same. However, in some situations surgery may be needed to the doctor may need to reposition the bones or repair torn ligaments. Your arm will then be in a sling for up to 6 weeks to allow healing before you begin rehabilitation exercises. You should consult an orthopedic surgeon if you have a severe grade III injury.

How long will the effects of a shoulder separation last?

Some separations heal by themselves in 2 to 4 weeks

without any loss of shoulder use. However, sometimes slight stiffness or loss of movement in the shoulder may occur, which may be temporary or, rarely, long-lasting.

A severe separation may take 2 months or more to heal, particularly if you have surgery to repair it.

You may have a permanent bump over your shoulder joint after a separation regardless of treatment. The bump does not normally cause other medical problems.

How can I take care of myself?

- Avoid participating in sports until the injury has healed.
- You should move your shoulder as the pain subsides to prevent a frozen or stiff shoulder.
- With your doctor's permission, work with a trainer or physical therapist to strengthen your shoulder.

When can I return to my sport or activity?

The goal of rehabilitation is to return you to your sport or activity as soon as is safely possible. If you return too soon you may worsen your injury, which could lead to permanent damage. Everyone recovers from injury at a different rate. Return to your sport will be determined by how soon your shoulder recovers, not by how

many days or weeks it has been since your injury occurred. You may safely return to your sport or activity when:

- Your injured shoulder has full range of motion without pain.
- Your injured shoulder has regained normal strength compared to the uninjured shoulder.

In throwing sports, you must gradually build your tolerance to throwing. This means you should start with gentle tossing and gradually throw harder. In contact sports, your shoulder must not be tender to touch and contact should progress from minimal contact to harder contact.

What can I do to help prevent recurring shoulder separation?

Exercise and lift weights under the supervision of a trainer or physical therapist to strengthen your shoulder muscles. Muscle-strengthening exercises will also help strengthen your ligaments and tendons. If you have symptoms, you should avoid activities that aggravate your pain, use ice packs, and take anti-inflammatory medication if needed.

Shoulder Separation Rehabilitation Exercises

PHASE I

1. Wand exercises

   A. Shoulder flexion: Stand upright and hold a stick in both hands. Stretch your arms by lifting them over your head, keeping your elbows straight. Hold for 5 seconds and return to the starting position. Repeat 10 times.

   B. Shoulder abduction and adduction: Stand upright and hold onto a stick with both hands. Rest the stick against the front of your thighs. While keeping your elbows straight, use your uninjured arm to push your injured arm out to the side and up as high as possible. Hold for 5 seconds and return to the starting position. Repeat 10 times.

   C. Horizontal abduction and adduction: Stand upright and hold a stick in both hands. Place your arms straight out in front of you at shoulder level. Keep your arms straight and swing the stick to one side, feel the stretch, and hold for 5 seconds. Then swing the stick to the other side, feel the stretch, and hold for 5 seconds. Repeat 10 times.

   D. Shoulder extension: Stand upright holding a stick in both hands behind your back. Move the stick away from your back, keeping your elbows straight. Hold the end position for 5 seconds then relax and return to the starting position. Repeat 10 times.

   E. Internal rotation: Stand upright holding a stick in both hands behind your back. Move the stick up and down your back by bending your elbows. Hold the bent position for 5 seconds and then return to the starting position. Repeat 10 times.

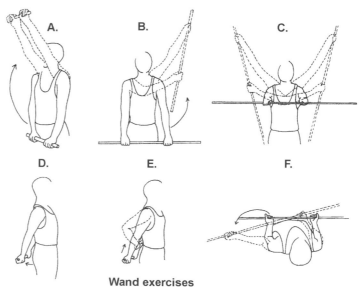

Wand exercises

   F. External rotation: Lying on your back, hold a stick with both hands, palms up. Your upper arms should be resting on the floor, your elbows at your sides and bent 90 degrees. Using your good arm, push your injured arm out away from your body while keeping your injured elbow at your side. Hold the stretch for 5 seconds. Return to the starting position. Repeat 10 times.

2. Active shoulder range of motion

   A. Flexion: Stand with your arms hanging straight down by your side. Lift both arms, thumbs up, over your head. Hold for 5 seconds. Return to the starting position. Repeat 10 times.

   B. Shoulder abduction and adduction: Stand with your arms at your sides. Bring your arms up, out to the side, and toward the ceiling. Hold for 5 seconds. Return to the starting position. Repeat 10 times.

Shoulder Separation Rehabilitation Exercises

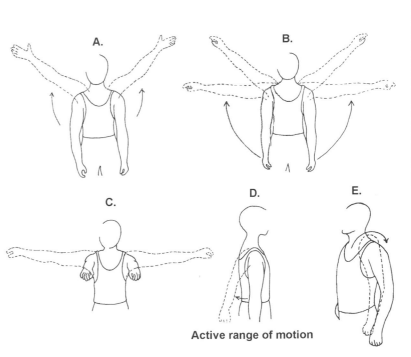

C. Horizontal abduction and adduction: Stand with your arms held straight out in front of you at shoulder level. Pull your arms apart and out to the sides as far as possible. Hold them back for 5 seconds, then bring them back together in front of you. Repeat 10 times. Remember to keep your arms at shoulder level throughout this exercise.

D. Shoulder extension: Standing, move your involved arm back, keeping your elbow straight. Hold this position for 5 seconds. Return to the starting position and repeat 10 times.

Active range of motion

E. Scapular range of motion: Shrug your shoulders up. Then squeeze your shoulder blades back and down, making a circle with your shoulders. Return to the starting position. Hold each position 5 seconds and do the entire exercise 10 times.

PHASE II

1. Sidelying horizontal abduction: Lie on your uninjured side with your injured arm relaxed across your chest. Slowly bring your injured arm up off the floor, elbow straight, so that your hand is pointing toward the ceiling. Repeat 10 times. Hold a weight in the hand as the exercise becomes easier.

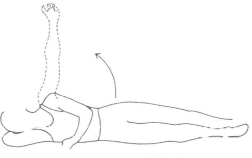

Sidelying horizontal abduction

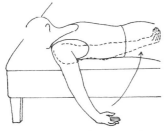

2. Prone shoulder extension: Lie on your stomach on a table or a bed with your involved arm hanging down over the edge. With your elbow straight, slowly lift your arm straight back and toward the ceiling. Return to the starting position. Repeat 10 times. As this becomes easier, hold a weight in your hand.

Prone shoulder extension

Shoulder Separation Rehabilitation Exercises

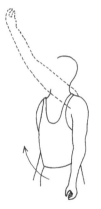

Biceps curls

3. Biceps curls: Standing, hold a weight of some sort (a soup can or hammer) in your hand. Bend the elbow of your involved arm and bring your hand, palm up, toward your shoulder. Slowly return to the starting position and straighten your elbow. Repeat 10 times.

4. Triceps: Lie on your back with your arms toward the ceiling. Bend your involved elbow completely, so that your hand is resting on the shoulder of the same side and your elbow is pointing toward the ceiling. You can use your other hand to help support your upper arm just below the elbow. Then straighten your elbow completely so that your hand is pointing toward the ceiling. Return to the starting position. Repeat 10 times. Hold a weight in your hand when this exercise becomes easy.

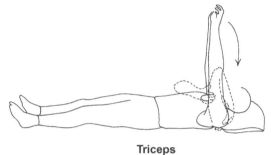

Triceps

5. Abduction: Stand with your injured arm at your side, palm resting against your side. With your elbow straight, lift your hand arm out to the side and toward the ceiling. Hold this position for 5 seconds. Repeat 10 times. Add a weight to your hand as this exercise becomes easier.

6. Shoulder flexion: Stand with your injured arm hanging down at your side. Keeping your elbow straight, bring your arm forward and up toward the ceiling. Hold this position for 5 seconds. Repeat 10 times. As this exercise becomes easier, add a weight.

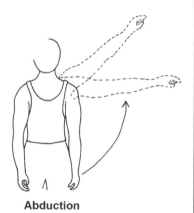

Abduction

Shoulder flexion

Shoulder Subluxation

What is a shoulder subluxation?

A shoulder subluxation is a temporary, partial dislocation of the shoulder joint. The shoulder is a ball and socket joint. The ball of the upper arm bone (humerus) is held into the socket (glenoid) of the shoulder blade (scapula) by a group of ligaments.

How does it occur?

A shoulder subluxation can occur from falls onto your outstretched arm, direct blows to your shoulder, or having your arm forced into an awkward position. If you have had a previous injury or if your shoulder ligaments are naturally loose you may sublux your shoulder doing simple activities like throwing or putting on a shirt or jacket.

What are the symptoms?

Symptoms of a shoulder subluxation include:

- the feeling that your shoulder has gone "in and out of joint"
- looseness in your shoulder
- pain, weakness, or numbness in your shoulder or arm

How is it diagnosed?

Your doctor will talk to you about your symptoms and perform a physical exam. Many times the diagnosis of a shoulder subluxation is made by your description of the injury. When your doctor examines you they may find that your shoulder is loose and may partially slip out of joint during the exam. Your doctor may order x-rays to see if you have had any fractures.

What is the treatment?

The pain from a shoulder subluxation is treated with ice packs for 20 to 30 minutes 3 to 4 times a day. You may take an anti-inflammatory medication, such as ibuprofen. You may need to avoid painful activities until the pain improves.

The most important treatment for the looseness in the shoulder that causes a subluxation is shoulder strengthening exercises.

Shoulders that continue to sublux and cause painful symptoms may require surgery to correct the joint looseness.

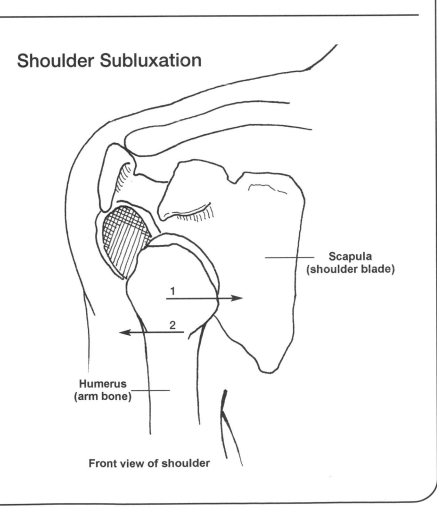

Shoulder Subluxation

Scapula (shoulder blade)

Humerus (arm bone)

Front view of shoulder

Shoulder Subluxation

When can I return to my sport or activity?

The goal of rehabilitation is to return you to your sport or activity as soon as is safely possible. If you return too soon, you may worsen your injury, which could lead to permanent damage. Everyone recovers from injury at a different rate. Return to your sport or activity is determined by how soon your shoulder recovers, not by how many days or weeks it has been since your injury occurred.

You may safely return to your sport or activity when:

- your injured shoulder has full range of motion without pain

- your injured shoulder has regained normal strength compared to the uninjured shoulder.

In throwing sports, you must gradually build your tolerance to throwing. This means you should start with gently tossing and gradually throw harder.

— *Shoulder Subluxation Rehabilitation Exercises* —

Do these exercises as soon as your doctor says you can.

PART I

1. Isometrics:

   A. Adduction: With a pillow between your chest and your arms, squeeze the pillow with your arms and hold 5 seconds. Release and repeat 10 times.

   B. Flexion: Stand facing a wall with your elbow bent at a right angle and held close to your body. Press your fist forward against the wall, hold this for 5 seconds, then rest. Repeat this 10 times.

   C. Extension: Standing facing away from the wall with your elbow touching the wall, press the back of your elbow into the wall and hold for 5 seconds. Rest. Repeat 10 times.

   D. Abduction: Standing with your injured side towards the wall and your elbow bent at a 90-degree angle, press the side of your arm into the wall as if attempting to lift it. Hold for 5 seconds. Rest. Repeat 10 times.

   E. Internal rotation: Standing in a doorway with your elbow bent at a 90-degree angle and your palm resting on the door frame, attempt to press your palms into the door frame and hold 5 seconds. Rest. Repeat 10 times.

   F. External rotation: Standing in a doorway with your elbow bent at a 90-degree angle and the back of your hand pressing against the door frame, attempt to press your hand outward into the door frame. Hold 5 seconds. Rest. Repeat 10 times.

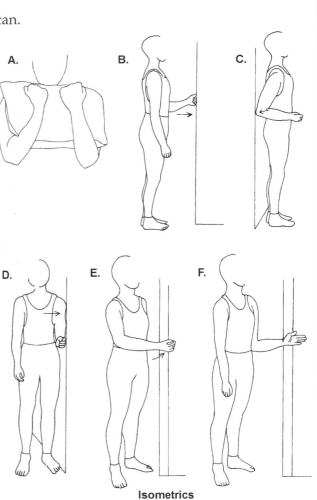

Isometrics

2. Careful range of motion:

   A. Flexion: Standing with your arms straight, raise your arm forward and up over your head. Hold this position for 5 seconds. Return to the starting position and repeat 10 times.

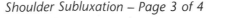

Careful range of motion

Shoulder Subluxation Rehabilitation Exercises

B. Extension: Standing with your arms straight, move your arm backward while keeping your elbow straight. Hold this position for 5 seconds. Repeat 10 times.

C. Abduction: Standing with your arms at your side, slowly raise your arms out away from your body and hold in position for 5 seconds. Return to the starting position. Repeat 10 times.

D. Elbow flexion: Standing, bend your elbow, bring your hand toward your shoulder. Return to starting position. Repeat 10 times. As this becomes easier, add a weight to your hand to give you some resistance.

PART II

3. Tubing exercises:

A. Internal rotation: Using tubing connected to a door knob or other object at waist level, keep your elbow in at your side and rotate your arm inward across your body. Make sure you keep your forearm parallel to the floor. Repeat 10 times. Do 2 sets of 10.

B. Adduction: Stand sideways with your injured side toward the door and out approximately 8 to 10 inches. Slowly bring your arm next to your body holding onto the tubing for resistance. Repeat 10 times. Do 2 sets of 10.

C. Flexion: Facing away from the door with the tubing connected to the door knob, keep your elbow straight and pull your arm forward. Repeat 10 times. Do 2 sets of 10.

D. Extension: Using the tubing, pull your arm back. Be sure to keep your elbow straight. Repeat 10 times. Do 2 sets of 10.

4. Latissimus dorsi strengthening: Sit on a firm chair. Place your hands on the seat on either side of you. Lift your buttocks off the chair. Hold this position for 5 seconds and then relax. Repeat 10 times. Do 2 sets of 10.

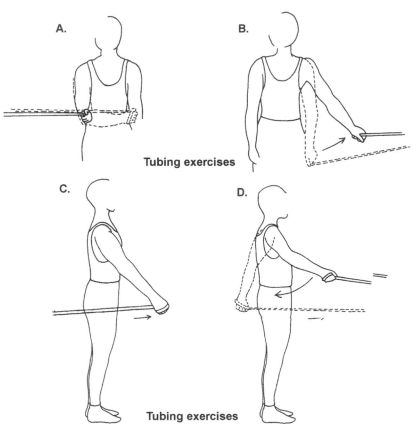

Tubing exercises

Tubing exercises

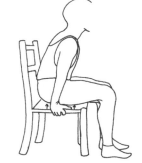

Latissimus dorsi strengthening

Triceps Tendonitis

What is triceps tendonitis?

Tendonitis is inflammation of a tendon, a strong band of connective tissue that attaches muscle to bone. Your triceps muscle, which acts to straighten your arm, is attached to the bony bump at the back of your elbow by a large tendon. Triceps tendonitis causes pain in the back part of the upper arm near the point of your elbow.

How does it occur?

Triceps tendonitis occurs from overuse of the upper arm and elbow, especially in activities like throwing and hammering. It may also be caused by a direct blow to the triceps muscle or tendon.

What are the symptoms?

Symptoms may include:
- pain when you straighten your elbow or fully bend your elbow
- tenderness at the triceps muscle and tendon
- swelling near the point of the elbow.

How is it diagnosed?

Your doctor will review your history and examine your arm and elbow. If the doctor thinks there may be a chip off the bone at the point of your elbow, he or she may order an x-ray.

How is it treated?

- Use ice packs on the painful area for 20 to 30 minutes 3 to 4 times a day until the pain goes away. You can also do ice massage: Freeze water in a cup and tear back the top of the cup. Rub the injured area with the ice for 5 to 10 minutes, 3 times a day. Be careful when icing your elbow. An important nerve runs just under the skin and can be damaged if you ice more than is recommended.
- Your doctor may recommend an anti-inflammatory medication such as ibuprofen.
- You may be given a strap to wear around the lower part of your triceps during activities that cause discomfort.

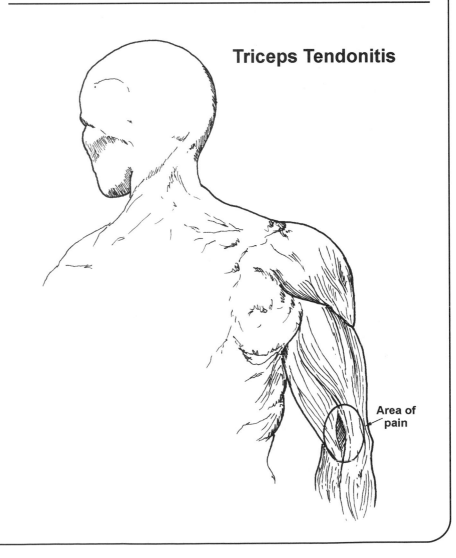

Triceps Tendonitis

Area of pain

Triceps Tendonitis

- Your doctor will give you rehabilitation exercises to help in your recovery.

When can I return to my sport or activity?

The goal of rehabilitation is to return you to your sport or activity as soon as is safely possible. If you return too soon you may worsen your injury, which could lead to permanent damage. Everyone recovers from injury at a different rate. Return to your activity will be determined by how soon your arm recovers, not by how many days or weeks it has been since your injury occurred. In general, the longer you have symptoms before you start treatment, the longer it will take to get better.

You may return to your sport or activity when:

- You no longer have tenderness or swelling at your triceps muscle or tendon.

- You have regained strength in your injured arm so that it is similar to the strength of your uninjured arm.

- You have full range of motion in your injured arm compared to your uninjured arm.

How is triceps tendonitis prevented?

The best way to prevent triceps tendonitis is to avoid overuse of your upper arm and elbow. It is important to recognize early symptoms so you do not make your injury worse by overactivity.

Triceps Tendonitis Rehabilitation Exercises

You may do all of these exercises right away.

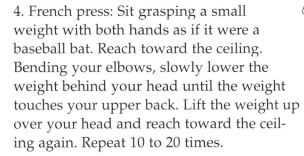

A.

B.

French stretch

1. French stretch: Stand with your fingers clasped together and your hands high above your head. Stretch by reaching down behind your head and trying to touch your upper back while keeping your hands clasped. Keep your elbows as close to your ears as possible. Hold this position for 15 to 20 seconds. Repeat 3 to 6 times.

2. Towel stretch: Stand with your injured arm over your head and your other arm down behind your back. Hold one end of a towel in each hand. Stretch your injured arm behind your head by pulling the towel down toward the floor with hand of your uninjured arm. Keep the elbow of your injured arm as close to your ear as possible. Hold for 15 to 20 seconds. Repeat 3 to 6 times.

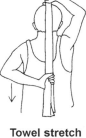

Towel stretch

3. Towel resistance exercise: Holding the towel as in the towel stretch above, lift the hand of your injured arm toward the ceiling while creating resistance by pulling down on the towel with your other hand. Keep the elbow of your injured arm as close to your ear as possible. Hold for 10 seconds. Repeat 10 times.

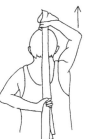

Towel resistance

A.   **B.**

French press

4. French press: Sit grasping a small weight with both hands as if it were a baseball bat. Reach toward the ceiling. Bending your elbows, slowly lower the weight behind your head until the weight touches your upper back. Lift the weight up over your head and reach toward the ceiling again. Repeat 10 to 20 times.

5. Palm-down curl: Stand with your hands at your side, holding a small weight palm down in the hand of your injured arm. Keeping your palm down and bending your elbow, slowly curl the weight up toward your shoulder as far as possible. For each repetition, move your hand down to the starting position more slowly than you lift your hand up toward your shoulder. Repeat 10 to 20 times.

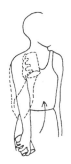

Palm-down curl

Triceps Tendonitis Rehabilitation Exercises

6. Triceps kick back: Lean forward with the hand of your uninjured arm resting on a table or chair for support. Hold a weight in the hand of your injured arm. Keep the elbow of your injured arm against your side. Your arm should be bent at a 90-degree angle with your upper arm parallel to the floor. Move the forearm of your injured arm backward until it is straight. Repeat 10 to 20 times.

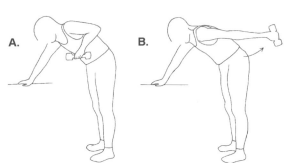

A. **B.**

Triceps kick back

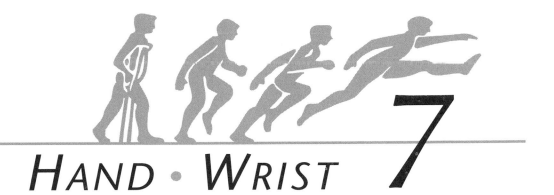

HAND · WRIST 7

Carpal Tunnel Syndrome

What is carpal tunnel syndrome?

Carpal tunnel syndrome is a common, painful disorder of the wrist and hand.

How does it occur?

Carpal tunnel syndrome is caused by pressure on the median nerve in your wrist. People who use their hands and wrists repeatedly in the same way (for example, illustrators, carpenters, and assembly-line workers) tend to develop carpal tunnel syndrome.

Pressure on the nerve may also be caused by a fracture or other injury, which may cause inflammation and swelling. In addition, pressure may be caused by inflammation and swelling associated with arthritis, diabetes, and hypothyroidism. Carpal tunnel syndrome can also occur during pregnancy.

What are the symptoms?

The symptoms include:
- pain, numbness, or tingling in your hand and wrist, especially in the thumb and index and middle fingers; pain may radiate up into the forearm
- increased pain with increased use of your hand, such as when you are driving or reading the newspaper
- increased pain at night
- weak grip and tendency to drop objects held in the hand
- sensitivity to cold
- muscle deterioration especially in the thumb (in later stages).

How is it diagnosed?

Your doctor will review your symptoms, examine you, and discuss the ways you use your hands. He or she may also do the following tests:
- The doctor may tap the inside middle of your wrist over the median nerve. You may feel pain or a sensation like an electric shock.
- You may be asked to bend your wrist down for one minute to see if this causes symptoms.
- The doctor may arrange to test the response of your

Carpal Tunnel Syndrome

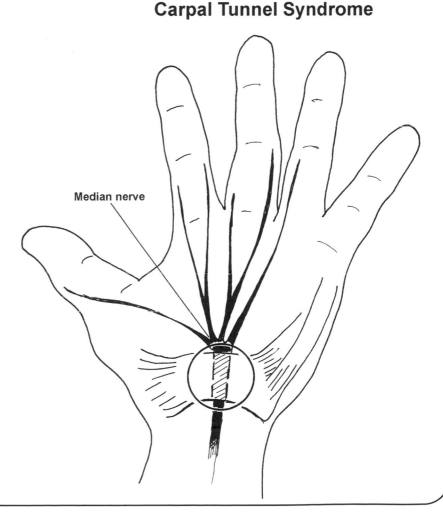

Median nerve

Carpal Tunnel Syndrome

nerves and muscles to electrical stimulation.

How is it treated?

If you have a disease that is causing carpal tunnel syndrome (such as rheumatoid arthritis), treatment of the disease may relieve your symptoms. Other treatment focuses on relieving irritation and pressure on the nerve in your wrist. To relieve pressure your doctor may suggest:

- restricting use of your hand or changing the way you use it
- wearing a wrist splint during sleep and physical activity involving the wrist
- exercises.

Your doctor may prescribe a cortisonelike medicine or a nonsteroidal anti-inflammatory medicine, such as ibuprofen. Your doctor may recommend an injection of a cortisonelike medicine into the carpal tunnel area. In some cases surgery may be necessary.

How long will the effects last?

How long the symptoms of carpal tunnel syndrome last depends on the cause and your response to treatment. Sometimes the symptoms disappear without any treatment, or they may be relieved by

nonsurgical treatment. Surgery may be necessary to relieve the symptoms if they do not respond to treatment or they get worse. Surgery usually relieves the symptoms, especially if there is no permanent damage to the nerve.

Symptoms of carpal tunnel syndrome that occur during pregnancy usually disappear following delivery.

How can I take care of myself?

Follow your doctor's recommendations. Also try the following:

- Elevate your arm with pillows when you lie down.
- Avoid activities that overuse your hand.
- Find a different way to use your hand by using another tool or try to use the other hand.
- Avoid bending your wrists down for long periods.

When can I return to my sport or activity?

The goal of rehabilitation is to return you to your sport or activity as soon as is safely possible. If you return too soon you may worsen your injury, which could lead to permanent damage. Everyone recovers from injury at a different rate. Return to your

sport will be determined by how soon your wrist recovers, not by how many days or weeks it has been since your injury occurred. In general, the longer you have symptoms before you start treatment, the longer it will take to get better.

You may return to your sport or activity when you are able to painlessly grip objects like a tennis racquet, bat, golf club, or bicycle handlebars. In sports such as gymnastics, it is important that you can bear weight on your wrist without pain. You must have full range of motion and strength of your wrist.

What can I do to help prevent carpal tunnel syndrome?

If you do very repetitive work with your hands, make sure that your hands and wrists are comfortable when you are using them. Take regular breaks from the repetitive motion. Avoid resting your wrists on hard or ridged surfaces for prolonged periods.

If you have a disease that is associated with carpal tunnel syndrome, effective treatment of the disease might help prevent this condition.

In some cases the cause is not known and carpal tunnel syndrome cannot be prevented.

© HBO & Company

— *Carpal Tunnel Rehabilitation Exercises* —

You may do all of these exercises right away.

1. Active range of motion
   A. Flexion: Gently bend your wrist forward. Hold for 5 seconds. Repeat 10 times. Do 3 sets.
   B. Extension: Gently bend your wrist backward. Hold this position 5 seconds. Repeat 10 times. Do 3 sets.
   C. Side to side: Gently move your wrist from side to side (a handshake motion). Hold for 5 seconds at each end. Repeat 10 times. Do 3 sets.

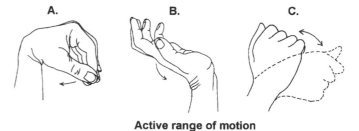

Active range of motion

2. Stretching: With your uninjured hand, help to bend the injured wrist down by pressing the back of your hand and holding it down for 15 to 30 seconds. Next, stretch the hand back by pressing the fingers in a backward direction and holding it for 15 to 30 seconds. Do this twice.

3. Tendon glides: Start with the fingers of your injured hand held out straight. Gently bend the middle joint of your fingers down toward your upper palm. Hold for 5 seconds. Repeat 10 times. Do 3 sets.

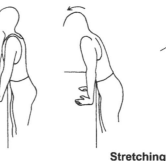

Stretching

4. Wrist flexion: Hold a can or hammer handle with your palm up. Bend your wrist upward. Hold this position for 5 seconds. Repeat 10 times. Do 3 sets. Gradually increase the weight of the object you are holding.

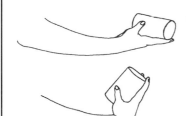

Wrist flexion

5. Wrist extension: Holding a can or similar object with the palm down, bend the wrist up. Hold this position for 5 seconds. Repeat 10 times. Do 3 sets.

6. Grip strengthening: Squeeze a rubber ball and hold for 5 seconds. Repeat 10 times.

Tendon glides

Wrist extension

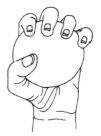

Grip strengthening

© HBO & Company

De Quervain's Tenosynovitis

What is de Quervain's tenosynovitis?

De Quervain's tenosynovitis is a painful condition affecting the tendons located on the thumb side of your wrist. A tendon is a strong band of tissue that attaches muscle to bone. A sheath, or covering, surrounds the tendons that go to your thumb. Tenosynovitis is an irritation of this sheath.

How does it occur?

De Quervain's tenosynovitis usually occurs from overusing your thumb or wrist, especially in activities that move your thumb directly away from your wrist such as skiing or hammering.

What are the symptoms?

Symptoms may include:

- pain when you move your thumb or wrist
- pain when you make a fist
- swelling and tenderness on the thumb side of your wrist
- feeling or hearing creaking as the tendon slides through its sheath.

How is it diagnosed?

Your health care provider will examine your wrist and thumb and find the areas that are tender and painful to move. An x-ray may be taken to be sure you don't have a broken bone.

How is it treated?

The initial treatment for de Quervain's tenosynovitis is a splint that will cover your wrist and thumb. It is important that you protect your thumb and wrist from activities that worsen your pain.

Treatment may also include:

- placing an ice pack on your thumb and wrist for 20 to 30 minutes every 3 or 4 hours until the pain goes away
- doing ice massage for 5 to 10 minutes several times a day
- taking an anti-inflammatory medication such as ibuprofen
- having an injection of a medication like cortisone.

You will be given rehabilitation exercises to help speed your recovery and prevent the problem from returning.

When can I return to my sport or activity?

The goal of rehabilitation is to return you to your sport or activity as soon as is safely possible. If you return too soon you may worsen your injury, which could lead to permanent damage. Everyone recovers from injury at a different rate. Return to your activity will be determined by how soon your wrist recovers, not by how many days or weeks it has been since your injury occurred. In general, the longer you have symptoms before you start treatment, the longer it will take to get better.

You may return to your sport or activity when it is no longer painful to move your thumb or wrist. You may need to do activities wearing a supportive splint until you no longer have symptoms.

How can I prevent de Quervain's tenosynovitis?

Avoiding activities that overuse your thumb or wrist may prevent de Quervain's tenosynovitis.

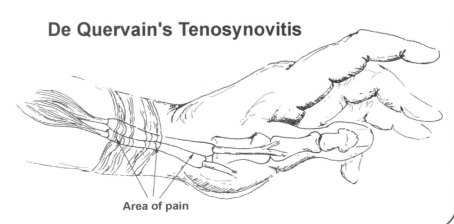

De Quervain's Tenosynovitis

Area of pain

— De Quervain's Tenosynovitis Rehabilitation Exercises —

You may do all of these exercises when the initial pain is gone.

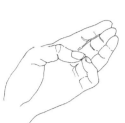

1. Opposition stretch: Rest your injured hand on a table, palm up. Touch the tip of your thumb to the tip of your little finger. Hold this position for 6 seconds. Repeat 10 to 12 times.

Opposition stretch

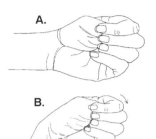

A.

B.

Wrist rock

2. Wrist rock stretch: Hold your injured hand out in front of you in the handshake position. Make a fist with your injured hand, but tuck your thumb inside your palm. Move your wrist down, hold for 5 seconds, then move your wrist up and hold for 5 seconds. Repeat 10 to 12 times.

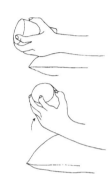

3. Thumb extension: Hold a small weight (a soup can, for example) in your injured hand. Rest your forearm on a table with your wrist and hand hanging over the edge of the table. Starting with your hand in the handshake position (thumb up), move your wrist up and down. Repeat 10 to 20 times.

Thumb extension

4. Wrist extension: Start in the same position as for the thumb extension (holding a small weight, resting your forearm on the table), but this time turn your hand palm down. Bend your wrist up, hold for 2 to 3 seconds, then bend your wrist down and hold for 2 to 3 seconds. Repeat 10 to 20 times.

Wrist extension

5. Palm-down curl: Stand with your hands at your side, holding a small weight palm down in your injured hand. Keeping your palm down and bending your elbow, slowly curl the weight up toward your shoulder as far as possible. For each repetition, move your hand down to the starting position more slowly than you lift your hand up toward your shoulder. Repeat 10 to 20 times.

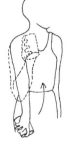

Palm-down curl

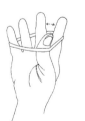

Finger spring

6. Finger spring: Place a large rubber band around the outside of your thumb and the rest of your fingers. Open your fingers to stretch the rubber band. Repeat 10 to 20 times.

Finger Dislocation

What is a finger dislocation?

A finger dislocation is a displacement of the bones of the finger from their normal position.

How does it occur?

A dislocation usually occurs when there is an accident such as a ball striking the tips of the finger or a person falling forcefully onto a finger or getting a finger hooked into a piece of equipment like a football mask or a basketball net.

What are the symptoms?

In a dislocation there is immediate pain and swelling. The finger looks swollen and crooked. You will usually be unable to bend or straighten the dislocated joint.

How is it diagnosed?

Your doctor will examine your finger. An x-ray will be taken to confirm the dislocation and to determine if there is also a break in your finger.

How is it treated?

Your doctor will realign the dislocated bones. Your finger will be placed in a protective splint for several weeks.

Your finger will most likely be swollen after the dislocation. You should apply ice packs to your finger for 20 to 30 minutes every 3 to 4 hours for 2 or 3 days or until the pain goes away. Your hand should be elevated on a pillow while you are lying down or on the back of a chair or couch while you are sitting. Your doctor may prescribe an anti-inflammatory medication. You will be given exercises to strengthen your finger during the healing process.

When can I return to my sport or activity?

The goal of rehabilitation is to return you to your sport or activity as soon as is safely possible. If you return too soon you may worsen your injury, which could lead to permanent damage. Everyone recovers from injury at a different rate. Return to your

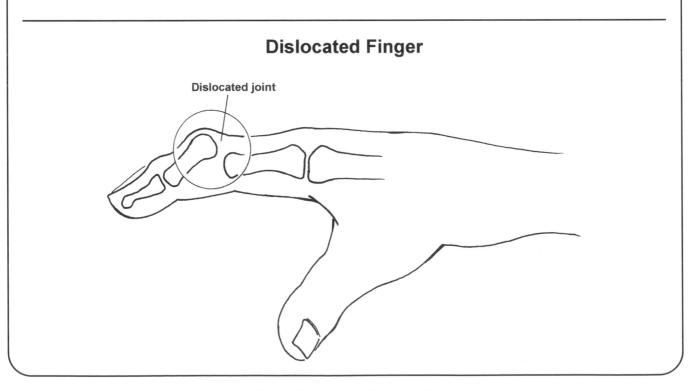

Dislocated Finger

Dislocated joint

Finger Dislocation

activity will be determined by how soon the your finger recovers, not by how many days or weeks it has been since your injury occurred.

Your doctor will recommend that your dislocated finger be splinted or "buddy taped" (taped to the finger next to it) for 3 to 6 weeks after your injury. In many cases, you will be able to return to your sport or activity as long as you are wearing your splint or have your finger taped.

Your finger may remain swollen with decreased range of motion and strength for many weeks. It is important to continue your rehabilitation exercises during this time and even after you return to your sport or activity.

How can I prevent finger dislocation?

Finger dislocations are usually the result of accidents that are not preventable. However, whenever possible you should try to avoid getting your finger stuck in objects such as helmets, nets, or athletic jerseys.

© HBO & Company

Finger Dislocation Rehabilitation Exercises

You may do all of these exercises right away.

1. Passive range of motion: Gently assist the injured joint by helping to bend it with your other hand. Gently try to straighten out the injured joint with your other hand. Repeat slowly, holding for 5 seconds at the end of each motion. Do this 10 times. Do these exercises 3 to 5 times per day.

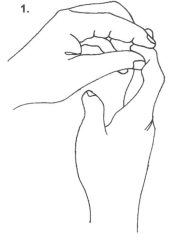 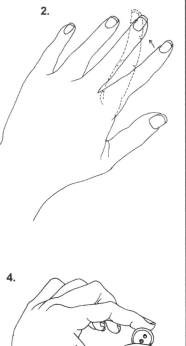

2. Finger lift: With your palm flat on a table and your fingers straight, lift each finger up individually and hold 5 seconds. Then put it down and lift the one next to it until you have done all 5 fingers individually. Hold each one 5 seconds and repeat 10 times.

3. Fist making: Make your hand into a fist. If the injured finger will not bend into the fist, assist it with your uninjured hand and try to help it bend into the fist. Hold this position for 5 to 10 seconds. Repeat 10 times.

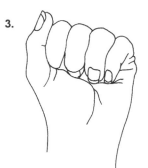

4. Object pick-up: Practice picking up small objects such as coins, marbles, pins, or buttons with the injured finger and the thumb.

Finger Sprain

What is a finger sprain?

A sprain is an injury to a joint that causes a stretch or tear in a ligament, a strong band of tissue connecting one bone to another.

How does it occur?

A sprain usually occurs when there is an accident such as a ball striking the tip of your finger or you fall forcefully onto your finger.

What are the symptoms?

There will be pain, swelling, and tenderness in your finger.

How is it diagnosed?

Your doctor will examine your finger and will order an x-ray to be sure you have not broken any bones in your finger.

How is it treated?

Treatment may include:
• applying ice packs to your finger for 20 to 30 minutes every 3 to 4 hours for 2 or 3 days or until the pain goes away
• elevating your hand on a pillow while you are lying down or on the back of a chair or couch while you are sitting
• taking an anti-inflammatory or other pain medication prescribed by your doctor
• doing exercises to strengthen your finger during the healing process.

When can I return to my sport or activity?

The goal of rehabilitation is to return you to your sport or activity as soon as is safely possible. If you return too soon you may worsen your injury, which could lead to permanent damage. Everyone recovers from injury at a different rate. Return to your activity will be determined by how soon your finger recovers, not by how many days or weeks it has been since your injury occurred. In general, the longer you have symptoms before you start treatment, the longer it will take to get better.

Your doctor will recommend that your sprained finger be splinted or "buddy taped" (taped to the finger next to it) for 1 to 4 weeks after your injury. In many cases, you will be able to return to your activities as long as you are wearing your splint or have your finger taped.

Your finger may remain swollen with decreased range of motion and strength for many weeks. It is important to continue your rehabilitation exercises during this time and even after you return to your sport.

How I prevent a finger sprain?

Finger sprains are usually the result of injuries that are not preventable.

Finger Sprain Rehabilitation Exercises

You may do all of these exercises right away.

1. Passive range of motion: Gently assist the injured joint by helping to bend it with your other hand. Gently try to straighten out the injured joint with your other hand. Repeat slowly, holding for 5 seconds at the end of each motion. Do this 10 times. Do these exercises 3 to 5 times per day.

2. Finger lift: With your palm flat on a table and your fingers straight, lift each finger up individually and hold 5 seconds. Then put it down and lift the one next to it until you have done all 5 fingers individually. Hold each one 5 seconds and repeat 10 times.

3. Fist making: Make your hand into a fist. If the injured finger will not bend into the fist, assist it with your uninjured hand and try to help it bend into the fist. Hold this position for 5 to 10 seconds. Repeat 10 times.

4. Object pick-up: Practice picking up small objects such as coins, marbles, pins, or buttons with the injured finger and the thumb.

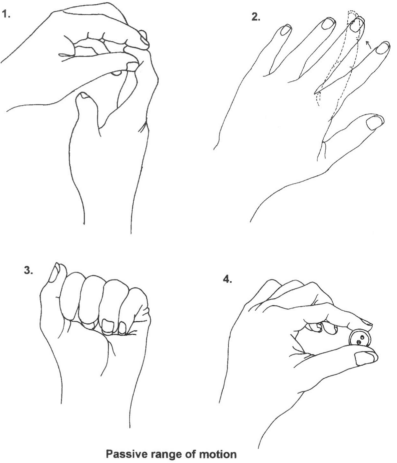

Passive range of motion

Ganglion Cyst

What is a ganglion cyst?

A ganglion cyst is a swollen, closed sac under the skin. The sac is attached to the sheath of a tendon or may be attached to a joint. The cyst contains fluid similar to joint fluid. It can vary in size from a small pea to a golf ball. Ganglion cysts are the most common type of mass that occurs in the hand or wrist. They may also occur in the foot.

How does it occur?

The cause of ganglion cysts is not known.

What are the symptoms?

You may feel discomfort or pain. Sometimes the area of the cyst becomes swollen or disfigured.

How is it diagnosed?

The doctor may stick a needle into the cyst to take a sample of the fluid inside it.

How is it treated?

Unless a cyst hurts, it does not need to be treated. If it does hurt, put ice on it for 20 to 30 minutes three or four times a day, or at least once daily, until it becomes less painful. Taking aspirin or other anti-inflammatory drugs may also help.

The fluid can be removed with a needle, but the cysts tend to fill up again with fluid. Do not try to smash the cyst with a heavy object. Even if this home remedy succeeds at first, the cyst will almost always fill up again with fluid. In addition, you could seriously damage your wrist.

If the cyst is painful or unsightly, it can be surgically removed. Surgery to remove the cyst requires making a small cut through the skin. The cut usually heals quickly and leaves a small scar.

How long will the effects last?

Sometimes cysts go away whether they are treated or not. If your cyst is painful or continues to get bigger, you may need to have surgery.

How can I take care of myself?

Follow the treatment recommended by your doctor.

When can I return to my sport or activity?

The goal of rehabilitation is to return you to your sport or activity as soon as is safely possible. If you return too soon you may worsen your injury, which could lead to permanent damage. Everyone recovers from injury at a different rate. Return to your sport will be measured by how soon your wrist recovers, not by how many days or weeks it has been since your injury occurred. In general, the longer you have symptoms before you start treatment, the longer it will take to get better.

Ganglion Cyst

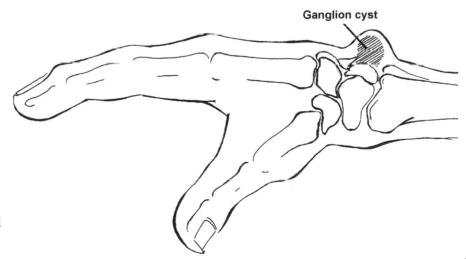

Ganglion Cyst

Your may return to your sport or activity when you have a wrist ganglion if you can do your activities without pain. You may need to wear a wrist brace or have your wrist taped. In sports such as gymnastics, you will not be able to participate fully until you can bear weight on your wrist while tumbling without pain. In sports such as baseball or tennis, it is important that your wrist does not hurt when you are holding the bat or racquet while doing your swing.

How can I help prevent ganglion cysts?

There is no known way to prevent these cysts because their cause is not known.

Ganglion Cyst Removal
(Ganglionectomy)

What is a ganglion cyst removal?

Ganglion cyst removal, called a ganglionectomy, is a procedure in which the doctor removes a cyst from your hand, wrist, foot, or other part of your body. A ganglion cyst is a swollen, closed sac under the skin. The sac is attached to the sheath of a tendon or may be attached to a joint. The cyst contains fluid similar to joint fluid.

Alternatives to this procedure include:
• taking out the fluid with a needle or a syringe, with or without a cortisone injection
• choosing not to have treatment, recognizing the risks of your condition.
You should ask your doctor about these choices.

How do I prepare for a ganglionectomy?

Plan for your care and recovery after the operation, especially if you are to have general anesthesia. Allow for time to rest and try to find other people to help you with your day-to-day duties.

Follow the instructions your doctor gives you. Do not eat or drink anything after midnight or the morning before the procedure. Do not even drink coffee, tea, or water after midnight.

What happens during the procedure?

You will be given a general, regional, or local anesthetic. Local and regional anesthetics numb part of the body while you remain awake. A general anesthetic relaxes your muscles and puts you to sleep. All three types of anesthesia should keep you from feeling pain during the operation.

Your doctor will cut around the cyst and remove it. Your doctor will then close the cut with stitches or special surgical strips.

What happens after the procedure?

You can go home the day you have the surgery. A bulky dressing, with or without a splint, may cover the area where you had the cyst to protect it. See your doctor in a week to get the stitches out.

You should ask your doctor what steps you should take and when you should come back for a checkup.

What are the benefits of this procedure?

The hand, wrist, foot, or other part of your body that had the cyst may return to normal function. The area may also feel and look better.
What are the risks associated with this procedure?

• There are some risks when you have general anesthesia. Discuss these risks with your doctor.

• A local or regional anesthetic may not numb the area quite enough and you may feel some minor discomfort. Also, in rare cases, you may have an allergic reaction to the drug used in this type of anesthesia. Local or regional anesthesia is considered safer than general anesthesia.

• The cyst may come back.

• There is a small risk of infection and bleeding. However, the cut usually heals quickly without any problems.

• In rare cases, nerves or blood vessels in the area may be damaged.

• The healing cut could form an unsightly scar. Usually the scar is not noticeable in the long run.

Ganglion Cyst Removal (Ganglionectomy)

You should ask your doctor how these risks apply to you.

When should I call the doctor?

Call your doctor immediately if:

- You have increasing pain despite taking the pain medicine recommended by your doctor.
- You notice pus; drainage; or increasing redness, swelling, and tenderness near the cut and stitches.

Call your doctor during office hours if:

- You have questions about the procedure or its result.
- You want to make another appointment.

Mallet Finger
(Baseball Finger)

What is mallet finger?

Mallet finger, also known as baseball finger, is an injury to the fingertip caused by a blow to the end of the finger. In mallet finger, the tendon that straightens the tip of the finger is injured and you may lose the ability to straighten your finger.

How does it occur?

There is usually a jamming injury to the tip of the finger.

What are the symptoms?

You may have pain and swelling at the tip of the finger. You may be unable to straighten the tip of your finger. If the injury is old or if you do not seek medical care soon enough, you may permanently lose the ability to straighten your finger.

How is it diagnosed?

Your doctor will examine your finger and review your symptoms. An x-ray may be taken to see if there is also a fracture. Commonly, the tendon will pull off a piece of the bone to which it is attached at the end of your finger.

How is it treated?

Your finger will be straightened and placed in a splint for about 6 weeks to allow the tendon to reattach to the finger bone or, if a piece of bone has been pulled off, to allow the bone to heal. It is important to keep this splint on to permit healing. Because your finger probably will be swollen, you should apply ice packs to your finger for 20 to 30 minutes every 3 to 4 hours for the first 2 or 3 days or until the pain goes away. Your hand should be elevated on a pillow when you are lying down or placed on the back of a chair or couch when you are sitting.

When can I return to my sport or activity?

The goal of rehabilitation is to return you to your sport or activity as soon as is safely possible. If you return too soon you may worsen your injury, which could lead to permanent damage. Everyone recovers from injury at a different rate. Return to your sport or activity will be determined by how soon your finger recovers, not by how many days or weeks it has been since your injury occurred.

It is important that you wear a splint for your mallet finger for at least 6 weeks after your injury. If you wear your

Mallet Finger

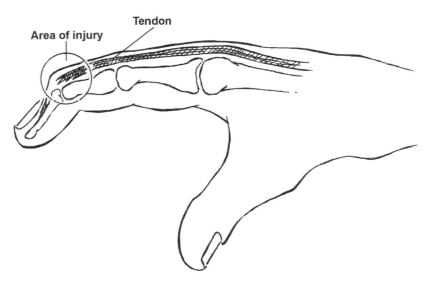

Mallet Finger (Baseball Finger)

splint as your doctor has recommended you may return to your activities immediately. NOT wearing your splint can lead to permanent injury or deformity of your finger.

How can I prevent mallet finger?

Mallet finger is caused by a direct blow to the end of the finger during an accident that is usually not preventable.

Mallet Finger (Baseball Finger) Rehabilitation Exercises

You may do all of these exercises when your doctor says you can remove your splint.

1. Passive range of motion: Gently assist the injured joint by helping to bend it with your other hand. Gently try to straighten out the injured joint with your other hand. Repeat slowly, holding for 5 seconds at the end of each motion. Do this 10 times. Do these exercises 3 to 5 times per day.

2. Finger lift: With your palm flat on a table and your fingers straight, lift each finger up individually and hold 5 seconds. Then put it down and lift the one next to it until you have done all 5 fingers individually. Hold each one 5 seconds and repeat 10 times.

3. Fist making: Make your hand into a fist. If the injured finger will not bend into the fist, assist it with your uninjured hand and try to help it bend into the fist. Hold this position for 5 to 10 seconds. Repeat 10 times.

4. Object pick-up: Practice picking up small objects such as coins, marbles, pins, or buttons with the injured finger and the thumb.

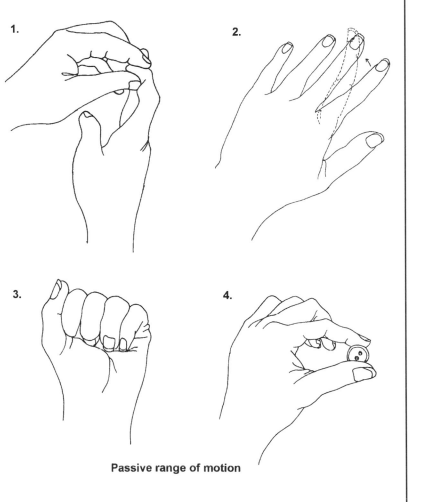

1. **2.**

3. **4.**

Passive range of motion

Navicular (Scaphoid) Fracture

What is a navicular or scaphoid fracture?

Your wrist is made up of eight bones that attach to the bones in the forearm and the bones in the hand. One of the wrist bones near your thumb has two different names: it is called the scaphoid bone or navicular bone. A fracture is a break through a bone. Because this wrist bone does not have a good blood supply, fractures to this bone sometimes have a healing problem.

How does it occur?

A navicular fracture is caused by a fall or a direct blow.

What are the symptoms?

You have pain and swelling in your wrist, usually just below the thumb. If you hold your hand in the "hitchhiking position," the thumb tendons are visible on the back of your hand and thumb. The tendons make an area called the "snuff box." When the navicular bone is fractured, there will be tenderness in the "snuff box."

How is it diagnosed?

Your doctor will examine your wrist and review your symptoms. An x-ray will be ordered and may show a break in the navicular bone. Sometimes a fracture may not show up in the first x-ray and your doctor

may recommend that you have a repeat x-ray in 1 to 2 weeks.

How is it treated?

You will need to wear an arm cast that will include your thumb. The cast may or may not extend above your elbow and may be left in place for up to 12 weeks to be sure the bone heals.

In some cases healing does not occur and the pieces of bone do not grow back together. This may require surgery to fix. Sometimes the failure of the pieces of bone to grow back together leads to a problem called avascular necrosis. In avascular necrosis, part of the bone dies because it does not get enough blood. In these cases, an operation is necessary to remove part of the injured bone, insert bone to help heal the fragment, or insert an artificial bone. Complete recovery may occur or you may have some permanent stiffness or loss of range of motion.

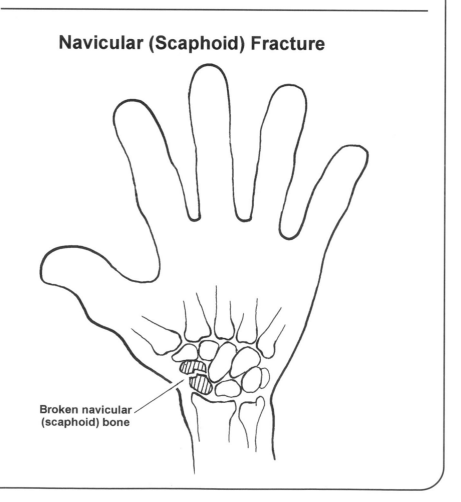

Navicular (Scaphoid) Fracture

Broken navicular
(scaphoid) bone

Navicular (Scaphoid) Fracture

When can I return to my sport or activity?

The goal of rehabilitation is to return you to your sport or activity as soon as is safely possible. If you return too soon you may worsen your injury, which could lead to permanent damage. Everyone recovers from injury at a different rate. Return to your sport or activity will be determined by how soon your wrist recovers, not by how many days or weeks it has been since your injury occurred.

You may return to your sport or activity when you have full range of motion in your wrist without pain. You doctor may allow you to return to competition with your wrist taped or in a brace. Your injured wrist, hand, and forearm need to have the same strength as the uninjured side. You must not have any pain when you do activities such as swinging a bat or a racquet or tumbling in gymnastics.

If you return to a sport or activity too soon after a navicular fracture there still could be problems with healing. It is very important to be sure that none of your activities cause wrist pain and that you do not develop tenderness over the "snuff-box" area of your wrist.

How can I prevent a navicular fracture?

A navicular fracture usually occurs during an accident that is not preventable. When you do activities such as rollerblading be sure to wear protective wrist guards.

Navicular (Scaphoid) Fracture
Rehabilitation Exercises

You may do stretching exercises 1 and 2 when your cast is removed. You may do strengthening exercises 3 through 7 when stretching is nearly painless.

1. Active range of motion

   A. Flexion (forward bending): Bend your wrist as far forward as you can, trying to touch your fingers to your wrist.

   B. Extension (backward bending): Try to bend your wrist backward as far as you can.

   C. Side to side: Move your wrist from side to side.

2. Stretching

   A. Wrist flexion and extension: With your hand bent forward stretching into the flexion position, apply pressure with your other hand to push it farther. Next, with your palm up, apply pressure on your fingers with your other hand to bend your hand and fingers backward.

   B. Wrist flexion stretch: Standing with the back of your hand on the table, your fingers and palms facing up and your elbows straight, lean away from the table. Hold this position for 15 to 30 seconds.

   C. Wrist extension stretch: Standing at a table with your palms down, your fingers flat, and your elbows straight, lean your body weight forward and hold this position for 15 to 30 seconds.

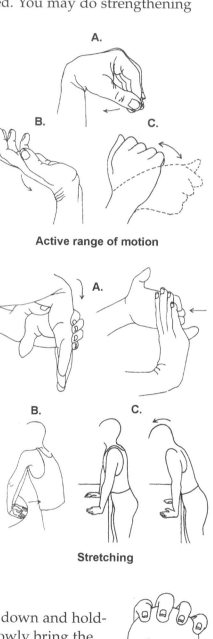

Active range of motion

Stretching

3. Wrist flexion: Holding a soup can or hammer handle with the palm facing up, bend your wrist upward. Slowly lower the weight and return to the starting position. Repeat 10 times. Do 3 sets of 10.

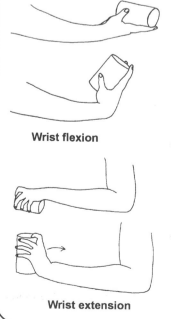

Wrist flexion

Wrist extension

4. Wrist extension: With your palm facing down and holding a can of soup or hammer handle, slowly bring the wrist and hand up. Slowly lower the weight down again to the starting position. Repeat 10 times. Do 3 sets of 10.

5. Finger flexion: Using a rubber ball or other object that you can grasp in your hand, squeeze as tight as you can with your fingers and hold for 5 seconds. Release and repeat this 10 times. Do 3 sets of 10.

Finger flexion

© HBO & Company

Navicular (Scaphoid) Fracture Rehabilitation Exercises

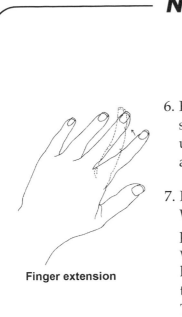

Finger extension

6. Finger extension: With your palm flat on a table and your fingers straight out, lift each finger straight up one at a time. Hold your finger up for 5 seconds then and put it down. Continue until you have done all 5 fingers. Repeat 10 times.

7. Pronation and supination of the forearm: With your elbow bent 90 degrees, turn your palm up and then turn your palm down without letting your elbow move. To challenge yourself, hold a hammer by the end of the handle and slowly turn the palm up. Then turn the palm down. Repeat 10 times. Do 3 sets of 10.

Pronation and supination of the forearm

Triangular fibrocartilage complex injuries

What is the triangular fibrocartilage complex?

The triangular fibrocartilage complex (also called the TFCC) is a small piece of cartilage and ligaments on the little finger side of the wrist located just past the end of the forearm bone (ulna). Cartilage is a tough rubbery tissue that acts as a cushion for the joint. The ligaments are connective tissue that attach the cartilage to bones in the wrist.

How do triangular fibrocartilage complex injuries occur?

These usually occur by:

- a fall onto the outstretched hand
- a direct blow to the little finger side of the wrist or hand
- swinging a bat or a racquet
- a violent twist to the wrist at work or in sports

What are the symptoms?

- Pain on the little finger side of the wrist
- Clicking or catching when moving the wrist

How is it diagnosed?

Your doctor will examine your wrist and hand. There will be tenderness at the little finger side of the wrist. There may be clicking or catching.

Your doctor may order an x-ray, an arthrogram (an x-ray done after special dye is injected into the wrist to outline the injured structures) or an MRI (magnetic resonance image).

Arthroscopy may be necessary to diagnose the tear.

What is the treatment?

The early treatment of TFCC injuries include:

- protective support such as a splint or a cast
- ice for 20 to 30 minutes 3 to 4 times a day
- anti-inflammatory medications such as ibuprofen
- wrist rehabilitation exercises
- an injection of a cortisone-like medication

A complete tear may require surgery. Many tears become painless with rest and time even if they don't actually heal.

When can I return to my sport or activity?

The goal of rehabilitation is to return you to your sport or activity as soon as is safely possible. If you return too soon you may worsen your injury, which could lead to permanent damage. Everyone recovers from injury at a different rate. Return to your sport or activity will be determined by how soon your wrist recovers, not by how many days or weeks it has been since your injury occurred. In general, the longer you have symptoms before you start treatment, the longer it will take to get better.

You may return to your sport or activity after your wrist injury when the injured wrist has full range of motion with-

---

Triangular fibrocartilage complex injuries

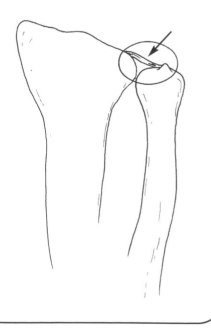

Triangular fibrocartilage complex injuries

out pain. Your doctor may allow you to return to competition with your wrist taped or in a brace. Your injured wrist, hand, and forearm need to have the same strength as the uninjured side. There must not be any pain when you do activities such as swinging a bat or a racquet or tumbling in gymnastics.

How can I prevent a TFCC injury?

Many injuries are caused by falls or blows that cannot be prevented. In racquet sports it is important to use good technique to prevent injury.

Triangular fibrocartilage complex Rehabilitation Exercises

You may do stretching exercises 1 through 5 when the sharp wrist pain goes away. You may do strengthening exercises 6 through 8 when stretching is nearly painless.

1. Active range of motion:

    A. Flexion: Gently try to bend your wrist forward. Hold for 5 seconds. Repeat 10 times. Do 3 sets.

    B. Extension: Gently bend your wrist backward. Hold this position for 5 seconds. Repeat 10 times. Do 3 sets.

    C. Side to side: Gently move your wrist from side to side, holding 5 seconds at each end. Repeat 10 times. Do 3 sets.

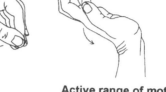
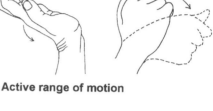

A.   **B.**   **C.**

Active range of motion

2. Stretching: With your uninjured hand, help to bend the wrist down by pressing the back of your hand and holding for 15 to 30 seconds. Next, stretch it backward by pressing the fingers in a backward direction and holding for 15 to 30 seconds.

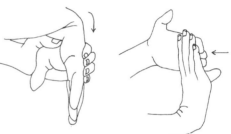

Stretching

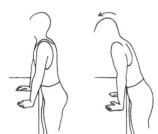

Wrist extension stretch

3. Wrist extension stretch: Stand at a table with your palms down, fingers flat, and elbows straight. Lean your body weight forward. Hold this position for 15 to 30 seconds.

4. Wrist flexion stretch: Stand with the back of your hands on a table, palms facing up, fingers pointing toward your body, and elbows straight. Lean away from the table. Hold this position for 15 to 30 seconds.

Wrist flexion stretch

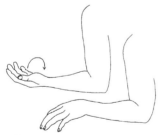

Pronation and supination of the forearm

5. Pronation and supination of the forearm: With your elbow bent 90 degrees, turn your palm upward and hold for 5 seconds. Slowly turn your palm downward and hold for 5 seconds. Make sure you keep your elbow at your side and bent 90 degrees throughout this exercise. Repeat this 10 times.

6. Wrist flexion exercise: Holding a can or hammer handle with your palm up, bend your wrist upward. Slowly lower the weight and return to the starting position. Repeat 10 times. Do 3 sets of 10. Gradually increase the weight of the can or weight that you are holding.

Wrist flexion

Triangular fibrocartilage complex Rehabilitation Exercises

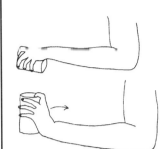

Wrist extension

7. Wrist extension: Holding a can or hammer handle with your palm facing down, slowly bend your wrist upward. Slowly lower the weight down to the starting position. Repeat 10 times. Do 3 sets of 10. Gradually increase the weight of the object you are holding.

8. Grip strengthening: Squeeze a rubber ball and hold for 5 seconds. Repeat 10 times.

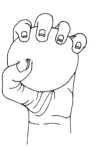

Grip strengthening

Trigger Finger

What is trigger finger?

Trigger finger is a condition in which it is difficult to straighten a finger (or fingers) once bent. The medical term for trigger finger is stenosing tenosynovitis.

How does it occur?

Trigger finger results from inflammation or swelling of the fibrous sheath that encloses the tendons. A tendon is a band of strong fibrous tissue that connects a muscle to a bone.

The straightening mechanism hesitates for a few moments before the tendon suddenly overcomes the resistance. The finger then straightens with a sudden jerk or triggering motion.

What are the symptoms of trigger finger?

Symptoms include:

- a snapping sensation (triggering) in the affected finger or fingers
- inability to extend the finger smoothly or at all (it may lock in place while bent)
- tenderness to the touch over the tendon, usually at the base of the finger or palm
- soreness in the affected finger or fingers.

How is trigger finger diagnosed?

Your doctor will review your symptoms and examine you.

How is trigger finger treated?

Sometimes it is helped by ice and anti-inflammatory medication, such as ibuprofen. If this does not work, your doctor may give you an injection of a local anesthetic to keep you from feeling pain in the area and a corticosteroid (cortisonelike medicine) to reduce the inflammation of the tendon sheath.

If necessary, the doctor will use surgery to remove the part of the tendon sheath that is causing the tendon to get stuck.

When can I return to my sport or activity?

You may return to your sport or activity when your finger no longer catches or locks.

How long do the effects of trigger finger last?

The severity of trigger finger varies from person to person. Although response to treatment varies, results are usually good.

Trigger Finger

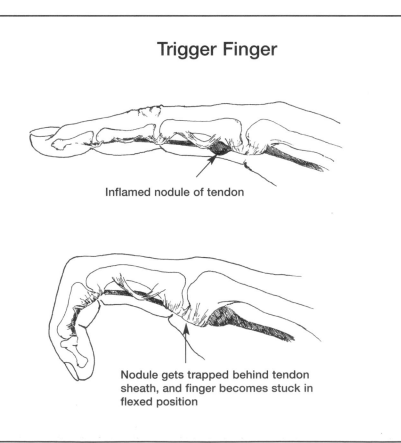

Inflamed nodule of tendon

Nodule gets trapped behind tendon sheath, and finger becomes stuck in flexed position

Trigger Finger

It is best to discuss progress with your doctor on a regular basis. Surgery for this condition is usually very successful.

How can I take care of myself?

It is important to follow your doctor's instructions. In addition, rest and limit the activity of the affected finger or fingers and of the hand and wrist.

What can I do to help prevent trigger finger?

Since the cause of trigger finger is unknown, there is no reliable way to prevent this condition from developing.

Ulnar Collateral Ligament Sprain
(Skier's Thumb)

What is an ulnar collateral ligament sprain of the thumb?

A sprain is a joint injury that causes a stretch or tear in a ligament. A ligament is a strong band of tissue connecting one bone to another. An ulnar collateral ligament sprain of the thumb is a painful injury that may cause looseness of the thumb joint at the base of the thumb where it attaches to the hand.

Sprains are graded I, II, or III, depending on the severity of the sprain:

- grade I sprain: pain with minimal damage to the ligament
- grade II sprain: more ligament damage and mild looseness of the joint
- grade III sprain: complete tearing of the ligament and the joint is very loose or unstable.

How does it occur?

A sprain of the ulnar collateral ligament in the thumb is a common injury in skiing. It may occur when you fall onto your outstretched thumb, bending it back toward your arm. This stretches and injures the ulnar collateral ligament. It may also be caused by catching your thumb on your ski pole strap. It may occur in other activities when you fall onto your outstretched thumb or when your thumb gets hooked onto another player's jersey or face mask.

What are the symptoms?

You usually have pain, swelling, and tenderness at the inner part of the base of your thumb where it attaches to your hand. It may be difficult to hold an object in your hand and apply force with your thumb. Moving your thumb causes pain.

How is it diagnosed?

Your doctor will review your symptoms, examine your thumb, and check to see if your thumb joint is loose. Your doctor may order an x-ray of your thumb to see if it is broken.

How is it treated?

A grade III sprain with a very loose joint requires surgery to repair the ligament. Grade I and grade II sprains may be treated with a cast, taping, or splinting so that the thumb does not move for up to 6 weeks.

**Ulnar Collateral Ligament Tear
(Skier's Thumb)**

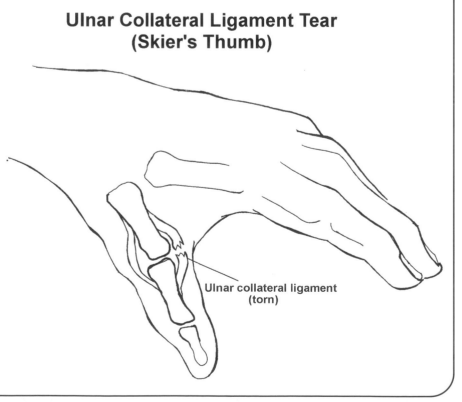

Ulnar collateral ligament
(torn)

— Ulnar Collateral Ligament Sprain (Skier's Thumb) —

Initially, the hand with the injured thumb should be kept elevated on a pillow when you are lying down or on the back of a chair or couch when you are sitting. Place ice on your thumb for 20 to 30 minutes every 3 to 4 hours for 2 to 3 days or until the pain goes away. Your doctor may prescribe an anti-inflammatory medication or other pain medication.

When can I return to my sport or activity?

The goal of rehabilitation is to return you to your sport or activity as soon as is safely possible. If you return too soon you may worsen your injury, which could lead to permanent damage. Everyone recovers from injury at a different rate. Return to your sport or activity will be determined by how soon your thumb recovers, not by how many days or weeks it has been since your injury occurred. In general, the longer you have symptoms before you start treatment, the longer it will take to get better.

After you have sprained the ulnar collateral ligament of your thumb you may return to your activity when your injured thumb has gained full strength compared to the uninjured thumb. Swelling must be gone and you must have full range of motion.

In sports such as skiing be sure that you are able to grasp a ski pole with full strength. In sports such as baseball or tennis be sure that you are able to grasp the bat and racquet with full strength and without pain. Your doctor may advise you to wear a thumb or wrist brace or tape your thumb before your activities.

How can I prevent an ulnar collateral ligament sprain?

Ulnar collateral ligament sprains are caused by falling onto an outstretched thumb. Many times this happens during accidents that are not preventable. However, in skiing you may be able to avoid this injury by using ski poles that do not have straps.

© HBO & Company

— Ulnar Collateral Ligament Sprain (Skier's Thumb) — Rehabilitation Exercises

If you have had surgery or if you have been in a cast or splint, you may do these exercises when your doctor says you are ready.

1. Thumb range of motion: With your palm flat on a table or other surface, move your thumb away from your hand as far you can. Hold this position for 5 seconds and bring it back to the starting position. Rest your hand on the table in a handshake position. Move your thumb out to the side away from your palm as far as possible. Hold for 5 seconds. Return to the starting position. Next, bring your thumb across your palm toward your little finger. Hold this position for 5 seconds. Return to the starting position. Repeat this entire sequence 10 times. Do 3 sets.

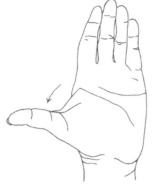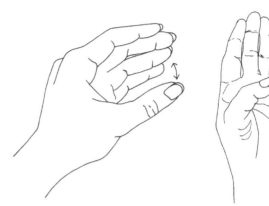

Thumb range of motion

2. Wrist range of motion: Move your wrist up and down and side to side. Move through each position until you feel a stretch. Hold the stretched position for 5 seconds. Repeat each position 10 times. Do 3 sets.

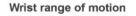

Wrist range of motion

3. Thumb strengthening: Pick up small objects such as paper clips, pencils, and coins using your thumb and each of your other fingers one at a time. Practice this exercise for about 5 minutes.

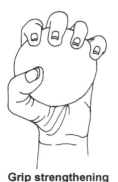

4. Grip strengthening: Grasp a rubber ball or similar round object and squeeze it as tightly as you can. Hold this position for 5 seconds. Repeat 20 times.

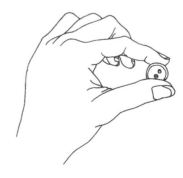

Thumb strengthening

Grip strengthening

Ulnar Neuropathy
(Handlebar Palsy)

What is ulnar neuropathy?

Ulnar neuropathy is an inflammation of the ulnar nerve, a major nerve in your arm that runs down into your hand. It supplies movement and sensation to your arm and hand. Ulnar neuropathy causes numbness, tingling, or pain into the arm and hand on the side of the little finger. Bicyclists call this condition handlebar palsy.

How does it occur?

The ulnar nerve may get inflamed in several areas as it travels from your neck to your hand. The ulnar nerve is commonly inflamed during bicycling from repeated shocks or bouncing while your hand is holding onto the handlebar. The nerve may be stretched when held in the lower position of a drop handlebar. Other activities that involve repetitive movements of the wrist may cause ulnar neuropathy.

What are the symptoms?

The symptoms include numbness, tingling, or pain in the forearm or hand on the side of the little finger.

How is it diagnosed?

Your doctor will ask about your symptoms and examine your neck, shoulder, arm, and wrist. Your doctor may refer you to a specialist to have tests done, such as a nerve conduction study (NCS) and electromyogram (EMG).

How is it treated?

It is important to try to find and eliminate the cause of your ulnar neuropathy. You may be prescribed wrist splints to reduce the discomfort. When you are bicycling, it might help to wear padded gloves. You might also try adjusting the position of your

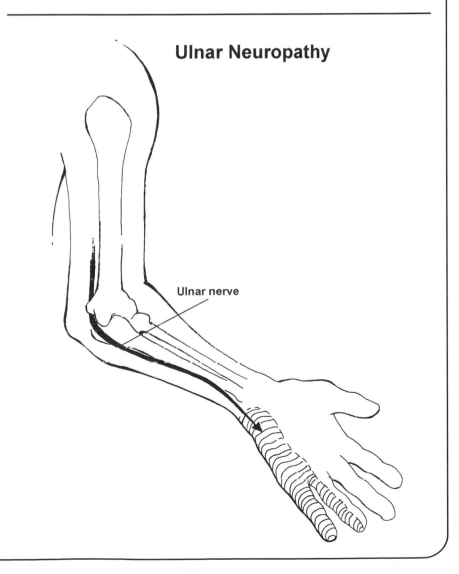

Ulnar Neuropathy

Ulnar nerve

Ulnar Neuropathy (Handlebar Palsy)

hands on the handlebar, such as by changing your grip from the top to the sides of the handlebar. Your doctor may prescribe anti-inflammatory medications or B vitamins.

When can I return to my sport or activity?

The goal of rehabilitation is to return you to your sport or activity as soon as is safely possible. If you return too soon you may worsen your injury, which could lead to permanent damage. Everyone recovers from injury at a different rate. Return to your sport or activity will be determined by how soon your nerve recovers, not by how many days or weeks it has been since your injury occurred. In general, the longer you have symptoms before you start treatment, the longer it will take to get better.

You may return to your sport or activity when you are able to forcefully grip your tennis racquet, bat, or golf club, or do activities such as working at a keyboard without pain or tingling in your elbow or hand.

How can I prevent ulnar neuropathy?

Ulnar neuropathy is caused by activities that inflame the ulnar nerve. Try to eliminate activities that cause repetitive motion of the wrist, which can irritate your ulnar nerve. When you are bicycling, change your hand position on the handlebar frequently.

Ulnar Neuropathy (Handlebar Palsy)
Rehabilitation Exercises

You may do all of these exercises right away.

1. Cervical range of motion exercises (neck):

A. Rotation: Slowly turn your head toward your shoulder, keeping your chin level. Hold for 10 seconds. Bring your head back to the neutral position. Then turn your head to the opposite shoulder.

B. Neck flexion: Bend your neck so that your chin touches your chest. Hold for 10 seconds. Bring your head back to the neutral position.

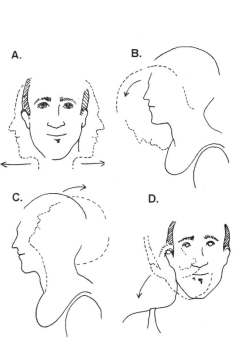

C. Neck extension: Slowly tilt your head backward so that your chin is pointing towards the ceiling. Hold for 10 seconds. Note: If this position causes you to be dizzy or if it brings on symptoms in your arm, do not do this exercise.

D. Side bend: Looking straight ahead, bring your ear toward your shoulder. Hold for 10 seconds. Return your head to the upright position. Repeat on the opposite side.

Cervical range of motion exercises

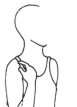

Shoulder Depression

2. Shoulder depression: Facing straight ahead, pull your shoulder blades down and back. Hold for 10 seconds. Relax. Repeat 10 times.

3. Elbow range of motion: Slowly bend your elbow and bring your hand toward your shoulder. Then straighten your elbow. Repeat 10 times.

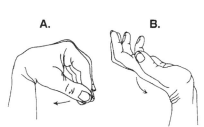

4. Wrist range of motion: Bend your wrist forward and backward. Repeat 10 times.

Wrist range of motion

Elbow range of motion

5. Straight finger flexion: Make a right angle with your knuckles and keep your fingers straight. Hold this position for 10 seconds. Repeat 5 times.

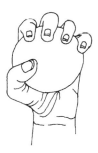

6. Finger squeeze: Practice squeezing items between each of the fingers on your involved hand. You can use paper, pens, and sponges. Hold for 10 seconds. Repeat 5 times for each finger.

7. Finger flexion: Practice squeezing a rubber ball and hold 10 seconds. Repeat 10 times.

Finger flexion

Finger squeeze

Wrist Sprain

What is a wrist sprain?

A sprain is an injury to a joint that causes a stretch or tear in a ligament. A ligament is a strong band of tissue connecting one bone to another. Your wrist is made up of eight bones that are attached to your hand bones and the bones of your forearm. The wrist joint is covered by a joint capsule and the bones are connected by ligaments.

How does it occur?

A wrist sprain can happen when you fall on your wrist or hand, when you are struck by an object, or during a forced motion of the wrist.

What are the symptoms?

You have pain, swelling, and tenderness in your wrist.

How is it diagnosed?

Your doctor will review your symptoms and examine your wrist. He or she may order an x-ray to be sure you have not broken any bones in your wrist.

How is it treated?

Treatment may include:
• putting ice packs on your wrist for 20 to 30 minutes every 3 to 4 hours for 2 or 3 days or until the pain goes away

• elevating your wrist on the back of a chair or couch while sitting or on a pillow while sleeping
• taking an anti-inflammatory or other pain medication prescribed by your doctor
• wearing a splint or cast on your wrist to prevent further injury
• doing exercises to help your wrist recover.

While you are recovering from your injury you will need to change your sport or activity to one that does not make your condition worse. For example, you may need to run instead of playing basketball.

When can I return to my sport or activity?

The goal of rehabilitation is to return you to your sport or activity as soon as is safely possible. If you return too soon you may worsen your injury, which could lead to permanent damage. Everyone recovers from injury at a different rate. Return to your sport or activity will be determined by how soon your wrist recovers, not by how many days or weeks it has been since your injury occurred. In general, the longer you have symptoms before you start treatment, the longer it will take to get better.

You may return to your sport or activity when the injured wrist has full range of motion without pain. Your doctor may allow you to return to competition with your wrist taped or in a brace. Your injured wrist, hand, and forearm need to have the same strength as the uninjured side. You must not have any pain when doing activities such as swinging a bat or a racquet or performing tumbling in gymnastics.

How can I prevent a wrist sprain?

A wrist sprain usually occurs during an accident that is not preventable. However, when you are doing activities such as rollerblading be sure to wear protective wrist guards.

Wrist Sprain Rehabilitation Exercises

You may do stretching exercises 1 through 5 when the sharp wrist pain goes away. You may do strengthening exercises 6 through 8 when stretching is nearly painless.

1. Active range of motion:

   A. Flexion: Gently try to bend your wrist forward. Hold for 5 seconds. Repeat 10 times. Do 3 sets.

   B. Extension: Gently bend your wrist backward. Hold this position for 5 seconds. Repeat 10 times. Do 3 sets.

   C. Side to side: Gently move your wrist from side to side, holding 5 seconds at each end. Repeat 10 times. Do 3 sets.

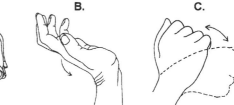
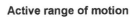

Active range of motion

2. Stretching: With your uninjured hand, help to bend the wrist down by pressing the back of your hand and holding for 15 to 30 seconds. Next, stretch it backward by pressing the fingers in a backward direction and holding for 15 to 30 seconds.

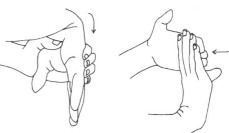

Stretching

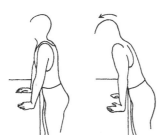

Wrist extension stretch

3. Wrist extension stretch: Stand at a table with your palms down, fingers flat, and elbows straight. Lean your body weight forward. Hold this position for 15 to 30 seconds.

4. Wrist flexion stretch: Stand with the back of your hands on a table, palms facing up, fingers pointing toward your body, and elbows straight. Lean away from the table. Hold this position for 15 to 30 seconds.

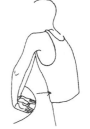

Wrist flexion stretch

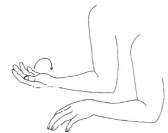

Pronation and supination of the forearm

5. Pronation and supination of the forearm: With your elbow bent 90 degrees, turn your palm upward and hold for 5 seconds. Slowly turn your palm downward and hold for 5 seconds. Make sure you keep your elbow at your side and bent 90 degrees throughout this exercise. Repeat this 10 times.

6. Wrist flexion exercise: Holding a can or hammer handle with your palm up, bend your wrist upward. Slowly lower the weight and return to the starting position. Repeat 10 times. Do 3 sets of 10. Gradually increase the weight of the can or weight that you are holding.

Wrist flexion

Wrist Sprain Rehabilitation Exercises

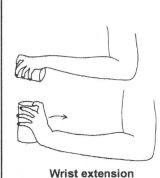

Wrist extension

7. Wrist extension: Holding a can or hammer handle with your palm facing down, slowly bend your wrist upward. Slowly lower the weight down to the starting position. Repeat 10 times. Do 3 sets of 10. Gradually increase the weight of the object you are holding.

8. Grip strengthening: Squeeze a rubber ball and hold for 5 seconds. Repeat 10 times.

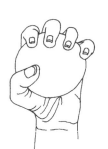

Grip strengthening

Wrist Tendonitis

What is wrist tendonitis?

Tendons are bands of connective tissue that attach muscle to bone. Tendonitis occurs when a tendon is inflamed from overuse. Your wrist moves in many directions, including down, up, in, and out. The muscles and tendons that perform these movements may become overused and inflamed. The muscles and tendons that cross your wrist and attach to your thumb may also become inflamed.

How does it occur?

Tendonitis is a problem caused by repetitive use. Possible overuse activities include throwing, catching, bowling, hitting a tennis ball, typing, or sewing.

What are the symptoms?

You have pain with repetitive activity. The tendon that is inflamed is tender to the touch. You may have swelling around the inflamed tendon.

How is it diagnosed?

Your doctor will review your symptoms and examine your wrist.

How is it treated?

Treatment may include the following:

- applying an ice pack for 20 to 30 minutes every 3 to 4 hours for the first 2 to 3 days or until the pain goes away
- elevating your wrist on a pillow while sleeping or on the back of a chair or couch while sitting
- wearing a splint that immobilizes the wrist or thumb or taping the wrist or thumb
- taking anti-inflammatory medication prescribed by your doctor
- doing stretching and strengthening exercises.

In many cases of tendonitis, the injury occurs because of poor technique in a sporting activity. Your doctor may review your technique and try to help you change it.

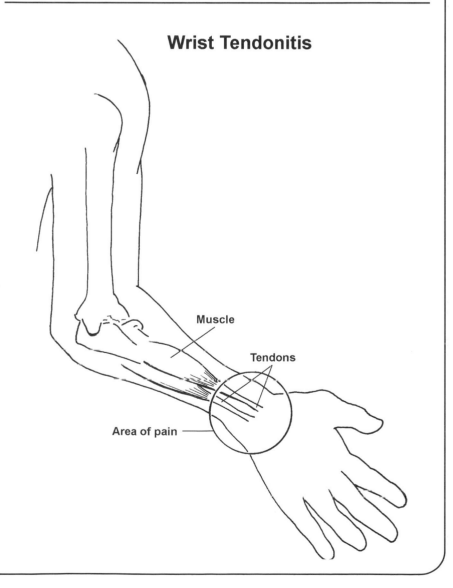

Wrist Tendonitis

Muscle

Tendons

Area of pain

Wrist Tendonitis

While you are recovering from your injury you will need to change your sport or activity to one that does not make your condition worse. For example, you may need to run instead of play racquet sports. The most important treatment for tendonitis is to change your activity.

When can I return to my sport or activity?

The goal of rehabilitation is to return you to your sport or activity as soon as is safely possible. If you return too soon you may worsen your injury, which could lead to permanent damage. Everyone

recovers from injury at a different rate. Return to your sport or activity will be determined by how soon your wrist recovers, not by how many days or weeks it has been since your injury occurred. In general, the longer you have symptoms before you start treatment, the longer it will take to get better.

You may return to your sport or activity after your wrist injury when the injured wrist has full range of motion without pain. You doctor may allow you to return to competition with your wrist taped or in a brace. Your injured wrist, hand, and forearm need to

have the same strength as the uninjured side. There must not be any pain when you do activities such as swinging a bat or a racquet or tumbling in gymnastics.

How can I prevent wrist tendonitis?

Tendonitis is caused from overuse. Use proper technique in activities such as throwing, hitting a tennis ball, and typing. You should not continue to do these activities when the warning signs of tendonitis begin.

© HBO & Company

Wrist Tendonitis Rehabilitation Exercises

1. Active range of motion

   A. Flexion (forward bending): Gently try to bend your wrist forward. Hold for 5 seconds. Repeat 10 times. Do 3 sets.

   B. Extension (backward bend): Gently bend your wrist backward. Hold this position for 5 seconds. Repeat 10 times. Do 3 sets.

   C. Side to side: Gently move your wrist from side to side, holding it for 5 seconds at each end. Repeat 10 times. Do 3 sets.

A. **B.** **C.**

Active range of motion

2. Stretching: With your uninjured hand, help to bend your wrist down by pressing the back of your hand and holding for 15 to 30 seconds. Next, stretch it backward by pressing the fingers in a backward direction and holding for 15 to 30 seconds.

Stretching

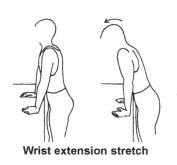

Wrist extension stretch

3. Wrist extension stretch: Stand at a table with your palms down, fingers flat, and elbows straight. Lean your body weight forward. Hold this position for 15 to 30 seconds.

4. Wrist flexion stretch: Stand with the back of your hands on a table, palms facing up, fingers pointing toward your body, and elbows straight. Lean away from the table. Hold this position for 15 to 30 seconds.

Wrist flexion stretch

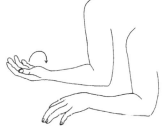

Pronation and supination of the forearm

5. Pronation and supination of the forearm: With your elbow bent 90 degrees, turn your palm upward and hold for 5 seconds. Slowly turn your palm downward and hold for 5 seconds. Make sure you keep your elbow at your side and bent 90 degrees throughout this exercise. Repeat 10 times.

6. Wrist flexion exercise: Hold a can or hammer handle in your hand with your palm facing up. Bend your wrist upward. Slowly lower the weight and return to the starting position. Repeat 10 times. Do 3 sets of 10. Gradually increase the weight of the can or weight you are holding.

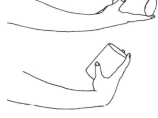

Wrist flexion

Wrist Tendonitis Rehabilitation Exercises

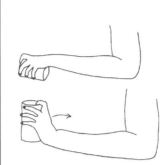

Wrist extension

7. Wrist extension: Hold a can or hammer handle in your hand with your palm facing down. Slowly bend your wrist upward. Slowly lower the weight down into the starting position. Repeat 10 times. Do 3 sets of 10. Gradually increase the weight of the object you are holding.

8. Grip strengthening: Squeeze a rubber ball and hold for 5 seconds. Repeat 10 times.

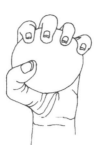

Grip strengthening

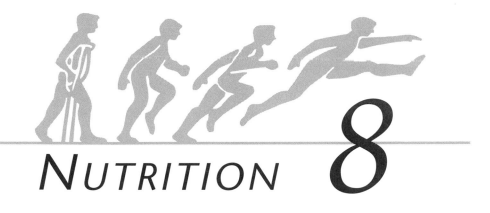

NUTRITION 8

Caffeine and Athletic Performance

How does caffeine affect athletic performance?

Many people like caffeine because it makes them feel more alert, gives them more energy, improves their mood, and makes them more productive. Athletes often use caffeine to help them perform better, both in routine workouts and in competition.

Like other drugs, caffeine can provide some benefits but too much can lead to problems. While one or two cups of coffee may give you short-term bursts of energy or improvement in concentration, it usually takes very high levels of caffeine to produce a real improvement in athletic performance. And at those high levels you can experience sleeplessness, anxiety, stomach upset, headache, and a wired or jittery feeling.

Caffeine works by stimulating your central nervous system. In the past, researchers thought that caffeine improved endurance performance by stimulating a greater use of fat for energy so that less of the stored energy in your muscles (glycogen) was burned. However, more recent caffeine studies don't support this theory. When caffeine improves endurance, it does so by acting as a stimulant.

Is there a limit on how much caffeine I can have?

Too much caffeine can not only produce ill effects but can deprive an athlete of the chance to compete.

The current list of drugs banned by the International Olympic Committee (IOC) contains more than 40 different stimulants, including caffeine over a certain limit. Coffee, tea, chocolate, and colas, as well as NO DOZ and some nonprescription painkillers contain caffeine. Because caffeine is a common ingredient in foods and drinks, the IOC allows an upper limit of 12 mcg/mL of urine tested.

Over a 2- to 3-hour period, a dose of 100 mg of caffeine results in a urine concentration of 1.5 mg/mL. So, for example, if in a 3-hour period you consumed 800 mg of caffeine (5 to 6 cups of strong coffee or a couple of espresso drinks), you could exceed the legal dose.

To improve your endurance by saving the energy in your muscles, you would have to take in so much caffeine that you would come close to exceeding the legal limit.

What are the sources of caffeine?

The table below lists items that contain caffeine and the urine levels they produce.

What should I keep in mind?

1. Be aware of the caffeine in your food, drinks, and medication, including nonprescription drugs.

2. Know how much caffeine you consume during the course of a day.

3. Listen to your body. Know how caffeine affects you. If

Product	Amount/Dose	Equivalent in urine within 2 to 3 hours
1 cup of coffee	100 mg	1.50 mcg/mL
1 Coke, Diet Coke	45.6 mg	0.68 mcg/mL
1 NO DOZ	100 mg	1.50 mcg/mL
1 Anacin	32 mg	0.48 mcg/mL
1 Excedrin	65 mg	0.97 mcg/

Caffeine and Athletic Performance

you have ill effects from caffeine, cut back.

4. Don't try using caffeine to give you a boost during competition if you haven't used caffeine before.

5. If you feel like coffee improves your performance, be sure you don't consume so much that you exceed the legal limit.

MODERATION - Use caffeine carefully. Too much caffeine may be bad for you and could cause you to be disqualified from competition.

Calcium

What is calcium?

Calcium is a mineral that is very important for:

- teeth
- nerves
- muscles
- bone health
- blood clotting.

If you do not get enough calcium in your diet you may be at risk for losing calcium from your bones and developing a condition called osteoporosis.

How much calcium do I need ?

How much calcium you need depends on your age and whether you are male or female. The recommendations are shown in the first table.

What are good sources of calcium?

Dairy products are one of the best sources of calcium. Calcium may also be found in a variety of other foods.

Many brands of orange juice, cereal, and bread are fortified with extra calcium. Check the labels.

Do I need a calcium supplement?

If you can get enough calcium in your diet, you do not need to take calcium supplements.

Calcium Recommendations

Group	mg calcium/day
Children	800
Teenagers (up to age 24)	1200
Adult men	800
Premenopausal women (over age 24)	1000
Postmenopausal women	1000-1500
Pregnant and breast-feeding women (age 18 or less)	1300
Pregnant and breast-feeding women (age 19-50)	1000

Dairy products are the easiest source of calcium. It is difficult to get enough calcium without consuming these products. Some people cannot digest most dairy products because their bodies lack the enzyme needed to break down milk sugar (lactose). They must follow a lactose-free diet. There

Sources of Calcium

Food	Serving size	mg calcium (approximate)
Milk, whole, 2%, 1%, or skim	8 oz	300
Yogurt	8 oz	300
Cheddar cheese	1 oz	200
Ice cream	1/2 cup	100
Frozen yogurt	1/2 cup	100
Cottage cheese	1/2 cup	90
Tofu, firm	4 oz.	250
Soy milk, unfortified	8 oz	80
Greens (collard, kale, mustard)	1/2 cup	80-150
Red beans, chickpeas	3/4 cup	60
Sardines (with bones)	3 oz	350
Salmon, canned (with bones)	3 oz	180
Molasses, blackstrap	1 tablespoon	125
Corn tortilla	2	90
Seaweed, dry	1/2 cup	100

Calcium

are enzyme replacement products available to aid in digestion of dairy products. Ask your doctor, nutritionist, or pharmacist about these products.

If you do need calcium supplements, many types are available. The calcium is usually combined with carbonate, citrate, lactate, gluconate, or phosphate. The body absorbs all forms of calcium equally well. However, avoid bone meal, dolomite, and oyster shell calcium because they may contain lead or other toxic metals. Check the label to see how much "essential calcium" is in each pill.

Too much calcium from supplements may cause a problem with kidney stones in some people.

Does anything affect the body's ability to absorb calcium?

Caffeine can decrease absorption, as can too much dietary fiber, phosphates (soft drinks), and taking medicines like tetracycline (an antibiotic) and antacids that contain aluminum. Vitamin D increases calcium absorption.

Creatine

What is creatine?

Creatine monohydrate is a dietary supplement used for increasing muscle mass and improving performance in short-duration, high-intensity exercise. It is popular with athletes, weight lifters, and body builders, and has been in use for the past 5 to 10 years.

The long-terms risks of using creatine are not known. Its use is not banned by the International Olympic Committee or other sports regulatory organizations.

Creatine is similar to an amino acid. It is made naturally in your liver and then stored in your muscles. In your diet it is found in red meat. As a supplement it is usually sold in powder or tablet form.

How does it work?

When muscles contract they use a substance called adenosine triphosphate (ATP), which is broken down into adenosine diphosphate (ADP). Creatine helps turn ADP back into ATP for the working muscles, giving them a greater energy source for short bursts of exercise such as sprinting. Creatine has been shown to be especially effective in performance of repeated bursts of exercise because it enhances recovery.

Studies show that creatine increases the amount of water stored in muscle and increases muscle volume. Almost all studies have been done in men.

Most athletes taking creatine will gain between 2 and 10 pounds over 4 to 10 weeks. Creatine makes athletes bigger but not more skillful or agile. Between 20% and 30% of people don't benefit from creatine, and nobody knows why. Athletes who compete in sports dependent on weight, power, and short bursts of intense activity (football, basketball) may benefit from creatine, while those in sports such as long-distance running may not. Most studies have shown no improvement in swimming or cycling performance.

How do I take it?

When you start taking creatine you need to take loading doses for 5 days. This dose is 20 to 25 grams per day. During this phase, it is important to eat lots of carbohydrates because this will help bring the creatine into your muscles and reduce its excretion into the urine. Creatine loading should be done in the preseason or several weeks before an important athletic event.

The maintenance dose of creatine is 2 to 5 grams a day. Most sports medicine experts believe you should stop taking it after 2 months. For most people, there is no increased benefit after 2 months, and the weight and performance benefits gained can usually be maintained through training. Many people take multiple cycles of it, taking it for 2 months, going off it for several months, and then going back on it again. Nobody knows how long it is safe to take it.

What are the side effects and risks?

The side effects of short-term use are minimal. Some people may have stomach upset or muscle cramping. To avoid dehydration and possible muscle cramping, drink lots of fluids while you are taking creatine.

The risks of long-term use of creatine are not known, but some doctors believe that it could lead to kidney damage.

Fluids and Hydration

How important are fluids?

Fluid replacement is probably the most important nutritional concern for athletes. Approximately 60% of your body weight is water. As you exercise, fluid is lost through your skin as sweat and through your lungs when you breathe. If this fluid is not replaced at regular intervals during exercise, you can become dehydrated.

When you are dehydrated, you have a smaller volume of blood circulating through your body. Consequently, the amount of blood your heart pumps with each beat decreases and your exercising muscles do not receive enough oxygen from your blood. Soon exhaustion sets in and your athletic performance suffers.

If you have lost as little as 2% of your body weight due to dehydration, it can adversely affect your athletic performance. For example, if you are a 150-pound athlete and you lose 3 pounds during a workout, your performance will start to suffer unless you replace the fluid you have lost. Proper fluid replacement is the key to preventing dehydration and reducing the risk of heat injury during training and competition.

How can I prevent dehydration?

The best way to prevent dehydration is to maintain body fluid levels by drinking plenty of fluids before, during, and after a workout or race. Often athletes are not aware that they are losing body fluid or that their performance is being impacted by dehydration.

If you are not sure how much fluid to drink, you can monitor your hydration using one of these methods.

1. Weight: Weigh yourself before practice and again after practice. For every pound you lose during the workout you will need to drink 2 cups of fluid to rehydrate your body.

2. Urine color: Check the color of your urine. If it is a dark gold color like apple juice, you are dehydrated. If you are well hydrated, the color of your urine will look like pale lemonade.

Thirst is not an accurate indicator of how much fluid you have lost. If you wait until you are thirsty to replenish body fluids, then you are already dehydrated. Most people do not become thirsty until they have lost more than 2% of their body weight. And if you only drink enough to quench your thirst, you may still be dehydrated.

Keep a water bottle available when working out and drink as often as you want, ideally every 15 to 30 minutes. High school and junior high school athletes can bring a water bottle to school and drink between classes and during breaks so they show up at workouts hydrated.

What about sport drinks?

Researchers have found that sports drinks containing between 6% and 8% carbohydrate (sugars) are absorbed into the body as rapidly as water and can provide energy to working muscles that water cannot. This extra energy can delay fatigue and possibly improve performance, particularly if the sport lasts longer than 1 hour. If you drink a sports drink, you can maintain your blood sugar level even when the sugar stored in your muscles (glycogen) is running low. This allows your body to continue to produce energy at a high rate.

Drinks containing less than 5% carbohydrate do not provide enough energy to improve your performance. So, athletes who dilute sports drink are most likely not getting enough energy from their drink to maintain a good blood sugar level. Drinking

Fluids and Hydration

beverages that exceed a 10% carbohydrate level (most soda pop and some fruit juices) often have negative side effects such as abdominal cramps, nausea, and diarrhea and can hurt your performance.

What does the sodium in sports drinks do?

Sodium is an electrolyte needed to help maintain proper fluid balance in your body. Sodium helps your body absorb and retain more water. Researchers have found that the fluid from an 8-ounce serving of a sports drink with 6% carbohydrates (sugars) and about 110 mg of sodium absorbs into your body faster than plain water.

Some parents, coaches, and athletes are concerned that sports drinks may contain too much sodium. However, most sports drinks are actually low in sodium. An 8-ounce serving of Gatorade has a sodium content similar to a cup of 2% milk. Most Americans do get too much sodium, but usually from eating convenience-type foods, not from sports drinks.

What are guidelines for fluid replacement?

- Drink a sports drink containing 6% to 8% carbohydrate to help give you more energy during intense training and long workouts.

For example, 240 mL (a 1 cup serving) of a drink with 24 grams of carbohydrate per serving would have a 10% carbohydrate concentration. Almost all drinks have the grams of carbohydrate per serving and the volume in mL somewhere on the container.

- Drink a beverage that contains a small amount of sodium and other electrolytes (like potassium and chloride).
- Find a beverage that tastes good; something cold and sweet is easier to drink.

- Drink 10 to 16 ounces of cold fluid about 15 to 30 minutes before workouts. Drinking a sports drink with a 6% to 8% carbohydrate level is useful to help build up energy stores in your muscles.
- Drink 4 to 8 ounces of cold fluid during exercise at 10 to 15 minute intervals.
- Start drinking early in your workout because you will not feel thirsty until you have already lost 2% of your body weight; by that time your performance may have begun to decline.
- Avoid carbonated drinks, which can cause gastrointestinal distress and may decrease the fluid volume.
- Avoid beverages containing caffeine and alcohol due to their diuretic effect.
- Practice drinking fluids while you train. If you have never used a sports drink don't start during a meet or on race day. Use a trial-and-error approach until you find the drink that works for you.

Formula for percentage of carbohydrate in your drink

$$\frac{\text{grams of carbohydrate/serving}}{\text{mL of drink/serving}} \times 100 = \text{\% of carbohydrate in drink}$$

The Healthy Diet

For a healthy diet you need to eat a wide variety of foods in moderate-sized portions that give your body the nutrients and energy it needs. You also need to limit foods in your diet that can be harmful to your body.

The Foods to Limit

Some foods contain very little nutritional value or have ingredients that can cause disease. Eating healthy doesn't mean giving up all sweets, salt, and snacks. It means eating such foods in moderation. The foods and food ingredients you need to limit include fat, cholesterol, sodium, alcohol, and sugar.

Eating foods high in cholesterol and saturated fat can cause atherosclerosis (narrowing of blood vessels from buildup of fatty deposits). This is critical for everyone but especially important if you have a family history of high cholesterol levels or diabetes. Atherosclerosis can lead to heart disease and strokes. Cholesterol is a substance found in animal products such as meat, eggs, dairy products, and baked goods made with eggs and milk. Vegetables do not contain cholesterol.

Of the various types of fats, saturated fats are the least healthy. They tend to increase the level of cholesterol in your blood. In fact, the amount of saturated fat in food is at least as important as the amount of cholesterol. Foods labeled "No Cholesterol" sometimes contain high saturated fat. Saturated fats are generally solid at room temperature. Foods that contain saturated fat include butter, cheese, margarine, shortening, tropical oils such as coconut and palm oil, and the fats in meat and poultry skin.

To reduce the saturated fat in your diet, limit the amount of butter and margarine you eat. Drink nonfat or low-fat milk. Choose lean cuts of meat and take the skin off poultry before you eat it. If you use cooking oil, avoid tropical oils such as palm or coconut oil as well as peanut oil. Better oils to use are sunflower, canola, soy, or olive oil.

Sodium, one of the ingredients in table salt, can contribute to high blood pressure if it is eaten in excess. Sodium is found in many foods, not just in table salt. Fast foods usually contain high amounts of sodium. An average healthy person should have no more than 2400 mg (milligrams) of sodium a day and no less than 500 mg a day. Read the labels on food packaging to check how much sodium is in the food. Table 3 shows some examples.

On food labels, "low sodium" means each serving contains less than 140 mg of sodium. "Moderate sodium" is 140 to 400 mg per serving. "High sodium" is more than 400 mg of sodium per serving.

Excess alcohol consumption can lead to weight gain, liver disease, brain damage, and other disorders. Women should have no more than one drink a day. Men should not have more than two drinks a day. A drink equals about 5 ounces of wine, one can of beer, or one ounce of distilled spirits.

Sugar and foods that contain a lot of sugar supply a large

Some Sodium Contents

Food	Approximate mg of Sodium
Big Mac or Whopper	1000
Bread (2 slices)	200 to 600
Cheese, cheddar (1.5 oz)	300
Fruit (1)	2 to 5
Milk (1 cup)	120
1 teaspoon of salt	2100

The Healthy Diet

number of calories but very little nutrition. Sugar also causes tooth decay.

The Foods You Need

A healthy diet depends on eating a variety of foods. If you eat a variety of foods you are more likely to get all the necessary nutrients. Your diet should contain the following nutrients:

- Proteins
  Proteins form the basic structure of body tissue and organs. The body uses proteins for growth and repair of cells. Proteins are found in eggs, milk, cheese, tofu, nuts, meat, fish, poultry, dried beans, split peas, and lentils. About 15% of your daily calories should come from protein.

- Carbohydrates
  Carbohydrates are the body's main source of energy. Carbohydrates are found in potatoes, bread, cereals, grains, pasta, milk, yogurt, vegetables, and fruit. They should make up at least half of your daily calories.

- Fats
  Fats provide energy and are used for growth and repair of tissues. They are found in olives, nuts, cheese, meat, fish, poultry, butter, oils, avocado, and mayonnaise. Saturated fats are less

healthy than polyunsaturated and monounsaturated fats. Saturated fats are found mostly in butter, margarine, meat, cheese, poultry with skin, tropical oils, and whole-milk dairy products. Monounsaturated fats are found in olive oil, canola oil, and avocados. Polyunsaturated fats are found in fish and some vegetable oils.
Fats should contribute no more than 30% of your daily calories. Only 10% of the fat you eat should be saturated fat. There are nine calories in a gram of fat. So, to calculate the maximum grams of fat you should eat each day, use these formulas:

1. Multiply the maximum number of calories you should eat in a day by 0.30 (30%) to calculate the maximum number of calories you should get from fat.

Number of calories a day x 0.30 = Number of calories from fat in a day

2. Divide the daily number of calories from fat (the answer from the calculation above) by 9 to find the maximum number of grams of fat you should eat each day.

Number of calories from fat / 9 = Number of fat grams a day
  For example, if you need 1800 calories per day, no more than 30% of those calories

should come from fat: 1800 x 0.30 = 540 calories from fat. Divide 540 by 9 to find out the maximum number of grams of fat you should consume each day: 540/9 = 60 grams of fat.

- Fiber
  Fiber is found in plants and is not digested by the body. It provides what is considered "bulk," which is used by the large intestine to help remove waste through bowel movements. Lack of fiber in your diet can worsen intestinal problems, such as constipation. Fruit, vegetables, bran, whole grains, and cereals are good sources of fiber. It is recommended that you get 20 to 35 grams of fiber a day. A diet high in fiber may help reduce your cholesterol levels.

- Vitamins and Minerals
  Vitamins are important nutrients that help to regulate metabolism and help the brain, nerves, muscles, skin, and bones function properly. The major vitamins are A, B, C, D, E, K, B-12, and seven B complex vitamins. Minerals are necessary in very small amounts for the body to function properly. For example, calcium is necessary for healthy teeth and bones, and zinc and magnesium are needed to control cell metabolism. Iron is important for healthy blood and

The Healthy Diet

many chemical reactions in your body. Vitamins and minerals are found in many foods, especially milk, cheese, green leafy vegetables, fish, meat, and poultry. They are also added to milk and cereal.

- Water

  Water is necessary to replace the fluid your body loses every day when you breathe, go to the bathroom, and sweat. You should drink six to eight glasses of water or other liquids (including soups and other beverages) every day.

  You can use the following chart as a guideline for choosing the types and amounts of foods you eat in a day. Remember that carbohydrates (grains, fruits, vegetables) should make up at least half of your daily calories and variety is important.

Meat versus Vegetarian Diet

Meat, including poultry and fish, is a very nutrient-rich food. Meat is one of the best sources of iron and protein. Most people get much more protein than they need, however. You should limit the amount of meat you eat, but you don't have to eliminate meat altogether. Choose lean cuts of meat and try to use the meat as a side dish rather than

Daily Food Serving Recommendations

servings	Number of serving size	Examples of Food Group
Meat, poultry, fish, dried beans, eggs	2 to 3	2 to 3 oz of lean meat, 1 egg, 1/2 cup cooked beans
Grains	6 to 11	1 slice of bread, 1/2 cup pasta or rice, 1 oz of cereal
Fruits	2 to 4	1 fruit, 3/4 cup fruit juice
Vegetables	3 to 5	1/2 cup nonleafy vegetable, 1 cup leafy vegetable
Milk, cheese, yogurt	2 to 3	1 cup milk or yogurt, 1 to 2 oz cheese

a main course. You can include meat in a casserole or stew, using the meat as a flavoring for the main dish without overeating the meat portion.

It is possible to have a healthy diet without eating meat. Vegetarians do have to be careful to make sure they get enough iron and protein, however.

Guidelines for Eating Healthfully

For best nutrition, choose foods containing high-fiber, complex carbohydrates and monounsaturated or polyunsaturated fats instead of refined, low-fiber carbohydrates and saturated fats.

Learn more about nutrition and healthy living. Read the ingredients on all packaged and canned foods you buy. Some contain more fat, sodium, sugar, and preservatives than you expect.
In addition:

- Bake or broil food instead of frying it.
- Don't eat more than four egg yolks a week. Egg whites are healthy, but egg yolks are not.
- Have a green leafy salad at least once a day. (Leaf lettuces and spinach are much more nutritious than iceberg lettuce.) Use oily dressings sparingly on the salads or try nonfat dressings.
- Eat fresh foods instead of canned foods.
- Eat more whole-grain products.
- Cook vegetables only slightly or eat them raw.
- Limit the amount of red meat you eat; eat more fish.
- Remove the skin from poultry before eating it.
- Limit fat, cholesterol, sugar, alcohol, salt, and caffeine in your diet.

The Healthy Diet

- Avoid pre-prepared foods as much as possible.

- Limit dining at fast food restaurants. If you do dine there, leave off the bacon, cheese, sour cream, mayonnaise, and fatty salad dressings. Order broiled instead of fried items.

Eating Healthy Snacks

Is snacking harmful?

Americans say they are very concerned about nutrition. Fifty-eight percent of those surveyed believe fat in food is a serious health problem. However, according to some food surveys, only 35% say they are doing all they can to eat a balanced diet. A great majority admit they eat between meals. The top-selling snack food in America is potato chips. The number-one snack from vending machines is the Snickers candy bar.

While many people complain they want healthier snacks in vending machines, far fewer people actually buy them. Most Americans feel guilty about picking high-fat, high-calorie snacks, but guilt isn't enough to change their eating habits. Should we feel guilty? Not always. There are times when snacking is important and good for your body.

Who should eat snacks?

- Infants and toddlers need to snack because they have such high energy demands and small stomachs.
- Teenagers who are rapidly growing and developing also need to snack because they require more calories and nutrients to sustain their growth spurts.
- Athletes involved in sports or endurance training need to snack to meet their increased energy demands. Carbohydrates (stored as a substance called glycogen in the liver and muscles) are used up during exercise and must be replenished.
- Laborers and construction workers have very high energy demands that cannot be met in three meals per day so they may need a snack.
- People who may not have time to sit down for a meal should snack so they don't have an energy letdown in the late afternoon.
- People who don't eat breakfast should carry a snack with them so they will have fuel flowing to their brains when they need to focus on their work.

If you do not fit into one of the above categories, it is still all right to snack on healthy foods. Just think twice before snacking on high-calorie, high-fat foods. Candy bars and ice cream between meals can lead to weight gain.

What snacks are good?

Well-planned snacks can help most people reach their dietary goals. Picking snacks to complement your meals or your diet is the key to snacking. Make sure you eat food from all five food groups during the day.

The five food groups are:

1. Meat, poultry, fish, dried beans, eggs
2. Grains
3. Fruits
4. Vegetables
5. Milk, cheese, yogurt

Carbohydrates (grains, fruits, and vegetables) should make up at least half of your daily calories.

For example, if all you had for breakfast was a bowl of cereal with low-fat milk and you became hungry at 10:00 a.m., pick a snack from the food groups that you missed. Because you had only two of the five food groups for breakfast, you should pick a snack from one or more of the other three, like fruits, fruit juice, vegetables, peanut butter on celery, apples, or bagels. Because most Americans do not eat enough complex carbohydrates you are always safe choosing snack foods like breads, cereals, bagels, fruits, and vegetables.

For active athletes or growing children who sometimes need foods with more calories, you can add these items to the list of snack foods: peanut butter sandwiches, low-fat milk-

Eating Healthy Snacks

shakes (with skim milk and low-fat ice cream), dried fruit, cottage cheese, and pasta with sauce.

Can I eat high-fat, high-calorie foods occasionally?

Indulging once in a while is normal and healthy. People who swear off all sweets and high-fat foods can begin to crave sweets and fatty foods, which can lead to overeating. Instead, sit down and enjoy the taste and pleasant feelings you get from having that high-fat, high-calorie snack. If guilt overcomes you or you want to enjoy this kind of snack more often, prepare for the extra calories and fat by skipping that extra serving of food at dinner or by exercising a little longer. The fear of having to give up a favorite snack is one of the main reasons most Americans exercise. You can have your cake and eat it, too, as long as you maintain a regular and consistent exercise program.

Snacks You Can Eat Every Day

Snack	Grams of fat	Calories
Nonfat yogurt with fruit (1 cup)	0	100
Baby carrots (3 oz)	0	40
Fresh fruit: Banana (small)	0	100
Apple (medium)	0	60
Pear (medium)	0	60
Orange (medium)	0	60
Kiwi (2)	0	40
Bagel (1)	1.4	165
Cold cereal	1.0	110
Fig Newtons (2)	2.0	100
Graham crackers (2)	1.5	60
Instant oatmeal (1 oz)	1.7	100
Rice cakes (2)	0.2	70
Pretzels (1 oz)	1.0	110
Skim milk (8 oz)	1.0	110

Iron

What is iron?

Iron is a mineral that is important to all body cells. It is particularly important for blood cells because iron is needed to make hemoglobin. Hemoglobin is the protein in blood cells that carries oxygen to body tissues.

If you don't have enough iron you may develop iron deficiency anemia, a condition in which your blood contains less hemoglobin than normal. People who have iron deficiency anemia are often tired and lack energy.

Iron deficiency anemia may result from:

- a diet that lacks enough iron
- blood loss
- body changes during pregnancy.

How much iron do I need?

How much iron you need depends on your age and whether you are male or female. The recommendations are:

What foods are good sources of iron?

Iron is found in a variety of foods. Heme iron is found in meat, poultry, and fish. Non-heme iron is found in fruits, vegetables, grains, nuts, and legumes. The body absorbs heme iron better than non-heme iron.

Many cereals and breads are fortified with extra iron. Check the labels.

Do I need an iron supplement?

If you get enough iron in your diet you don't need a supplement. Taking unnecessary sup-

Food sources of iron

Food	Serving size	mg iron (approximate)
beef	3 oz	2.5
chicken, white	3 oz	0.8
chicken, dark	3 oz	1.1
lamb	3 oz	1.5
pork, loin	3 oz	0.7
pork, shoulder	3 oz	1.0
pork, leg	3 oz	0.6
turkey, white	3 oz	1.1
turkey, dark	3 oz	2.0
fish	3 oz	1.1
clams, raw	2 oz	8.0
shrimp	3 oz	2.6
liver, beef	3 oz	5.0
liver, chicken	3 oz	7.2
tofu, extra firm	4 oz piece	1.0
navy beans	1/2 cup	2.5
black-eyed peas	1/2 cup	4.0
garbanzo beans	1/2 cup	4.5
green peas	1 cup	2.5
lentils	1/2 cup	3.3
apricots, dried	10	1.7
dates	10	1.0
raisins	1/4 cup	1.0
prune juice	8 oz	2.7
green beans	1 cup	1.6
spinach	1/2 cup	3.2
potato, baked with skin	1	2.7
bagel	1	2.5
molasses, blackstrap	1 tablespoon	2.5
macaroni, enriched cooked	1 cup	2.0
wheat germ, toasted	2 tablespoons	1.0

Iron

Daily Recommended Requirement for Iron

Group	mg Iron/day
Children 1 through 10 years old	10
Males 11 through 18 years old	12
Men over 18 years old	10
Premenopausal females over 11 years old	15
Postmenopausal women	10
Pregnant and breast-feeding women	15 to 30

plements may be harmful. You can accumulate too much iron in your body, which can damage various organs.

If you have iron deficiency anemia your doctor may recommend a supplement. Some supplements cause constipation. Make sure you drink enough fluid and have enough fiber in your diet.

Does anything affect the way the body absorbs iron?

Vitamin C (found in citrus fruits and tomatoes) helps the body absorb nonheme iron. Eating heme-iron-rich foods with nonheme-iron-rich foods helps increase absorption. Consuming coffee and tea (even decaffeinated), excess dietary fiber, or calcium supplements within 2 hours of eating iron-rich foods can decrease iron absorption.

Precompetition meals

What's the purpose of the precompetition meal?

The precompetition meal serves two purposes:

- to keep you from feeling hungry before and during the event
- to maintain the levels of sugar in your blood for your
- muscles to use during training and competition.

Many athletes often skip meals before they train or workout, especially if the workout is in the early morning. Skipping meals or not eating before an early morning workout lowers the stored energy in your body and can impair your performance. This is particularly true if your workout involves endurance training that lasts for 30 minutes or longer.

When should I eat my precompetition meal?

Your stomach should not be full during your event. In general, it takes 1 to 4 hours for your stomach to digest a meal and empty it into your intestines. If you are nervous, that process may take even longer. Food that remains in your stomach during an event may cause stomach upset, nausea, and vomiting. If you

eat your meal 1 to 3 hours before the start of your competition, your stomach will be almost empty during the event.

What is a good precompetition meal?

Your pre-event meal should include foods that are high in carbohydrates, such as breads, pasta, fruits, or vegetables. Your stomach and intestines digest these foods quickly. Carbohydrates also help build up stored energy in your body for use later during your event.

To avoid stomach upset or nausea, the closer you are to the time of your event the less you should eat. You can have a liquid meal closer to your event than a solid meal because your stomach digests liquids faster. This is especially useful if you are nervous and tense.

If you compete at all-day events such as track meets, swimming meets, or tournaments, you may be tempted by whatever is available at concession stands. Consider the amount of time you have between your events, bring healthy foods, and plan accordingly. Suggested pre-event menus include the following: 1 hour or less before competition

- fruit or vegetable juice such as orange, tomato, or V-8, and/or
- fresh fruit such as apples, watermelon, peaches, grapes, or oranges and/or
- up to 1 and a half cups of a sports drink, such as Gatorade.

2 to 3 hours before competition

- fresh fruit, fruit or vegetable juices, and/or
- bread; bagels; English muffins with limited amounts of
- butter, margarine, or cream cheese; or low-fat yogurt; and/or
- up to 4 cups of a sports drink, such as Gatorade.

3 to 4 hours before competition

- fresh fruit, fruit or vegetable juices, and
- bread; bagels; baked potatoes; cereal with low-fat milk;
- low-fat yogurt; sandwiches with a small amount of peanut
- butter, lean meat, or low-fat cheese; and/or
- up to 7 and one-half cups of a sports drink.

Precompetition meals

Does eating sugary foods before exercise improve performance?

Athletes sometimes consume simple carbohydrates such as honey, candy, or soft drinks right before exercise in hopes of getting quick energy. Unfortunately, eating sugary foods won't provide it. Most of the energy for exercise comes from foods eaten several hours or even days before the start of the race or event.

If you are an endurance athlete, recent evidence suggests that eating some sugary foods (like energy bars, some types of candy bars, or sports drinks) 35 to 40 minutes before an event may benefit you by providing energy (glucose) to your exercising muscles when your other energy stores have dropped to low levels. However, athletes are sensitive to having their blood sugar levels go up and down quickly. Eating sugary foods right before an event could harm their performance. Try different things and find out what works best for you.

Does caffeine improve performance?

Caffeine works by stimulating your central nervous system. In the past, researchers thought that caffeine improved endurance performance by stimulating a greater use of fat for energy so that less of the stored energy in your muscles (glycogen) was burned. However, more recent caffeine studies don't support this theory. When caffeine improves endurance, it does so by acting as a stimulant.

Caffeine does not help everyone. Some people are very sensitive and have side effects that include nausea, muscle tremors, and headaches. Too much caffeine can cause you to produce more urine and lose more water, especially in hot weather. You could become dehydrated and hurt your performance.

The International Olympic Committee has placed limits on the amount of caffeine an athlete in international competition may use. Tablets containing caffeine taken before or during exercise should be used with caution due to their high levels of caffeine and the possibility of overdosing. What should I avoid for my precompetition meal? The hot dogs, doughnuts, nachos, potato chips, and candy bars found at most concession stands are very high in fat and not digested quickly. If you eat these foods as pre-event meals, they will likely be in your stomach much of the morning or afternoon. Avoid or limit eating these foods for your pre-event meal.

Strategies for Weight Gain

Why is weight management important?

Proper diet and a good conditioning program play a vital role in athletic performance. Athletes who are under their ideal playing weight will not perform as well as they might.

What about weight gain?

How many calories you need depends on your age, sex, weight, and activity level. To maintain your weight, you have to take in the same number of calories you burn. It takes about 3,000 calories a day for the average 165-pound man who is 19 to 24 years old to maintain his weight. From ages 25 through 49, the daily calorie requirement for maintenance drops to 2,700. An average 127-pound woman, 19 through 24 years old, will have to consume 2,100 calories daily for weight maintenance. From ages 25 through 49, it takes 1,900 calories per day. Your body weight will change when there is a difference between calories in and calories out.

To gain weight, athletes need to consume more calories than they expend. This sounds simple but may not be easy. Most research shows that it takes longer to gain weight than to lose it.

Since the goal is to increase muscle mass, be sure to increase your exercise level. Consuming more calories without exercise will increase body fat stores.

How many calories do I burn during exercise?

In planning your calorie needs, consult the following table. It gives the average calories burned for different activities. Multiply the number of calories burned per minute by the number of minutes that you exercise to get the number of calories you need to replace after exercise.

Family history plays a major role in an athlete's build. Athletes from naturally thin fami-

Calories Burned per Minute of Activity

120-lb person	160-lb person	Activity
2.5	3.4	Walking 2 miles an hour Bicycling 5 miles an hour
3.3	4.4	Walking 3 miles an hour Bicycling 6 miles an hour Badminton
5.1	6.8	Walking 4 miles an hour Dancing Calisthenics Bicycling 10 miles an hour Roller skating
6	8	Tennis (singles) Water skiing Basketball (recreational) Swimming (35 yards/minute)
6.5	8.7	Walking briskly 5 miles an hour
7.3	9.7	Jogging 5 miles an hour Bicycling 12 miles an hour
7.8	10.5	Downhill skiing Basketball (vigorous competition) Mountain climbing
9.2	12.3	Jogging 7 miles an hour Cross-country skiing Squash and handball
12.9	17.3	Running 9 miles per hour

From "The Ultimate Sports Nutrition Handbook" by Ellen Coleman and Suzanne Nelson Steen, Bull Publishing, 1996, Palo Alto, CA.

Strategies for Weight Gain

lies are less likely to be able to transform their bodies from slight, slender figures to bulky, muscular ones. With improved diet and suitable weight training, however, they can increase their chances of gaining weight. Many people naturally gain weight as they age because their metabolism slows down.

What are the keys to gaining muscle mass?

Muscle mass can be gained through moderate to intense strength training several times each week, coupled with taking in extra calories.

For each pound gained as muscle in a week, you will need to consume about 500 extra calories each day. The extra calories should come from a variety of foods: milk, meat, fruits, vegetables, and grains.

The key is to be consistent. Eating three meals a day with snacks in between is an essential part of gaining lean body mass. If you sleep in and skip breakfast, you miss a chance to add extra calories to your diet.

Eat enough to satisfy your appetite and then try to eat a little more. This can be done by:

- eating larger than normal portions
- eating an extra snack or meal

- drinking commercial liquid meals or milkshakes with regular meals or as snacks.

Some good snacks if you are trying to gain weight are:

- peanut butter sandwich
- low-fat milkshake (with skim milk and low-fat ice cream)
- dried fruit
- cottage cheese
- pasta with sauce.

Commercial protein supplements will not help you gain weight and will probably add too much protein to your diet. If you need a liquid supplement, make sure it provides the extra calories you need as carbohydrates, not protein.

Strategies for Weight Loss

Why is weight management important?

Proper diet and a good conditioning program play a vital role in athletic performance. Athletes who are not at their ideal playing weight will not perform as well as they might.

What about fad diets and crash diets?

Fad diets are popular because they promise rapid weight loss. However, fad diets and crash diets actually result in a loss of lean muscle mass, water, and stored energy, not a loss of excess body fat. As a result, most athletes on such diets become tired early in the day or game and have a hard time finding the energy they need.

How does weight loss occur?

How many calories you need depends on your age, sex, weight, and activity level. To maintain your weight, you have to take in the same number of calories you burn. It takes about 3,000 calories a day for the average 165-pound man who is 19 to 24 years old to maintain his weight. From ages 25 through 49, the daily calorie requirement for maintenance drops to 2,700. An average 127-pound woman, 19 through 24 years old, will have to consume 2,100 calories daily for weight maintenance. From ages 25 through 49, it takes 1,900 calories per day. Your body weight will change when there is a difference between calories in and calories out.

How can I lose weight?

To lose weight you must eat less, exercise more, or both. Combining diet with exercise is a healthier, more balanced, and more successful way of losing weight than by dieting alone.

One pound of body weight is equal to 3,500 calories. Eating 500 fewer calories per day will result in a weight loss of 1 pound per week. Eating 250 fewer calories per day combined with a 250-calorie deficit from exercise will also result in a weight loss of 1 pound per week. Athletes should lose no more than 2 to 3 pounds per week.

Calories Burned per Minute of Activity

120-lb person	160-lb person	Activity
2.5	3.4	Walking 2 miles an hour Bicycling 5 miles an hour
3.3	4.4	Walking 3 miles an hour Bicycling 6 miles an hour Badminton
5.1	6.8	Walking 4 miles an hour Dancing Calisthenics Bicycling 10 miles an hour Roller skating
6	8	Tennis (singles) Water skiing Basketball (recreational) Swimming (35 yards/minute)
6.5	8.7	Walking briskly 5 miles an hour
7.3	9.7	Jogging 5 miles an hour Bicycling 12 miles an hour
7.8	10.5	Downhill skiing Basketball (vigorous competition) Mountain climbing
9.2	12.3	Jogging 7 miles an hour Cross-country skiing Squash and handball
12.9	17.3	Running 9 miles per hour

Strategies for Weight Loss

Good High-Carbohydrate Foods to Eat

Food	Calories	Carbohydrates (grams)
Potato	220	50
Bagel	165	31
Biscuit	103	13
White bread, 1 slice	61	12
Cereal, 1 cup	110	24
Oatmeal, 1/2 cup	66	12
Graham crackers, 2	60	11
Rice, 1 cup	223	50
Noodles, 1 cup	159	34
Pizza, cheese, 1 slice	290	39
Pretzels, 1 oz	106	21

Making Proper Food Choices

Food Type	Choose	Decrease
Meats	Fish, poultry without skin, lean cuts of beef, lamb, pork, shellfish cold cuts, sausage,	Fatty cuts of beef, lamb, pork; spare ribs, organ meats, regular hot dogs, bacon
Dairy	Skim or 1% milk, buttermilk	Whole or 2% milk, whipped toppings, cream
	Nonfat or low-fat yogurt or cottage cheese	Whole-milk yogurt or cottage cheese
	Low-fat cheeses, farmer or pot cheeses (no more than 2 to 6 grams of fat per ounce)	All natural cheeses (blue, cheddar, Swiss, Roquefort)
	Sherbet, sorbet	Ice cream
Eggs	Egg whites (2 whites = 1 whole egg in recipes)	Egg yolks
Fruits Vegetables	Fresh, frozen, canned, dried	Vegetables prepared in butter, cream, or other sauces
Breads Cereals	Homemade baked goods, using unsaturated oils sparingly, angel food cake, low-fat crackers, low-fat cookies.	Commercial baked goods: pies, cakes, doughnuts, croissants, muffins, biscuits, high-fat cookies, high-fat crackers.

From "The Ultimate Sports Nutrition Handbook" by Ellen Coleman and Suzanne Nelson Steen, Bull Publishing, 1996, Palo Alto, CA.

Exercise

You should exercise 3 to 6 times per week for 30 to 60 minutes at 60% to 80% maximum heart rate. The goal is to expend at least 300 calories per exercise session. This would be about a 3-mile jog, 12-mile bicycle ride, or a 1-mile swim. See the chart below for more examples of calories burned during different types of exercise.

You may also burn off calories simply by being more active during the day:

- Take the stairs instead of the elevator.
- Park farther away from the store and walk briskly through the parking lot.
- Do your errands on foot or on a bicycle instead of driving.

Diet

To lose weight safely, it is important to eat a wide variety of foods. You should eat enough carbohydrates to fuel your body for exercise. You should reduce your fat intake to reduce calories, rather than follow a very low calorie diet. Because everyone is different, there are no general guidelines as to how much or how little you should eat or exercise. Use the charts below to help guide you in your food choices.

© HBO & Company

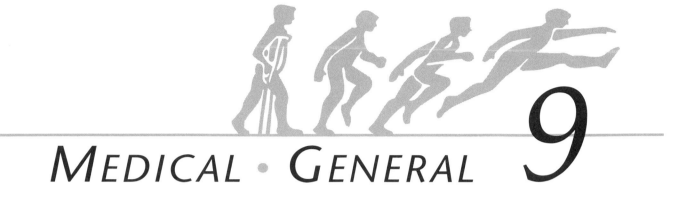

MEDICAL · GENERAL 9

Altitude Sickness

What is altitude sickness?

Altitude sickness is a problem that can occur when you travel to a high altitude, usually over 8000 feet above sea level. It is also called mountain sickness.

Especially serious types of altitude sickness are:

- high-altitude pulmonary edema (fluid in the lungs)
- high-altitude cerebral edema (swelling of the brain).

How does it occur?

The air at high altitudes contains less oxygen than at sea level. Your body has to work harder to get the oxygen it needs. Over several days at high altitude, your body adjusts to the lower amount of oxygen in the air.

Many people fly from sea level to mountain altitudes of 6,000 to 10,000 feet and start vigorous physical activity right away. Not giving the body time to adjust to the higher elevation can cause altitude sickness.

Certain health factors increase the risk of altitude sickness. These include:

- dehydration
- heart disease
- smoking
- diabetes
- anemia
- high blood pressure

- chronic lung problems such as asthma
- drinking too much alcohol.

Many athletes assume they won't get altitude sickness because they are in good shape. However, some people tend to get altitude sickness regardless of their condition.

Pulmonary or cerebral altitude edema may start out as a milder form of altitude sickness. It may then worsen into one of these more serious problems. But sometimes the edema occurs without the usual symptoms of mountain sickness.

What are the symptoms?

With altitude sickness, you may first feel like you have flu or a hangover. You may have:

- headache
- tiredness
- loss of appetite
- nausea
- trouble sleeping
- trouble breathing during exercise.

If you have pulmonary edema, excess fluid builds up in your lungs. You may become short of breath and start coughing. It may become very hard for you to breathe. You may cough up pink mucous.

When you have high-altitude cerebral edema, your brain swells. You may become confused and disoriented. You may feel weak, loose your sense of balance, or have trouble seeing.

How is it diagnosed?

Your health care provider will ask about your medical history and do a physical exam. If you do not have one of the more serious types of altitude sickness, the results of your exam will probably be normal. If you have fluid in your lungs, your health care provider will hear the sounds it makes. If you have brain swelling, your provider will probably see that you are having problems with your balance, vision, or ability to think clearly.

How is it treated?

The most important treatment for altitude sickness is to return to a lower elevation. For example, if you are at an altitude of 8,000 to 9,000 feet, you may need to travel down to an elevation of 5,000 feet or lower to help your symptoms go away. If this is not possible, you may be given oxygen for 12 to 24 hours. Your health care provider may prescribe medications.

If your symptoms go away at a lower altitude, you may try to return to a higher elevation after your body adjusts.

Altitude Sickness

This may take 1 to 3 days.

Both types of high-altitude edema are very serious and can be fatal. If you have had fluid in your lungs or brain swelling, you should not go back to the higher altitude.

How can I prevent altitude sickness?

To prevent altitude sickness:

- Begin your climb into the mountains a little at a time. Spend the first night at an altitude of 5,000 to 6,000 feet if possible.

- Ease into your physical activity by taking it easy the first day or two.
- Drink plenty of fluids such as water or sports drinks.
- Avoid drinking a lot of alcohol, coffee, or tea. They will cause you to urinate more often and become dehydrated.
- Avoid smoking. Smoking makes it more difficult for your body to get oxygen.
- Avoid sleeping pills. They may cause shallow breathing at night, making it more difficult for your body to absorb oxygen while you sleep.

Your health care provider may prescribe medications to help prevent altitude sickness. Take the medication before you get to a high altitude. Continue to take it while you are at high altitude.

© HBO & Company

Anorexia Nervosa

What is anorexia nervosa?

Anorexia nervosa is an eating problem that occurs when a person is extremely afraid of becoming overweight and therefore eats as little as possible. This condition is both a physical illness and a psychiatric illness. Hormone changes result from the low weight and low levels of body fat. In young women menstruation stops. Anorexia nervosa can be a very severe illness. Death may occur from starvation or suicide.

This illness occurs most often in young women. However, about 5% to 10% of people with anorexia nervosa are men.

How does it occur?

The cause of anorexia nervosa isn't clear. A contributing factor in many cultures is the emphasis on equating female beauty with thinness. Factors that increase the risk of developing anorexia nervosa include:

- a family history of anorexia nervosa or other eating disorders
- a family or personal history of mood disorders, such as major depression and bipolar disorder (manic depression).

What are the symptoms?

Symptoms may include:

- weight loss, usually severe
- binge eating (eating large amounts of food in a short time) and/or purging (using laxatives or making yourself throw up)
- tiredness
- depressed or anxious mood
- insomnia
- if you are a woman, a loss of your monthly periods when your weight drops below a certain level.

How is it diagnosed?

Your doctor does a physical exam and medical history. Your doctor will investigate eating and other behavior patterns, such as:

- extreme selectiveness in choosing food that is low in calories
- binge eating
- purging, taking laxatives
- ritualistic eating
- overexercising
- denial of hunger and denial of any problem at all.

How is it treated?

This can be a very difficult condition to treat. Individual psychotherapy and family therapy are usually necessary. Medication (especially medica-

tion effective in mood disorders) may be prescribed to help reduce the fear of becoming fat, reduce depression and anxiety, and aid in weight gain. You may need to be hospitalized if your condition is severe and life-threatening.

How long will the problem last?

If you have anorexia, you may have symptoms for many years and will probably need ongoing treatment. Any stressful situation can cause a relapse. After you have reached a normal weight, you may need to continue psychotherapy or medication for months or years. In addition, you may be weighed regularly to make sure you continue eating properly.

How can I take care of myself?

In addition to following your doctor's treatment plan and developing a support network, you can:

- Eat a nutritious, well-balanced diet.
- Moderate your exercise program.
- Get plenty of rest and sleep.
- Maintain a realistic weight for your height and body frame.

Anorexia Nervosa

- Take mineral and vitamin supplements.
- See your doctor regularly to have your weight checked.
- Keep an optimistic outlook.
- With your therapist, work out areas of conflict in your life.
- Balance your work with recreation and social activities.

- Learn to communicate your feelings.

What can be done to help prevent anorexia nervosa and maintain good physical health?

Acceptance of yourself and your body can help prevent this problem. In addition you can:

- Keep appointments with your doctor or therapist.
- Avoid skipping meals.
- Avoid using laxatives.
- Avoid drinking alcohol.
- Avoid smoking cigarettes.

Athletic Amenorrhea

What is amenorrhea?

Amenorrhea is not having a menstrual period.

There are two main kinds of amenorrhea, primary and secondary. Primary amenorrhea is when a young woman has not had a period by the age of 16. Secondary amenorrhea is when a woman begins missing periods and has only two periods in a year or doesn't have a period for 4 to 6 months.

What is athletic amenorrhea?

Athletic amenorrhea is when a woman does not have periods because she exercises very intensely and is very lean. Some women with athletic amenorrhea stop having periods. Some young women with athletic amenorrhea may delay their first period for years, even into their 20s.

How does athletic amenorrhea occur?

Intense exercise and extreme thinness may reduce the levels of hormones that regulate a woman's periods. These hormones, estrogen and progesterone, are important for overall body health. Estrogen is especially vital for healthy bones.

Athletic amenorrhea is often seen in sports that emphasize thinness, such as gymnastics, figure skating, and long-distance running. When thinness is heavily emphasized, some young women may develop eating disorders such as anorexia or bulimia. A person with anorexia diets excessively, sometimes to the point of starvation. People with bulimia binge (eat a lot at one time) and then purge, either by vomiting, using laxatives, or exercising excessively.

What are the symptoms?

You will not have periods.

A lack of estrogen leads to a lack of calcium in your bones. This makes the bones brittle and weak, a condition called osteoporosis. Intense exercise puts extra stress on weak bones, leaving athletes with osteoporosis at risk for stress fractures. Young women who have osteoporosis may never get enough calcium in their bones as they grow and mature. As they get older, their bones may break easily.

When a woman has a combination of athletic amenorrhea, an eating disorder, and osteoporosis, it is called the female athlete triad.

How is it diagnosed?

Your doctor will do various tests, including a pregnancy test, to find out why your periods have stopped or why they never started. (Pregnancy is the most common reason women miss periods.) He or she will talk to you about your exercise patterns and eating habits.

Your doctor may order a DEXA scan, a special type of x-ray that measures the density of your bones.

How is it treated?

Athletic amenorrhea needs to be treated in several ways because it often is a problem involving:

- too much exercise
- poor diet
- hormone imbalance.

To treat it:

- You may need to exercise less.
- Eat enough food to take in enough calories for your workouts.
- Make sure you have enough calcium in your diet.
- You may need to take birth control pills or other forms of estrogen to restore hormone balance.

If you are sexually active you can become pregnant, even if you have amenorrhea. Take precautions if you do not want to become pregnant.

Athletic Amenorrhea

How is it prevented?

A well-balanced diet with enough calories helps prevent athletic amenorrhea. It is important to recognize when you are exercising too much and eating too little. Eating disorders are serious problems and should be discussed openly with your health care provider.

Bulimia Nervosa

What is bulimia?

Bulimia nervosa is an eating disorder. It is characterized by binge eating (eating large amounts of food in a short time) followed by self-induced vomiting and/or use of laxatives.

Although most bulimics have a normal weight, they feel a lack of control over their eating behavior. After binging, they induce vomiting or use laxatives or diuretics because they are fearful of becoming overweight. They often feel that their lives are controlled by conflicts about eating. Although the disorder can affect men, most people with bulimia nervosa are female adolescents or young women.

How does it occur?

The exact cause of bulimia nervosa is not known. Some researchers believe that eating disorders may be related to malfunctioning of the part(s) of the brain regulating mood and appetite.

Factors that increase the risk of developing bulimia nervosa include:

- a family history of bulimia nervosa or eating disorders
- a family or personal history of mood disorders, such as major depression or bipolar disorder (manic depression).

What are the symptoms?

Symptoms of bulimia include:

- repeated episodes of binge eating
- strict dieting or fasting
- repeated weight loss and gain of more than 10 pounds
- dehydration
- weakness
- depression and guilt after binge eating
- damaged teeth from gastric acid contained in vomit
- swollen cheeks from repeated vomiting
- preoccupation with being thin
- depressed or anxious mood.

How is it diagnosed?

The doctor takes a medical history and does a physical exam. The doctor will ask about eating patterns, looking for such behavior as:

- repeated episodes of binge eating followed by self-induced vomiting or use of laxatives
- alternate binging and fasting
- secret eating and binging
- exercising excessively to prevent weight gain.

How is it treated?

People with this problem must recognize that they are suffering from a dangerous disorder. Treatment involves regulation of new eating habits. The doctor may recommend psychotherapy and family counseling and may prescribe medication used for mood disorders, such as antidepressants or mood stabilizers.

How long will the effects last?

The risk of relapse exists for years after treatment ends. Without treatment, a person with bulimia may become depressed and suicidal.

How can I take care of myself?

- Eat well-balanced, nutritious meals.
- Schedule meals regularly, but not too rigidly. Avoid irregular eating habits and avoid fasting.
- Take vitamin and mineral supplements.
- Avoid using laxatives and diuretics.
- Seek professional help if you need to lose weight so you can lose weight slowly and to a reasonable level.
- Exercise regularly and in moderation.

Bulimia Nervosa

What can be done to help prevent bulimia?

Many bulimics do not feel good about themselves. You can raise your self-esteem and thus prevent or minimize bulimia if you:

- Try to resolve areas of conflict in your life.
- Try to achieve a balance of work, social activities, recreation, rest, and exercise in your life.

- Create a support group of good friends.
- Keep a positive outlook on life.
- Stop judging yourself and others.

© HBO & Company

Cast Care

What is a cast?

A cast is a supportive structure that surrounds an injured body part to protect it, keep in from moving, and allow it to heal. Casts are made of fiberglass or plaster. They are most often used for broken bones. They are also used sometimes for torn ligaments or tendons and may be used after surgery.

How is a cast put on?

Your health care provider will first place padding around your injured body part. Casting material is rolled like a bandage over the padding. The casting material then hardens. While the casting material hardens, it will get warm.

How is a cast removed?

Your health care provider will remove the cast with a special cast saw. The special saw is designed so that it will not cut your skin. The cast should be removed only by your provider.

How long will I need to wear my cast?

How long you wear your cast depends on your injury. Some injuries heal within a few weeks and some take several months.

Can I get my cast wet?

Most casts should not get wet. A plaster cast will fall apart if it gets wet. A fiberglass cast won't fall apart but the padding underneath may start to smell if it gets wet. Wet padding may also hurt your skin.

When you shower or bathe, put your cast in a heavy plastic bag. Hold the bag in place with a rubber band. Even then, try not to get the bag wet. If your cast does get wet, you can dry it with a hair dryer.

Your doctor may give you a special cast and liner that allows you to get the cast wet and even swim.

After my cast is put on what problems should I watch for?

Your injury may continue to swell. To limit swelling, elevate the injured area at a level above your heart. Signs of problem swelling include:

- You have severe or persistent pain.
- Your fingers or toes feel numb or painful or can't move.
- The color of your fingernails or toenails changes.

Sometimes the body part inside a cast becomes infected. Signs of infection include:

- drainage from the skin under the cast
- pain
- fever.

After a while the cast may not fit well. It may feel too loose or too tight. It may weaken due to wear and tear.

Contact your health care provider immediately if you have any of these problems.

What can I do about itching?

Many people have itching inside a cast. Never reach inside a cast with your fingernails or another object to scratch. It may injure your skin and cause an infection. Sometimes shaking a small amount of talcum powder inside a cast or using a hair dryer on a cool setting helps relieve the itching.

How active can I be when I have my cast?

How active you can be depends on your injury. Be sure to ask your health care provider about this.

Crutches

What are crutches?

Crutches are supports that help you walk when you have an injured leg or foot.

How do I use crutches?

Walking: Bring the crutches forward evenly, keeping your injured leg off the ground. Lean forward, putting your weight on your hands against the grips of the crutches. Don't rest your armpits on the crutches. This can cause damage to a nerve that passes through the armpit. Swing your good leg forward, placing your foot just in front of the crutches. Repeat. (Note: In some cases your doctor may allow you to put some weight on your injured leg while you are using crutches.)

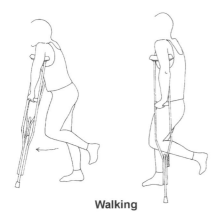

Walking

Getting up from a chair or bed: Hold both crutches by the grips in the hand on the side of the injured leg. Push up from the chair or bed with the other hand while pushing up on the crutches. Use your good leg to bring you to a standing position. Get your balance and bring your crutches into position before starting to walk.

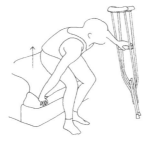

Getting up

Sitting down: Hold your crutches by the grips in the hand on the injured side. Hold onto the chair or bed with the other hand and lower yourself slowly. Unless you are allowed to put some weight on your injured leg, keep your injured leg off the ground and keep your weight on the good leg.

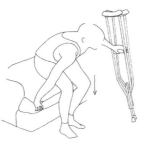

Sitting down

Stairs: Going up, get close to the stairs. Step up with the good leg, then bring the crutches and the injured leg up to the stair that the good leg is on. Repeat. Going down, first bring the crutches and the injured leg down to the lower step. Then step down with the good leg. Repeat. If there is a handrail, put both crutches under the opposite arm and use the rail for support. Remember: "Up with the good, down with the bad."

Going through doorways:

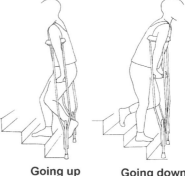

Going up   **Going down**

Be sure to give yourself enough room to allow your feet and crutches to clear the door. After opening the door, block it from swinging closed with a crutch tip. Walk through the doorway.

How can I take care of myself while I'm using crutches?

- Be careful not to slip on water or ice.
- Sometimes crutches rub against the skin between your arm and chest. You

Crutches

may want to use body lotion or talcum powder to prevent skin chafing.

- If your hands get sore or tired, you may want to put extra padding on the crutch grips.

- Be sure not to lean on the crutches and put pressure on your armpits. If there is pressure on your armpits even when you use the crutches correctly, they are too long and need to be shortened.

Exercise-Induced Asthma

What is exercise-induced asthma?

Asthma is a lung condition that causes wheezing, coughing, shortness of breath, and chest tightness. Exercise-induced asthma is a form of asthma that some people have during or after physical activity.

How does it occur?

In a person with asthma, the small airways of the lungs go into spasm or constrict. In exercise-induced asthma, this can occur:

- during or after physical activity and usually when breathing is hard, heavy, or fast
- when the air is cold
- when the humidity is very low or high
- when there is a lot of air pollution
- when there are a lot of allergens in the air.

For many people, winter sports such as cross-country skiing or bicycling in the cold air may trigger symptoms.

What are the symptoms?

The symptoms of exercise-induced asthma include:

- wheezing
- coughing
- shortness of breath
- chest tightness
- fatigue
- decreased athletic performance.

How is it diagnosed?

Your health care provider will ask about your history of breathing problems during or after exercise. He or she may ask you to run on a treadmill or to exercise outside the office. When you return, your health care provider will then listen to your lungs with a stethoscope to see if you are wheezing after the exercise.

Your health care provider may give you a small device called a peak-flow meter, which measures how fast you can exhale air in one breath. During a bout of exercise-induced asthma, this measurement will decrease from your normal measurement.

How is it treated?

Exercise-induced asthma can be successfully treated with medication. The kind of medication usually tried first is an inhaled bronchodilator. Examples of these medications are albuterol (Ventolin, Proventil) and pirbuterol (Maxair). Your health care provider will instruct you to take two puffs of this medication about 15 to 30 minutes before your activity. If your provider tells you to, you may also use this medication during your activity if you get symptoms.

How can I take care of myself?

Know what triggers your asthma. Some people have most symptoms during strenuous activity in cold, dry air. During the winter you may need to exercise indoors or to wear a mask when you exercise outside. Wearing a mask warms the air before you inhale it. Breathing through your nose warms the air more than mouth breathing and may help prevent exercised-induced asthma. You may also need to be aware of conditions such as air pollution or allergens such as dust or pollen.

Doing warm-up exercises before a vigorous workout may help prevent an asthma attack.

Many people, including successful athletes, have exercise-induced asthma. Proper education, use of medication, and activity modification should allow you to remain healthy and physically fit.

© HBO & Company

Frostbite

What is frostbite?

Frostbite is a problem where parts of your body are injured by freezing. The most common body parts to get frostbite are toes, feet, fingers, hands, nose, and ears.

How does it occur?

Frostbite occurs when the temperature of a body part drops below freezing. The skin and body tissues just below the skin become frozen and the blood flow decreases. Two types of frostbite can occur, superficial (mild) and deep (severe).

What are the symptoms?

Frostbitten skin may:

- feel cold
- feel like it is tingling or numb
- blister
- turn black in severe cases.

How is it diagnosed?

The doctor examines the frostbitten body part and will look for signs of frostbite.

How is it treated?

Frostbite is treated by rewarming the frostbitten skin. If your gloves or socks are wet, remove them. You can warm up and thaw mild frostbitten skin by placing your hands under your armpits or your feet against a warm person's belly.

Deep frostbite is treated best by rewarming the area in a hot water bath with a temperature of 104 to 108 degrees Fahrenheit. Once frostbitten areas are rewarmed and thawed, it is important that they do not get frozen again because worse tissue injury will occur. Sometimes body parts that have had severe frostbite may need to be amputated.

How long will the effects of frostbite last?

Frostbitten tissue may take time to get full sensation and strength back. Sometimes numbness at the tips of fingers or toes does not improve. A frostbitten body part will get colder faster than other body parts in the future.

How do I prevent frostbite?

Frostbite is best prevented by being prepared and dressing appropriately. It is important to wear several layers of clothes over one another rather than wearing a single, thick layer. The best layers are those that provide good insulation and keep moisture away from the skin. Materials that do this include polypropylene, polyesters, and wool. It is important to wear an outer garment that is waterproof but will also "breathe," such as Gore-Tex.

Heat Illness – Exercising in the Heat

What are heat illnesses?

When exercising in very hot or humid weather your body can become overheated and problems such as heat cramps, heat exhaustion, or heatstroke may occur.

How do they occur?

During exercise your body produces heat and your temperature rises. Your body has ways of cooling itself naturally, one of which is by sweating. When the sweat evaporates, it cools your skin. When the temperature is too hot or when there is too much humidity, sweating may no longer cool your body enough to keep your temperature from rising to dangerous levels. If your temperature goes above 104 degrees Fahrenheit, your body can lose the ability to cool itself.

Becoming dehydrated can also lead to heat illness.

What are the symptoms?

As your body gets hotter and is unable to cool down, symptoms progress. First, you may become dehydrated and get heat cramps. If not treated, your symptoms could become more severe and you could eventually develop a more serious problem, such as heat

exhaustion or heatstroke.

Symptoms of heat cramps:

- cramping or spasming of muscles during or after exercise.

Symptoms of heat exhaustion:

- rising body temperature
- dizziness
- weakness
- nausea
- vomiting
- muscle aches
- headaches
- increased sweating.

Symptoms of heatstroke:

- body temperature of 104 degrees F or higher
- no sweating
- confusion and disorientation
- erratic behavior
- agitation
- seizures
- coma
- injury to body organs.

How are they diagnosed?

Your doctor will examine you and ask you about your symptoms.

How are they treated?
HEAT CRAMPS:

Heat cramps are treated by drinking a lot of fluids, massaging the cramped area, and

stretching the cramping muscles. Heat cramps may improve more rapidly if you drink a sports drink that contains salt and other electrolytes, rather than water.

HEAT EXHAUSTION AND HEATSTROKE:

It is important that any exercising athlete with heat exhaustion or heatstroke immediately stop any activity. Follow the first aid procedures for heat exhaustion and heatstroke:

- Remove the person from the heat. Either bring the athlete inside or put him or her in the shade. Immediately cool the person down:
- He or she can be wet down with moist towels or a spray bottle and fanned.
- The person may be placed in a cool tub or packed in ice until his or her body temperature is below 102 degrees Fahrenheit.
- Have the person take in fluids, either by mouth or through a vein (intravenously). If the person cannot sip fluids, medical personnel may administer intravenous fluids in a first aid station or a hospital.

Heat Illness - Exercising in the Heat

A person with heatstroke needs to be brought to a hospital for further treatment and checked for organ damage. Heatstroke may cause damage to the kidneys, heart, lungs, muscles, liver, intestines, and brain.

How can I prevent heat illness?

It is very important for you to accustom yourself gradually to exercising in the heat. In hot or humid conditions, exercise early in the morning or later in the day.

It is very important to drink lots of fluids and avoid dehy-dration. Thirst or the lack of it is not an accurate indication of dehydration. You may lose up to 2 quarts of water for every hour that you exercise. It is a good idea to drink 2 cups of water about 30 minutes before exercising. While you are exercising, stop every 20 minutes and drink a cup of water.

If you are exercising for more than 1 hour, a sports drink may be useful before and during exercise. Sports drinks contain salt and potassium that is lost through sweating. It is important to avoid fluids that contain caffeine or alcohol because they will cause your body to lose more fluid through urination.

To be sure that you are drinking enough fluid during exercise, weigh yourself before and after your workout. If you have lost weight you have become dehydrated and need to drink more. Your urine should be light-colored. If it is dark and concentrated, you need to drink more.

Wear loose fitting, light colored clothes. If you take medications, talk to your doctor to see if these medications could make problems in the heat worse. Most importantly, if you feel ill while exercising in the heat, STOP EXERCISING.

— Groin (Inguinal) Hernia —

What is a groin (inguinal) hernia?

The internal organs are held in place by wide band of muscle that extends from the groin (the area joining the leg and the body) to the ribs. Because of a sudden strain, the muscle may separate at a weak point. Then an organ, most often the bowel but sometimes the bladder or an ovary, can squeeze through the gap, creating a bulge. This bulge is referred to as a groin (or inguinal) hernia. A complication of a groin hernia is that after the bowel has pushed through the muscle wall, its contents may become trapped. A further, more dangerous complication is that the blood supply to the bowel may be cut off or strangulated and the tissue may die, resulting in gangrene. This is a medical emergency. Surgery is often necessary to correct the hernia.

How does it occur?

Some people, especially men, are born with a weakness in their groin muscles. With or without this weakness, a hernia may be caused by any factor that increases pressure in the abdomen, such as the following:

- lifting heavy objects
- coughing or sneezing a lot
- straining for a bowel movement from being constipated
- being obese
- being pregnant
- in men, trying to urinate when there is a blockage due to an enlarged prostate.

What are the symptoms?

Symptoms associated with a groin hernia may include:

- pain or discomfort in lower abdominal or groin area
- a bulge that can be pushed back in
- a bulge that cannot be pushed back in; a potentially life-threatening problem because the bowel (or other organ) may be trapped or strangulated
- constipation
- blood in the stool.

How is it diagnosed?

To diagnose a groin hernia, your doctor will take your medical history, review your symptoms, and examine you.

How is it treated?

If the hernia bulge can be pushed back in and causes you few symptoms, you may not need surgery. Otherwise, treatment for groin hernias is elective surgery. Your doctor will usually suggest that you have the operation as soon as possible to avoid complications. The surgery is done under local or general anesthesia.

During the operation, the doctor will make a cut in the lower side of your abdomen. He or she will push your intestine back into the abdominal cavity and bring other tissue around the hernia to help cover the opening (the hernial defect). If there is not enough strong tissue available around

Groin (Inguinal) Hernia

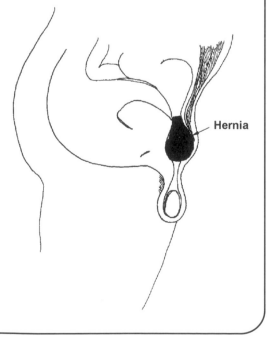

Hernia

Groin (Inguinal) Hernia

the hernia, the doctor may place a mesh over the weak spot in the abdominal wall. The doctor may make the opening between the abdominal wall and the groin, called the inguinal canal, smaller to try to prevent another hernia. Some doctors do hernia repair with a laparoscope, an instrument that requires only small incisions to perform the operation.

The doctor will decide whether you can go home the day of the operation or should stay in the hospital for one or more days. Your follow-up will depend on the severity of your symptoms and your related condition.

If symptoms continue, or if you develop new symptoms, tell your doctor immediately.

How long will the effects last?

The effects will last as long as you have the hernia.

How can I take care of myself?

Follow these guidelines:

- Follow your doctor's advice for losing weight if you are overweight.
- Be careful when you lift, pull, or push heavy objects.
- Stop smoking and avoid coughing.

- Take medication to reduce allergies and sneezing.
- Avoid constipation by eating foods that are high in fiber, using stool softeners, or drinking a natural stimulant beverage such as prune juice.
- Use laxatives or enemas only if recommended by your doctor.
- Wear a jock strap or similar groin support.

How can I help prevent a groin hernia?

Follow these guidelines:

- Be careful when you lift, push, or pull heavy objects.
- Adjust your occupational duties if necessary.
- Follow your doctor's advice for a nutritious, safe diet to lose weight if you are overweight.
- Avoid constipation.
- Avoid smoking.

Herpes Gladiatorum

What is herpes gladiatorum?

Herpes gladiatorum is a skin infection caused by the herpes simplex virus. It occurs often in wrestlers. It causes a rash that commonly appears on the face, neck, shoulder, and arms.

How does it occur?

An infected wrestler can pass the infection to an uninfected wrestler by skin contact.

What are the symptoms?

The herpes simplex rash is usually a cluster of blisters that may or may not be painful.

How is it diagnosed?

Your doctor will examine your skin. He or she may do a culture to test for the herpes virus. Knowing that the rash is from the herpes virus may help your doctor treat you.

How is it treated?

The rash usually lasts 7 to 10 days. It is important that you do not have skin contact with any uninfected person while you have the skin rash. Your doctor may prescribe a medicine called acyclovir (Zovirax) in a pill or an ointment form to speed your recovery.

How can it be prevented?

It is important for you to watch for any rashes so you don't spread them to others. In many athletic leagues, wrestlers who have rashes are not allowed to compete. It is also important to routinely clean and disinfect wrestling mats.

Hypothermia

What is hypothermia?

Hypothermia is a problem where your body's temperature becomes dangerously low. Many of your body's organs can be damaged by hypothermia.

How does it occur?

Your body temperature may gradually drop from increased exposure to cold or immediately from falling into cold water.

What are the symptoms?

The symptoms of hypothermia occur gradually and progress as follows:

- you feel cold and begin to shiver
- you have difficulty thinking and become mentally confused
- you lose the ability to shiver
- your heart starts beating irregularly
- you fall into a coma.

If not treated hypothermia can result in death.

How is it diagnosed?

Your body temperature is checked and will usually be less than 96 degrees Fahrenheit. The doctor will check for shivering, confusion, or other symptoms of hypothermia.

How is it treated?

A person with hypothermia needs immediate attention. First try to get medical help. If the person's clothes are wet, it is important that they are removed and that the person is placed in warm clothing, blankets, or a sleeping bag. A dry hat should be put on the person's head because the head is a primary source of heat loss. Let the person warm up gradually in a warm room.

Bring the person to a hospital to receive treatment. The treatment at the hospital depends on how low the person's temperature has become. Doctors may use warm oxygen, warm intravenous fluids, or a warming blanket. Specific treatment for injured organs is also given.

How long will the effects of hypothermia last?

How long the effects of hypothermia last depends upon how badly the individual organs were damaged. In many cases people are fine right after treatment. In other cases, hypothermia can result in death.

How do I prevent hypothermia?

Hypothermia is best prevented by being prepared and dressing appropriately. It is important to wear several layers of clothes over one another rather than wearing a single, thick layer. The best layers are those that provide good insulation and keep moisture away from the skin. Materials that do this include polypropylene, polyesters, and wool. It is important to wear an outer garment that is waterproof but will also "breathe." Wearing a hat is also important.

Hypothermia can occur when people least expect it. Follow these safety guidelines:

- Carry proper clothing in a backpack so you are prepared for bad weather.
- Do not begin an outing too late in the day when weather could suddenly change.
- Take off clothing when it gets wet and put on warm, dry clothes.
- Drink plenty of nonalcoholic fluids. People who get hypothermia are often dehydrated.

Ice and Heat Therapy

Why is ice used for sports injuries?

Ice is used after an injury to reduce swelling and decrease pain. Ice decreases blood flow to the injured tissue and reduces inflammation.

When should I use ice?

Ice should be used after an acute injury for the first 48 to 72 hours, or until the swelling goes away. For instance, if you have sprained your ankle 5 days ago but it is still swollen, you should still be using ice.

Some injuries come from overuse. For example, you may have pain in your knees after running or in your elbow after playing golf or tennis. You should use ice after doing the activity that causes the discomfort.

How should I use ice?

Ice packs can be made by placing ice cubes or crushed ice in a ziplock plastic bag, or by using a commercial frozen gel pack. Ice packs should not be placed directly on the skin to avoid frostbite; they should be placed over a wet washcloth or towel and can be held in place by an ace bandage. Ice packs should be used for 20 to 30 minutes for 3 to 4 hours.

To do ice massage, first freeze water in a paper or Styrofoam cup, then tear away the top lip of the cup, and massage the ice into the injury for 5 to 10 minutes. Ice massage works very well for overuse injuries.

When you first apply ice, you will feel coldness, then burning, and then after several minutes you will feel numbness.

Can there be any harmful effects from ice therapy?

If ice packs are put directly on the skin and left too long, frostbite may occur. The skin and tissue underneath (muscles, nerves, and fat) may be injured, either temporarily or permanently. Certain parts of the body (the elbow, outside of the knee and outside of the foot) can be injured by cold more easily because they don't have as much padding or insulation.

Why is heat used for sports injuries?

Heat can reduce muscle spasm, improve joint stiffness and make soft tissue more limber.

Heat can be used to help loosen tight muscles and joints during a warm-up period. Examples include: moist hot packs to tight leg muscles that are going to be stretched before running, or to a shoulder before throwing, or for stretching chronically tight neck or back muscles.

When should I use heat?

Heat should be used for stiff muscles and joints when you are trying to make them more limber. It is important not to use heat in the first few days after an injury or while your injury has any swelling.

How should I use heat?

Moist heat is more effective than dry heat as it penetrates deeper and has a better effect on muscles, joints and soft tissue. It should be used for 15-20 minutes, or longer if recommended by your doctor.

Moist heat in the form of towels soaked in hot water or warmed in a microwave are useful but usually lose their heat within 5 to 10 minutes. Commercial moist heat packs are more convenient and provide longer therapy. Hot tubs or whirlpools are also useful. Ultrasound is a form of deep heating that is used by therapists and trainers.

Heat creams and ointments are popular but don't provide

Ice and Heat Therapy

heat very deep into muscle tissue. The massaging effect of putting the cream on is helpful. Be careful not to get these creams into your eyes or in sensitive skin.

Can there be any harmful effects from heat therapy?

Heat increases the blood flow to an injury and can worsen swelling. Heat packs which are too hot or left in place too long may cause burns.

Impetigo

What is impetigo?

Impetigo is a contagious skin infection usually caused by staphylococcus or streptococcus bacteria. Epidemics can occur in sports with close body contact such as wrestling.

How does it occur?

Impetigo is common in sports because of the increased perspiration, body heat, and friction caused by sports equipment. The extra moisture and warmth create an environment that encourages growth of the bacteria and the friction provides breaks in the skin to allow the bacteria to enter. This infected skin rash occurs after a person has contact with this bacteria, usually over an area of broken skin. The bacteria may be on another person's skin or on equipment.

What are the symptoms?

The rash or lesions of impetigo are sores that usually have a weeping golden crust. They may be the size and thickness of a dime or become larger and deeper.

How is it diagnosed?

Your doctor will examine your skin.

How is it treated?

Impetigo is best treated by antibiotics taken by mouth. Some antibiotic creams are useful in treating impetigo. It is extremely important to keep your skin clean with soap and water. The condition is no longer contagious when the rash is gone.

How can impetigo be prevented?

It is important for coaches in sports such as wrestling, to keep mats and equipment clean. In sports such as wrestling where there may be close contact it is important that athletes not be allowed to participate while they have impetigo.

Magnetic Resonance Imaging (MRI)

What is magnetic resonance imaging (MRI?)

Magnetic resonance imaging (MRI) is a special test that produces very clear, detailed pictures of the organs and structures within your body. The test uses a powerful magnetic field, radio waves, and a computer to create images in cross-section. While an x-ray is very good at showing bones, an MRI lets your doctor see structures made of soft tissue such as ligaments and cartilage and organs such as your brain and heart.

When is it used?

Injuries show up well on an MRI. For example, an MRI may show whether you have torn ligaments or torn cartilage in your knee and help your doctor decide whether or not you need surgery. It is also useful for injuries involving the shoulder, back, or neck. Doctors use MRIs to see problems in the brain and spinal cord and to see the size and location of tumors.

How do I prepare for the procedure?

No special preparation is needed. You may eat normally and and take any usual medications. For the test, wear loose, comfortable clothing without metal fastenings such as zippers or clasps because metal will interfere with the test. Do not wear jewelry. If you have any metal in your body (such as plates or screws from a previous surgery) tell your doctor. If you have a pacemaker you cannot have an MRI because the test may damage it. If you have any metal fragments in your eyes you cannot have an MRI because the test may injure your eyes.

What happens during the procedure?

You lie down on a cushioned bed that moves into a dough-nut-shaped magnet that is open on both ends. If you get nervous when you are in small closed spaces you should talk to your doctor about this before you have your MRI. He or she may be able to give you a medication that will help you feel less nervous. You will have to be very still during the procedure so the pictures will not be blurry.

Most MRIs take between 30 and 60 minutes. You will hear loud knocking and a whirring sound while the pictures are being taken. You will wear earplugs or music will be provided so that the noise doesn't sound so loud.

When the test is over you may go home. Your doctor will schedule a visit with you to discuss the results.

What are the benefits and risks?

An MRI is painless. There is no radiation and there are no harmful side effects.

Mouth Guards

What is a mouth guard?

A mouth guard is a protective device that fits inside the mouth to protect the teeth. The most common type of mouth guard fits around the top teeth. The bottom teeth are protected when the mouth guard overlaps them. Some mouth guards fit both top and bottom teeth.

Mouth guards are available in sporting good stores and come in several sizes. Many mouth guards can be custom-fitted by boiling them and biting into the mouth guard or by pouring a gel into the mouth guard that solidifies when you bite into it. A mouth guard may also be custom-made by your dentist.

Why wear a mouth guard?

Your teeth are important. Mouth guards should always be worn in contact sports such as football, lacrosse, hockey, and rugby. It is recommended that they be worn in other sports such as basketball. A mouth guard not only protects your teeth but acts as a shock absorber during head contact. Mouth guards have been found to lower your risk of getting a concussion.

Exercise During Pregnancy

Exercise During Pregnancy

In this discussion of exercise during pregnancy you will learn which muscle groups you should concentrate on when you exercise. Tips for exercising during pregnancy are also offered. You will find out what kind of exercises you are allowed to do and when you should stop exercising.

When should I start exercising?

Childbirth is among the most physically stressful challenges a woman ever faces. Regular exercise during pregnancy:

- strengthens muscles needed for labor and delivery
- improves posture
- lessens some of the discomforts of pregnancy
- helps you feel less tired.

Exercise in preparation for pregnancy and childbirth should begin when you are planning to get pregnant. The sooner you begin exercising, the better you will feel. A big mistake many women make is not starting an exercise program until the last 3 months of pregnancy, when they start childbirth classes.

Before you begin an exercise program, discuss it with your health care provider. Make sure you follow his or her advice on an exercise program that is appropriate for you. If you are experiencing problems with your pregnancy, you should not exercise. Exercise can affect the amount of oxygen available to your baby. A baby that already has problems with getting enough oxygen may not tolerate even light exercise by the mother.

Which muscle groups are most important to exercise?

In addition to your heart, the three muscle groups you should concentrate on during pregnancy are the muscles of your back, pelvis, and abdomen.

- Strengthening your abdominal muscles will make it easier to support the increasing weight of your baby.
- Strengthening pelvic muscles will permit your vagina to widen more easily during childbirth. This will help prevent urinary problems (leaking urine when you cough or sneeze) after delivery.
- Strengthening back muscles and doing exercises to improve your posture will minimize the strain of pregnancy on your lower back. It will help prevent discomfort caused by poor posture.

What kinds of exercise can I do?

Many old ideas about strenuous exercise during pregnancy have been disproved in recent years. The type and intensity of sports and exercise you participate in during pregnancy depend on your health and on how active you were before you became pregnant. This is probably not a good time to take up a new strenuous sport. If you were active before you became pregnant, however, there is no reason you cannot continue, within reason.

- Walking. If you did not do any exercise before becoming pregnant, walking is a good way to begin an exercise program.
- Tennis. If you are an active tennis player, you can probably continue to play unless you have special problems or feel unusually tired. Just be aware of your change in balance and how it affects rapid movement.
- Jogging. If you jog, you probably can continue as long as you feel comfortable doing it. Avoid becoming overheated and stop if you feel uncomfortable or

Exercise During Pregnancy

unusually tired. Remember to drink plenty of water.

- Swimming. If you are a swimmer, you can continue to swim. Swimming is an excellent form of exercise. The water supports your weight while you tone and strengthen many different muscles. Scuba diving is not advised.

- Golf and bowling. Both of these sports are good forms of recreation. You will just have to adjust to your enlarged abdomen. Be careful not to lose your balance.

- Snow skiing, water skiing, and surfing. These sports can be dangerous because you can hit the ground or water with great force. Falling while traveling at such fast speeds could harm your baby. Talk to your health care provider before participating in these activities.

- Climbing, hiking, and skiing above 10,000 feet. Elevations above 10,000 feet can deprive you and your baby of oxygen. This can cause premature labor.

What are the guidelines for exercising during pregnancy?

- Warming up and cooling down are very important. Start slowly and build up to more demanding exercises. Toward the end of an exercise session, gradually slow down your activity. Try working back through the exercises in reverse order.

- Regular exercise (at least three times a week) is better for you than spurts of exercise followed by long periods of no activity.

- Check your pulse during peak activity. Slow down your activity if your heart starts beating faster than the target range recommended by your health care provider. Don't exceed a heart rate of 140 beats per minute. Exercise that is too strenuous may speed up the baby's heartbeat to a dangerous level. In general, if you are able to carry on a conversation comfortably while exercising, your heart rate is probably within the recommended limits. Check to make sure.

- Don't try to do too much. Remember that the extra weight you are carrying will make you work harder as you exercise. Stop immediately if you feel tired, short of breath, or dizzy.

- Drink water often before and after exercise to prevent dehydration. Take a break in your workout to drink more water if needed.

- Don't participate in sports and exercise in which you might fall or be bumped.

- Be very careful with your back. Avoid positions and exercises that increase the bend in your back. They put extra stress on the stretched abdominal muscles and compress your spinal joints. Deep knee bends, full sit-ups, double leg raises, and straight-leg toe touches also may injure the tissues that connect your back joints and legs.

- Do not get overheated. Avoid outdoor exercise in hot, humid weather. Also avoid hot tubs, whirlpools, or saunas.

- Do not exercise if you have an illness with a temperature of 100 degrees F (37.8 degrees C) or higher.

- Avoid jerky, bouncy, or high-impact motions that require jarring or rapid changes in direction. These may cause back, abdominal, pelvic, and leg pain. They could also cause you to lose your balance.

- Wear a good-fitting support bra to protect your enlarged breasts.

Make exercise a part of your daily life. Daily tasks can double as exercise sessions if you do the following:

Exercise During Pregnancy

- Tighten your abdominal muscles when you are standing or sitting.
- Squat when you lift anything, whether it is light or heavy.
- Rotate your feet and ankles anytime your feet are elevated.
- Check your posture each time you pass a mirror.

When should I stop exercising?

You should stop exercising and call your health care provider if you have any unusual symptoms, such as:

- pain, including pelvic pain
- bleeding
- faintness
- irregular heartbeat (skipped beats or very rapid beats)
- difficulty walking.

Remember that it is very important to discuss your plans for exercise with your health care provider. If you are experiencing problems with your pregnancy, exercise is not advised. Talk to your health care provider if you have any questions.

Sprains

What is a sprain?

A sprain is an injury that causes a stretch or a tear in a ligament. Ligaments are strong bands of tissue that connect bones at a joint.

Sprains may be classified as mild, moderate, or severe.

How does it occur?

A twisting or severe stretching of a joint is the usual cause of a sprain.

What are the symptoms?

- Your joint is swollen and painful.
- You may not be able to move the injured joint.
- The skin of the joint may be red at first. In a few hours to days, it may look bruised.

How are sprains diagnosed?

Your health care provider will examine your injury. You may have an x-ray to make sure you have not broken a bone.

How are sprains treated?

The general rule for treating sprains is R-I-C-E:

- Rest: At first you will need to avoid activities that cause pain. If you have an ankle sprain or knee sprain you may need crutches.
- Ice: Put ice packs on the sprained area for 20 to 30 minutes every 3 to 4 hours. Do this for 2 to 3 days or until the swelling goes away.
- Compression: Your health care provider may recommend that you wrap an elastic bandage around your injured joint to reduce swelling.
- Elevation: Keep the injured joint above the level of your heart as much as you can until the swelling stops.

Also:

- Your health care provider may give you a device to help support the joint, such as a splint, brace, or sling.
- Your health care provider may recommend anti-inflammatory medication or another pain reliever.
- You may be given exercises to help you recover faster.

Some sprains with complete tearing of ligaments may need surgery.

How can I prevent a sprain?

Most sprains occur from accidents that are not easily prevented. However, make sure you wear proper shoes for your activities. Watch for uneven surfaces when you are walking or exercising.

Strains

What is a strain?

A strain is a stretch or tear of a muscle or tendon. Tendons are strong bands of tissue that attach muscles to bones. People commonly call muscle strains "pulled muscles."

How does it occur?

The usual cause of muscle strain is forceful contraction (tightening) of the muscle during an activity. For example, it might happen when you run, jump, throw, or lift a heavy object.

What are the symptoms?

- You may feel a burning or a popping at the time of the injury.
- The injured muscle hurts.
- It is hard to use the injured muscle.
- The injured area may be swollen or bruised.

How is it diagnosed?

Your health care provider will examine the injured area and find that it is tender.

How is it treated?

The general rule for treating strains is R-I-C-E:

- Rest: At first you will need to avoid activities that cause pain. If you have a leg strain you may need crutches.
- Ice packs: Put ice packs on the strained muscle for 20 to 30 minutes every 3 to 4 hours. Do this for 2 to 3 days or until the pain goes away. You can also do ice massage: Freeze water in a cup and tear back the top of the cup. Rub the injured area with the ice for 5 to 10 minutes, three times a day. This is especially useful for strains you have had for more than a few days.

- Compression: Wrap an elastic bandage around your strained muscle to reduce swelling.
- Elevation: Keep the injured muscle elevated above your heart as much as possible.

Also:

- Depending on which muscle you have strained, you may be given crutches, a brace, or a sling.
- Your health care provider may recommend anti-inflammatory medication or another pain reliever.
- You may be given exercises to help you recover faster.

How can it be prevented?

The best way to prevent strains is to warm up properly and stretch your muscles before exercise. The more flexible and strong your muscles are, the less likely they will be strained.

Index